The Plague Years

The Plague Years collects scholarly and essayistic reflections on literary, visual, and sonic representations of the COVID-19 and other pandemics. These are placed alongside poetry and short fiction written in the first two years of quarantine or isolation. This range expresses the intellectual and imaginative struggle and ingenuity entailed in coming to terms with the rampant spread of disease and its emotional, cultural, and political consequences.

The contributions are from diverse contexts: Africa (from Egypt to South Africa), China, Japan, the US, and Scandinavia. They consider some of the array of contemporary engagements: poems translated from Mandarin about the traumas of the frontline, Chinese calligraphic poetry printed on cartons of PPE, comments on the literary history of representing epidemics and pandemics, political analyses of the post-truth present, and the role of life-writing and gaming in an interrupted world. Given the generative and creative obliquity of many of its parts, this collection shifts how one thinks about the diseased present and the archival pasts on which it draws.

The chapters in this book were originally published as a special issue of *English Studies in Africa*.

Michael Titlestad is Personal Professor in the Department of English at the University of the Witwatersrand, Johannesburg, South Africa. He has widely published in the fields of maritime, South African, and dystopian literature, and he is the editor of *English Studies in Africa*. His most recent book is *Shipwreck Narratives: Out of Our Depth* (2021).

Karl van Wyk is Lecturer at the University of the Witwatersrand, Johannesburg, South Africa. He began teaching in the English Department at the beginning of 2021. His research and publication interests include postmodern historiography. He is particularly concerned with WWII alternate history and South Africa's attitudes to, and representations of, apartheid history.

Grace A. Musila is Associate Professor in the Department of African Literature at the University of the Witwatersrand, Johannesburg, South Africa. She is the editor of *Wangari Maathai's Registers of Freedom* (2020), and the author of *A Death Retold in Truth and Rumour: Kenya, Britain and the Julie Ward Murder* (2015).

The Plague Years

Reflecting on Pandemics

Edited by
**Michael Titlestad, Karl van Wyk and
Grace A. Musila**

Routledge
Taylor & Francis Group

LONDON AND NEW YORK

First published 2023
by Routledge
4 Park Square, Milton Park, Abingdon, Oxon, OX14 4RN

and by Routledge
605 Third Avenue, New York, NY 10158

Routledge is an imprint of the Taylor & Francis Group, an informa business

British Library Cataloguing-in-Publication Data
A catalogue record for this book is available from the British Library

ISBN13: 978-1-032-28667-9 (hbk)
ISBN13: 978-1-032-28684-6 (pbk)
ISBN13: 978-1-003-29801-4 (ebk)

DOI: 10.4324/9781003298014

Typeset in Times New Roman
by codeMantra

Publisher's Note
The publisher accepts responsibility for any inconsistencies that may have arisen during the conversion of this book from journal articles to book chapters, namely the inclusion of journal terminology.

Disclaimer
Every effort has been made to contact copyright holders for their permission to reprint material in this book. The publishers would be grateful to hear from any copyright holder who is not here acknowledged and will undertake to rectify any errors or omissions in future editions of this book.

Contents

Citation Information

The chapters in this book were originally published in *English Studies in Africa*, volume 64, issue 1–2 (2021). When citing this material, please use the original page numbering for each article, as follows:

Chapter 1
The Plague Years: An Introduction
Michael Titlestad, Grace A. Musila and Karl van Wyk
English Studies in Africa, volume 64, issue 1–2 (2021) pp. 1–3

Chapter 2
Masked Masterpieces: *in R≡lational Folds*
Sally-Ann Murray
English Studies in Africa, volume 64, issue 1–2 (2021) pp. 4–23

Chapter 3
'As others feel pain in their lungs': Albert Camus's The Plague
Hedley Twidle
English Studies in Africa, volume 64, issue 1–2 (2021) pp. 24–40

Chapter 4
Self/isolation
Dan Wylie
English Studies in Africa, volume 64, issue 1–2 (2021) pp. 41–46

Chapter 5
Plague and Cultural Panic: Edgar Allan Poe's 'The Masque of the Red Death'
Laurence Wright
English Studies in Africa, volume 64, issue 1–2 (2021) pp. 47–58

Chapter 6
Two paintings
Ingrid Winterbach
English Studies in Africa, volume 64, issue 1–2 (2021) pp. 59–60

Chapter 25

Tick Tock
Sonia Fanucchi
English Studies in Africa, volume 64, issue 1–2 (2021) pp. 255

Chapter 26

Re-imagining a New Normal: COVID-19 Pandemic and the Changing Face of Social Interaction
Josiah Nyanda
English Studies in Africa, volume 64, issue 1–2 (2021) pp. 256–267

For any permission-related enquiries please visit:
http://www.tandfonline.com/page/help/permissions

Notes on Contributors

Kyle Allan is a South African writer, musician, researcher, and facilitator. He has published two books of poetry: *House Without Walls* (2016) and *The Space Between Us* (2018), with a third book coming out this year, *Remote Harbour*. He is the editor of *New Coin*, a Rhodes University-affiliated journal of poetry, which has 56 years of publication history. He is currently a Ph.D candidate at the University of KwaZulu-Natal, Pietermaritzburg, South Africa, under the supervision of Professor Cheryl Stobie. His topic is 'Sexual Pessimism: Eros and Embodiment in Selected Poems of South African Poets'. His M.A. dissertation (also under the same supervisor) focused on representations of precarity in selected poems of four South African poets (Mxolisi Nyezwa, Seitlhamo Motsapi, Angifi Dladla, and Ike Mboneni Muila). He is also currently Executive Director of Heartnet (Health Empowerment and Response Networks), an organization focused on youth and community development, founded in September 2020, based in Pietermaritzburg.

Taieb Belghazi earned his Ph.D in 1993 from the Centre for Critical and Cultural Theory at Cardiff University, UK, where he was a Chevening scholar. He later held a Fulbright postdoctoral scholarship at Duke University, Durham, USA, and was a member of the UNESCO-sponsored International Panel on Reading for All. He was Director of the Centre for Doctoral Studies: The Human and Space in the Mediterranean (2010–2015) and served as Professor of Cultural Studies and History of the present at the Faculty of Letters in Rabat for many years. He has also been Visiting Professor at a number of universities, including Duke University; the University of California, Irvine; and the Ferguson Centre for African Studies and Asian Studies at the Open University, England. He is currently a member of the research center The Human, Languages, Cultures & Religions at the Faculty of Letters in Rabat and the Academic Director of The School for International Training Program 'Multiculturalism and Human Rights' in Rabat. Prof. Belghazi has been a consultant for a number of projects, including the project Diaspora as a Social and Cultural Practice (The University of Southampton, UK) and the UNESCO project on reconceptualizing Mediterranean dialogues. He is a member of the editorial boards of the periodicals Time and Society (England), Current Writing (South Africa), and Al Azmina Al Haditha (Morocco). He has published a number of writings on social movements, the politics of identity, and global/local dynamics. His current research centers on the politics of social movement and emotions. His publications include *The Idea of the University* (editor), *Time and Postmodernism*, and *Dialogues Khatibi and Weber* (editor).

Eirikur Bergmann is Professor of Politics at Bifrost University, Iceland. As author of nine academic books and numerous journal articles he writes mainly on Nationalism, Populism, Conspiracy Theories and Participatory Democracy. Bergmann is also the author of *Samsæríð, Hryðjuverkamaður snýr heim* and *Glapræði* published in Icelandic.

Maren Bodenstein has published novels, short stories and flash fiction. She grew up in a small and relatively isolated German community in KwaZulu-Natal and has recently completed a family memoir which is largely based there. Maren is fairly new to poetry and relishes associative freedom and language puzzlings. (It's also a relief not to spend so much time on a piece.)

Devin William Daniels is a Ph.D candidate in the Department of English at the University of Pennsylvania, Philadelphia, USA. He is completing a dissertation titled 'Informatic States: Administration, Identity, and Surveillance in the U.S. Novel, 1940–1977'. His work is published or forthcoming in *Mediations, Contemporaries at Post45*, and *Hyped on Melancholy*.

Chatradari 'Chats' Devroop is Associate Professor and the Academic Leader for Research (ALR) in the School of Arts at the University of KwaZulu-Natal, South Africa. Chats is one of many artistic-cum-academics who draws on his practice for inspiration in his scholarly work. His performance-based music-making encompasses diverse music genres, including art music to commercial musics. His academic work spans diaspora studies, the South African music academy and areas of music and technology.

Sonia Fanucchi is Lecturer of Victorian and Medieval undergraduate and postgraduate modules at the University of the Witwatersrand, Johannesburg, South Africa. She has researched widely in the areas of Victorianism, Medievalism, anti-Catholicism as well as in Dante's language of memory. Among her recent articles are 'Newman's Callista: an Apologia for Ritual' published in the *SASMARS* journal in 2020 and 'Re-membering history: allegory as sacrament in Inferno's Prologue scene', is forthcoming in *Religion & Literature*.

Ute Fendler is Chair of Romance Literary and Comparative Studies at the University of Bayreuth, Germany, since 2006. She is Co-spokesperson of EXC Africa Multiple (since 2019). Her research interests include literatures and film cultures of the Caribbean, West Africa, the Indian Ocean and South America; comparative romance literary and film studies; iconographies; transmediality; popular culture; and memory. Some of her recent publications include 'Ghosts as Mediators: Memory, Healing, Knowing and the Negation of Time' in *Ghosts, Spectres, Revenants*; 'Lusophone Filmmaking in the Realm of Transnational African Cinemas: From 'Global Ethnic' to 'Global Aesthetics' in *Contemporary Lusophone African Film: Transnational Communities and Alternative Modernities*; 'SM Entertainment: From Stage Art to Neo Culture Technology (NCT)' in: *Culture and Empathy*; 'K-pop Fandom in Germany: A Macro and a Micro Perspective' in *Transcultural Fandom and the Globalization of Hallyu*; 'Superheroes for Africa?' in *Africa Today*.

Ronit Frenkel is Professor of English at the University of Johannesburg, South Africa, and the editor of the pan-African journal, *The Thinker*. She holds a Ph.D in Comparative Cultural and Literary Studies from the University of Arizona, USA, and an M.A. in African Literature from the University of the Witwatersrand, Johannesburg, South Africa. She mostly works on contemporary South African literary and cultural studies. She also has a strong interest in African literatures, public cultures, the Indian Ocean and transnational connectivity.

Yanbin Kang works as Research Fellow at JNU Collaborative Innovation Centre for the Communication of Chinese Culture in Hong Kong, Macao, Taiwan, and Overseas. She is also Professor of English at the School of Foreign Studies at Jinan University, Guangzhou, China, where she teaches British and American literature and comparative literature. She has published articles on poetry and comparative poetics in journals such as *Papers on Language and Literature, Visual Communication, Style, Renascence, Orbis Litterarum, English Studies* and *The Emily Dickinson Journal*. Her current project explores Dao in Ralph Waldo Emerson and related writers including Emily Dickinson, Wallace Stevens, A. R. Ammons, Anne Carson and the contemporary Chinese writer Mu Xin.

Leon Krige (b. 1962, Johannesburg, South Africa) studied architecture at the University of the Witwatersrand, Johannesburg, South Africa, 1981–86, and Staedelschule Frankfurt, Germany, 1987–89. He teaches architecture at the University of Johannesburg, South Africa, and photographs cities at night as research on urban transformation and people from communities in transformation. His work has been shown at Velo, Fada & Nirox galleries, Johannesburg, 2012, the Johannesburg FNB art fair, 2013 and 2015, 1–54 Art fair Somerset House, London, 2015, Courtauld Institute East Wing, London, 2015, Cape Town & Johannesburg art fair 2016/2017, Agog gallery, Johannesburg, 2016, University of Johannesburg GSA graduate school of architecture, 2017, Solo Gallery Agog, 2018, Johannesburg, Cities in Transition and ABC architecture museum, Haarlem, Netherlands, 2019.

Moulay Driss El Maarouf completed his Ph.D, 'The Local and Global Dynamics of Moroccan Music Festivals' in 2013 in Bayreuth University, Germany, where he was on the BIGSAS and DAAD scholarship recipients. After defending his thesis, he was awarded a three-year postdoctoral grant by the Volkswagen Foundation to complete his research project: *Remembering Childhood: Identity, Space, and Circulation in Childhood Playing Narratives*. Towards the end of this fellowship, he joined the DAAD research programme 'The Maghreb in Transition: Media, Knowledge and Power' as a coordinator and academic advisor from 2016 to 2019. In 2020, he co-founded AfriBIAN (Africa Bayreuth International Alumni Network) after a successful application to DAAD to fund a two-year project, entitled Rolling Religion on the African Map: Religion in times of Transition. El Maarouf's academic interests span several topics within Cultural Studies, including cultural theory, music festivals and sub-culture, childhood lives, social movements, scatology and popular culture. El Maarouf currently holds a teaching position at the English Department at Sidi Mohamed Ben Abdellah University (Sais), Fez, Morocco.

Phelelani Makhanya is a writer born in Stanger, South Africa. His work has been published in major South African literary journals such as *New Contrast, New Coin, Botsotso Journal* and *Avbob Poetry Project*. He was shortlisted for the 2021 Time of the Writer Poetry for Human Rights. He has two published poetry collections, *This Time I Shall Not Cry* and *My Father's Blazer*.

David Medalie is Professor in the Department of English and Director of the Unit for Creative Writing at the University of Pretoria, South Africa. He supervises postgraduate work in English and Creative Writing. He is a short story writer, novelist and anthologist. His recent publications include *Recognition*, an anthology of South African short stories, which he edited for Wits University Press.

Kobus Moolman is Professor of Creative Writing in the Department of English at the University of the Western Cape, South Africa. He has published seven collections of poetry and two plays, and has edited a collection of poetry, prose and art by South African writers living with disabilities. He has won numerous local and international awards for his work. His first collection of short fiction, *The Swimming Lesson and Other Stories*, was published in 2017. His latest collection of poetry, *The Mountain behind the House* (Dryad Press), was published in 2020.

Omar Moumni is Professor of English and Cultural Studies in the Department of English, Faculty of Letters and Human Sciences at Sidi Mohamed Ben Abdellah University, Fez, Morocco. He is the author of *Ruptures in the Western Empire: White Female Captives and Cinematic Orientalism* (2012), *Postcolonial Matters* (2013) and *The Objectification of Women in Moroccan Advertizing* (2015). He has a number of published articles and has contributed in scores of international conferences. He is a visiting research scholar at New York University (NYU, Steinhardt), Multinational Institute of American Studies: Department of Humanities and Social Sciences in the Professions (2016). His current research covers a variety of areas including Postcolonial Literature, Visual Culture and Gender Studies.

Zhiyong Mo is a National Senior Art Designer and Associate Professor at the School of Journalism and Communication at Jinan University, Guangzhou, China. He holds a Ph.D from Wuhan University and an M.A. from Tsinghua University, China. As a professional practitioner of Chinese traditional calligraphy and Lingnan painting, his artworks have been collected by major institutions. Prof. Mo has also contributed to leading journals, including *Visual Communication* and *PAJ: A Journal of Performance and Art*.

Sally-Ann Murray is Professor in the English Department at Stellenbosch University, South Africa, serving as Chair from 2015 to 2020. Her third poetry collection, *Otherwise Occupied* (Dryad Press, 2019), was nominated for a 2020 South African Literary Award, and her autobiographical novel *Small Moving Parts* (Kwela, 2009) won multiple prizes. She has published short stories, and her latest academic essays address examples of queer contemporary South African short fiction and autoethnography as method. Life being what it is (why ask *why*?), she veers between wry and awry.

Grace A. Musila is Associate Professor in the Department of African Literature at the University of the Witwatersrand, Johannesburg, South Africa. Her teaching and research center on Eastern and Southern African literatures, African popular cultures, and gender in Africa. She has published journal articles and chapters in these areas. She is also the editor of *Wangari Maathai's Registers of Freedom* (HSRC Press, 2020); author of *A Death Retold in Truth and Rumour: Kenya, Britain and the Julie Ward Murder* (Boydell & Brewer, 2015); and co-editor of *Rethinking Eastern African Intellectual Landscapes* (Africa World Press, 2012; with James Ogude and Dina Ligaga).

Josiah Nyanda holds a Ph.D in English from the University of the Witwatersrand, Johannesburg, South Africa, where he also lectures English and Critical Thinking in the Faculty of Engineering and the Built Environment, and in the School of Accountancy. His other publications can be found in *Scrutiny2*, *Social Dynamics*, *English Studies in Africa*, *Journal of African Languages and Literary Studies*, *Contracampo* and *Blackwell Companion of African Literature*, among others. His area of specialty is life-writing, especially political auto/biographies from Zimbabwe. He is also a Research Alumnus of the University of Tübingen, Germany.

Machiko Oike is Director of the Research Center for Diversity and Inclusion at Hiroshima University, Japan, managing a wide variety of projects concerning gender, ethnicity, culture, aging, illness and other topics. Her research interests include the representation of gender and sexuality in African literature and social activism through literature and other cultural works. Among her publications is *AIDS and Literature: African Women Writing Sexuality, Love and Death* (2013) (in Japanese).

Damian Shaw joined the University of Macau, China, in 2008. He has lectured in South Africa (1997–2002) and Quanzhou (2002–2008) in English Literature. He was a language researcher and specialist music editor for the Cambridge International Dictionary of English and enjoys writing occasional poetry. Damian's main research interests relate to colonial writing of the Romantic and Victorian eras, including poetry, travel writing, the gothic and anti-slavery literature. He is particularly interested in representations of China and Africa during this period.

Michael Titlestad is Personal Professor in the Department of English at the University of the Witwatersrand, Johannesburg, South Africa. He has widely published in the fields of maritime, South African and dystopian literature, and he is the editor of *English Studies in Africa*. His monograph, *Shipwreck Narratives: Out of Our Depth* (Palgrave), appeared at the end of 2021.

Hedley Twidle is a writer, teacher and researcher based at the University of Cape Town, South Africa. His essay collection, *Firepool: Experiences in an Abnormal World*, was published by Kwela Books in 2017. *Experiments with Truth*, a study of narrative non-fiction and the South African transition, appeared in the African Articulation series from James Currey in 2019.

Karl van Wyk is Lecturer at the University of the Witwatersrand, Johannesburg, South Africa. He began teaching in the English Department at the beginning of 2021. His research and publication interests include postmodern historiography. He is particularly concerned with WWII alternate history and South Africa's attitudes to, and representations of, apartheid history.

Crystal Warren has worked as a librarian and literary researcher and is now Curatorial Manager at Amazwi South African Museum of Literature in Makhanda, where she oversees the collections and research. Her research interests include poetry, contemporary South African literature, speculative fiction and youth literature.

Ingrid Winterbach is both a visual artist and a novelist. Her work has won most of the major prizes available for Afrikaans fiction and has been translated into English, French, and Dutch. Her latest novel, her thirteenth, *Voorouer. Pelgrim. Berg.* was published in Afrikaans in May 2021.

Laurence Wright is Extraordinary Professor at North-West University, Potchefstroom, South Africa. He was formerly H.A. Molteno Professor of English and Director of the Institute for the Study of English in Africa at Rhodes University, South Africa. He is Fellow of the English Academy of Southern Africa, a member of the South African Academy of Science and Honorary Life-President of the Shakespeare Society of Southern Africa. He has published widely on Shakespeare, on the future of the humanities, on South African language policy and on the country's educational crisis. Currently, he is writing about Conrad, Somerset Maugham, and V.S. Naipaul; about southern African railway poetry; and about Petina Gappah, Tom Sharpe, and Wulf Sachs.

Dan Wylie teaches English at Rhodes University, South Africa. He has published two books on the Zulu leader Shaka (*Savage Delight: White Myths of Shaka* and *Myth of Iron: Shaka in History*, both UKZN Press); a memoir, *Dead Leaves: Two Years in the Rhodesian War* (UKZN Press); and several volumes of poetry. Most recently, he has concentrated on Zimbabwean literature and on ecological and animal concerns in literature. He founded the annual Literature & Ecology Colloquium in 2004 and edited the collection of essays, *Toxic Belonging? Identity and Ecology in Southern Africa* (Cambridge Scholars Press). Related publications are *Elephant* and *Crocodile*, both in the Reaktion Books Animals Series, and *Slow Fires* (poems with etchings by Roxandra Britz; Fourthwall Books). Most recently published are his collection *Raven Games: New and Collected Poems*; a study of another South African poet, *Intimate Lighting: Sydney Clouts, Poet* (UNISA Press); and *Death & Compassion: The Elephant in Southern African Literature* (Wits University Press). He writes a blog at http//danwyliecriticaldiaries.blogspot.co.za.

Beth Wyrill is a heritage practitioner with a Ph.D from Rhodes University, South Africa, exploring theories of archive, South African literary history and museology. She has spent the past five years working as a Research Curator at the Amazwi South African Museum of Literature and is presently taking on a new position with the Museum of London. She has worked previously on historiographic metafiction in the novels of selected South African authors.

Introduction

Michael Titlestad, Karl van Wyk and Grace A. Musila

This is not the apocalypse. While some of the customary signs are there – deserted streets, masks and hazmat suits, empty supermarket shelves, hospitals and morgues overflowing – the four horsemen are not gathering at the horizon. Yet the pervasive register in reportage and on social media over the last two years has been biblical, as if eschatology dictates that we conceive of the COVID-19 pandemic as, paradoxically, an iteration of the last days. Without making the routine observation that the apocalypse is never *now* but always deferred, we might wonder why apocalypticism is the default script in relation to immanent disasters and future imaginaries.

Until recently, we largely lacked a lexicon and grammar for global contagion, its social and political consequences and its possible containment. Bubonic plague and even Spanish flu are too remote to be serviceable in this respect and, anyway, our epidemiological knowledge has meant that our experience of COVID-19 has been distinct from historical pandemics. HIV, the cause of one of our most recent pandemics, could have been comparable were it not for the medical developments of ARV therapy, which, in many cases, has turned the disease into a chronic illness. It has also proved less likely to mutate than coronaviruses. It is glib and unethical to suggest that this absence amounts to a 'crisis of representation,' for the only real 'crises' are infection, death and bereavement, in comparison with which the struggle to come to terms with the coronavirus and its effects is at least secondary. Yet, the humanities must concern itself with representation: how the virus, its spread and its effects have been inscribed and understood existentially and mobilized politically.

It is too brazen to suggest that the world will never be the same again because the pandemic has only exacerbated existing dynamics: it has fuelled populism, reinforced capitalism and increased the reach of hedge fund managers and others who profit off risk. And climate change – despite a short-lived lull in carbon emissions and a brief flourishing of wildlife in empty cities – is only becoming more evident in its effects and its outcomes increasingly predictable. Much has remained the same. But even as humanity marches unwaveringly (even triumphantly) towards its own destruction, we can acknowledge that representation is integral to both understanding and mobilization, even if not constitutive. It is in this that the current volume coheres: how has COVID-19 entered discourses; on what archives have we drawn in our accounts; and how has blindness and denial been contiguous with insight and the acknowledgement that our capacities are limited? As we journey through questions of epistemology, we pose new questions concerning the representation of what we know: has the virus, masking and vaccination been aestheticized; have writers cast the present as an exception; how is blame attributed to individuals and nations; how are the frontline and health workers rendered; has the virus impacted material and literary culture; and what ideologies are being articulated in representations? Obviously, no list of questions or collection of essays can be exhaustive. At most one can hope they are somewhat representative; that they offer insights into the questions, discourses and perspectives emerging from various geo-historical locations.

Coming to terms with the virus has stretched the imagination; it is invisible, known only through symptoms, vectors of infection, statistics and the distribution of cases. This results in interpretative latitude. At times it seems, in the words of Laurie Anderson, that language itself has been a virus.[1] Misrepresentation, galvanized by populism, conspiracy theories and regional rivalries, has detracted from science. A vocal constituency has embraced 'post-truth' and done the Enlightenment a fundamental disservice with fatal consequences. This is perhaps the best reason to dwell on COVID-19 among the discourses. This activity is not quaint, rarefied or apolitical. Partial or absolute misrepresentation is a matter of life or death.

These essays (generally assays) take different disciplinary approaches to the pandemic. They range from political and social analyses (Bergmann is concerned with the relation between COVID-19 and populism; Moumni explores aspects of the pandemic's intersection with racism; and Nyanda considers shifts in African sociality in the last two years), archives of representation (Wright on Edgar Allan Poe's 'The Masque of the Red Death' and Twidle on Camus's *The Plague*), dystopian literature and its tropes, which have been constitutive of representations (Warren's survey of South African dystopian literature; Daniels' examination of Deon Meyer's *Fever*; and Wyrill's comments on novels by Diane Awerbuck and Russel Brownlee), and the pandemic in particular fields (Yang on Chinese COVID-19 poetry; Mo's description of the use of Chinese calligraphy on cartons of PPE – including his magnificent, artistic rendering of this practice; Shaw on the depiction of COVID-19 themes on postage stamps; El Maarouf, Belghazi and Fendler on COVID-19 gaming; and Devroop and Titlestad on the sonification of the virus). Some of the essays are writerly, aesthetic enquiries: Murray on a poster campaign in Stellenbosch; Allan's reading of the present through the 2000s poetry of Angifi Dladla and Mxolisi Nyezwa; and Frenkel's use of Zadie Smith's *Intimations* as an affective mirror); while Oike describes an intimate practice of memory in Ugandan HIV memory books. We – the editors – decided that exegesis, even aestheticized, should be placed in counterpoint with creative engagement. The articles are punctuated with short stories by David Medalie and Kobus Moolman; COVID-19 poems by Dan Wylie; ten Chinese poems (translated by Yanbin Kang); additional poetry by Maren Bodenstein, Sonia Fanucchi, and Phelelani Makhanya; two paintings by Ingrid Winterbach; and the cover photographic image by Leon Krige. The term 'multi-modal' is mawkish, yet the variety of representational practices adopted in this issue gives us a wider view of the tropology of the virus, the lived reality and fear of infection, the experience of isolation, the obfuscation of reality in conspiracy theories, the social changes that have been wrought and the mobilization in the interests of personal and public health. The topic warrants a multiplicity of voices, speaking in different ways.

We owe a debt of gratitude to all the writers, who invested time, thought and emotion in these pieces under difficult circumstances – all were written under lockdown. This issue demanded patience and creativity in equal measure, for which we thank Jessica Jacobs, Mokheseng Buti and the dedicated staff of Taylor & Francis.

Note

1   Anderson, Laurie, 'Like a Virus'. https://www.youtube.com/watch?v=KvOoR8m0oms. Accessed on 31 July 2021.

Masked Masterpieces: in R≡lational Folds

Sally-Ann Murray

This paper creatively re-thinks *Masked Masterpieces*, a COVID-19 public art fundraising initiative for financially at-risk students, organized by Stellenbosch University (SU) and underwritten by donors. The project features five portraits by famous South African artists, re-purposed with protective masks, and installed in large-scale reproductions around Stellenbosch town. In the paper, *Masked Masterpieces* serves as a generative critical prompt: not for a simplistic 'unmasking,' but for a female scholar's process of thinking through 'the fold,' an 'en/folding' engagement that turns and returns, erratically reviewing difficult, overlapping subjects linked to masking and mastery. In exploring both the substance and the shape of my thought process, I draw loose inspiration from innovations in mixed-materials structural design, where 'folded surfaces … respond to spatial inquiries by transforming not into aggregates of fragments but into catalytically interconnected elements' (Vyzoviti and Sotiriou 524).

Masked Masterpieces is a Stellenbosch University COVID-19 bursary fundraising initiative that re-purposes portraits by famous South African artists. The campaign originates in the Major Gifts and Transformational Giving office of the University's Development and Alumni Relations Division and is funded by institutional partners in the private sector. These are notable patrons with 'a vested interest in art education' (Corrigall 2020): the Beck Family Philanthropy; the Fuchs Foundation; Investec; the Norval Foundation; the Rupert Art Foundation; and Strauss & Co. Plaques displayed alongside the artworks offer visitors information in isiXhosa, Afrikaans and English. They detail something of the artists' life stories, indicate where to view the unmasked originals in and around Stellenbosch, and how to donate to the bursary fund via SnapScan or EFT. Proceeds from the project are intended to assist students of the so-called missing middle in SU's Faculty of Arts and Social Sciences, 'students unable to access state funding and yet unable to afford university studies,' often 'talented and academically gifted students' who 'are vulnerable to dropping out' (plaque text) due to economic hardship exacerbated by the pandemic. The project is envisaged as a mode of concerned redress in the manner of corporate social responsibility, hoping to turn elite cultural capital and historical privilege into an engine of social justice. Yet there are anomalies that invite exploration.

The *Masked Masterpieces* images are five large-format reproductions of renowned portraits by celebrated South African artists, sited around the town of Stellenbosch: Gerard Sekoto's 'The Senegal Woman' (1973, on a purpose-made, free-standing billboard in front of the gabled wall of the Distell building facing the R44); Irma Stern's 'The Initiate' (1935, on the wall adjacent to the GUS gallery in Dorp Street); Maggie Laubser's 'Portrait of a Coloured Girl' (1930, in the Dorp Street alley off Bird Street); Vladimir Tretchikoff's 'Chinese Girl' (1952, on the gabled wall corner of Drostdy and Plein Streets); and Zanele Muholi's 'Aphelile IV, Durban, 2020' (on a customized free-standing billboard at the Stellenbosch taxi rank, corner of Bird and Merriman streets). The female subjects in four of the reprints now wear digitally-superimposed depictions of surgical masks, while the Muholi is a photographic reproduction of a black-and-white head-and-shoulders photo study by the artist, in which a black female persona performed by Muholi wears white disposable surgical gloves, a white medical mask across the nose and mouth and a white cloth mask angled awry upon the subject's up-coiled weave, as if in uncertain adjustment, with two dangling fabric ties framing the eyes' steady gaze.

≡

What am I to make of this?

≡

Under lockdown, my face-to-face university life goes remote; my mind is isolated and virtually stalled. The faces in *Masked Masterpieces* become familiar imaginative company, a generative cohort that prompts my thinking, providing a pretext for a thoughtful process of re-configuring this SU project through 'the fold' and 'en/folding'. This is an engagement that turns and returns, erratically reviewing difficult, overlapping subjects linked to identity, masking, mastery, femaleness, m/othering. Fold and folding, associated with the making of a mask, appear in the essay's content, but also inform its structure. This is apt, since language and thought are deeply 'folded into one another, through etymological derivatives of "implication," "explication," and "application,"' for '(un)folding is how thought interlaces itself' and is 'interlaced with itself' (Deleuze qtd. in Friedman and Schäffner 19). In finding the shape and substance of this paper, I draw figurative inspiration from innovations in mixed-materials structural design, where 'folded surfaces ... respond to spatial inquiries by transforming not into aggregates of fragments but into catalytically interconnected elements' (Vyzoviti and Sotiriou 524). This is considered an 'emergence property of folded forms' that has the potential to 'revoke the dualism of the intentional and the unintentional, the essential and the accidental' (524). Accordingly, some issues I consider (apparently) face-to-face; others effect a more obscure, slanted crease. Some elements, ambiguous, both hold and withhold intimacy, and shifts between point of view and person may prompt in a reader vertiginous moves of affiliation and distance. The paper offers an oblique, partial, layered portrait of *Masked Masterpieces* as public art in im/personal relation to aspects of (women's) life situations in the pandemic. A convolute. An aggregated form of fold.

≡

Folds are complex; contingent. Valley fold with hill fold, subversion layered with complicity. For Mary Corrigall, the masks in the five portraits 'inevitably provoke questions' about the sitters' identities, a questioning 'amplified by the fact' that four of the portraits are the work of painters 'we might classify as modernist artists,' meaning 'the identities of the sitters were not intended to be revealed' (2020). Despite my critical distance from the campaign, the five faces prove compelling. The supersized faces draw my close attention in these un-face-to-face times, especially outside the more usual art context of a gallery's white cube. While I meet the campaign's 'challenge' of correctly matching portrait and artist, it is the subjects' possible performativity that intrigues, even though three of them are anonymous faces. (Unnamed lives. Unidentified bodies.) The masks' partial concealment highlights the eyes. Are these subjects … tired, tolerant, poised, hostile, screened, knowing? Is any supposed mood an attribution of my own longing for connection, overlaid with traces of the artists' agency? Are portrait subjects, though passively reproduced, also expressing, even asserting, enfoldments of self? I cannot be certain. The young female face in Stern's 'Initiate' (Figure 1) seems reticent. Her downcast eyes deflect intimacy, withdraw from my musing. Do Stern's hesitant lines and delicate colouring imply something of her subject's culturally distanced self, and/or Stern's own apprehension of unequal folds of authority and persistent racial hierarchy? For the life of me, I cannot discern. Still, to my eyes, the girl's rendering is so faint as to imply an imminent vanishing. A life (a way of life?) impossible to hold.

≡

Pack of 50 3-ply disposable surgical face masks. Recommended as the leading face mask for use in the office, home, outdoors or anywhere indoors.

- Three layers of non-woven fabric in each mask ensure safe filtration and absorption of harmful air-borne particles
- Low breathing resistance and high filtration efficiency
- Non-woven lace loops for secure, optimized comfort
- One size fits all
- Available in black and blue

Buy yours now! While stocks last!

≡

One person in our family bubble signals compliance by buying for sole personal use a starter-pack of three blue disposable medical masks. Wears and washes, washes and wears; eventually replaces when folds have flattened, a compromised method that unevenly covers medical, functional and environmental obligations. (Aesthetics is not part of the equation.) When the elasticated ear-bands break loose from their short-lived dabs of cheap glue, as ever happens, I am asked to stitch the connections. This can take many minutes for the hopeless camel faced with the narrow needle. Even with good light, in this cabin-fevered house there is no clear-eyed I to be found big enough for when I need it.

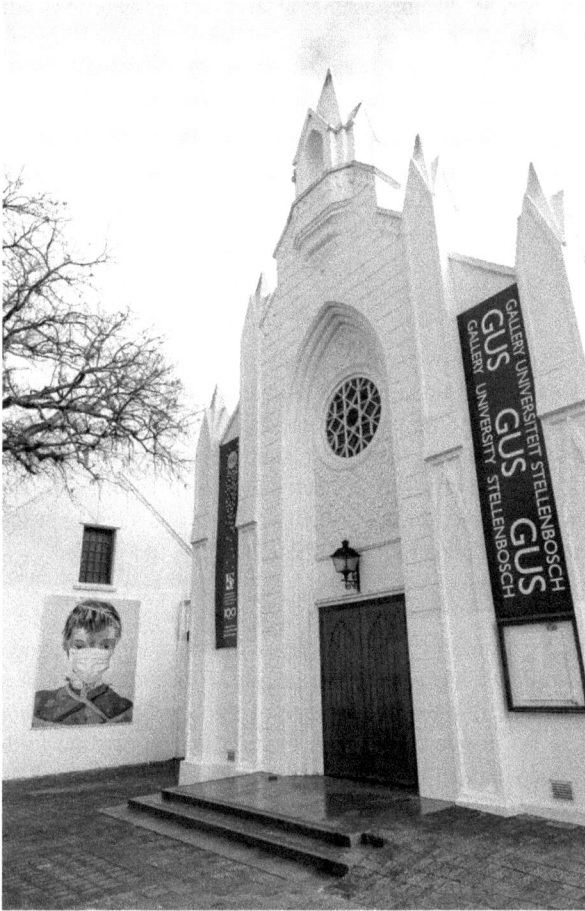

Figure 1.   Stern's 'The Initiate', photo SU campaign material.

One person gives scarce thought to face masks. Misplaces masks (' … s *NOT* FUCKING LOST!!!') as often as they must be worn. Quizzed – uuughhhh uhuhuh outraged exasperationnnnn – expects a miracle mask to materialize on demand. Since this *deus ex machina* is on endless repeat, the mask becomes the new missing sock.

Time and again, another close relation appropriates any mask to hand. Does not believe in masking, *ergo*, why acquire your own. (Statement, not question.) Speaks often and loudly about being too healthy to catch COVID-19 but also, maybe, let's all just get this virus already. Because: herd immunity, right? Not surprisingly, this same someone has many times had to buy a mask on the spot: in public. cops. caught short. Invariably these masks are misfits: I'm told the sizing is Chinese or the fabric is sweaty or the fabrication is crap. So out they go, worn but once or twice ('thrice' being a completely preposterous notion). The shortest life span.

Which is how we have an improbably tiny infant's mask abandoned on the rosewood dining room table for all the interminable months of the hard lockdown. So lost. Forlorn. Cupped empty as a mouthless breast on a dark blanket. I leave it there because it is beautiful and melancholy, life and death both, *modus vivendi* and *memento mori*. The black fabric is printed with a swirling mayhem of whirling planets. The entire universe, remembered and discarded in our house.

≡

At the pre-eminent local boys' high school, pupils are tasked to make masks for a community service project. It's inspiring to see the WhatsApp messages of a teenage boy cutting the patterns, measuring and pinning, folding and turning inside out. (Sent by proud mom to her book club). He is bent over his mother's sewing machine, giving it his all. Would I be so moved if he were a girl?

≡

Zimbabwean scholar Tinashe Mawere argues that the 'urgency of the viral plague can offer a convenient pretext' for views and practices that enable 'state repression, gender violence, toxic and patriarchal nation-building projects and many forms of physical, structural and symbolic violence' (2020). He writes to '(un)mask' some of the 'other dangerous pandemics' that 'require urgent questioning and critique' but that have been side-lined by the world's collective focus on managing the pandemic (2020). The COVID-19 crisis has exposed existing structural fault-lines in the social fabric, showing the abnormality of 'the normal'.

≡

When curfew permits, I get out of the house, get in the car and drive away, mask-less. Downtown: no tourists; no students. Many destitute people. *Haweloos*: without safe harbour, haven or shelter. Cars are scarce. I draw alongside one of the *Masked Masterpieces*, no traffic from behind, the light red in my pondering favour. Framed by the pristine folds and unbent edges of a gargantuan but hyper-realistic blue safety mask, the eyes of Sekoto's Senegalese woman seem heavy, burdened with more than a woman can bear. (Figure 2.) I think, in passing,

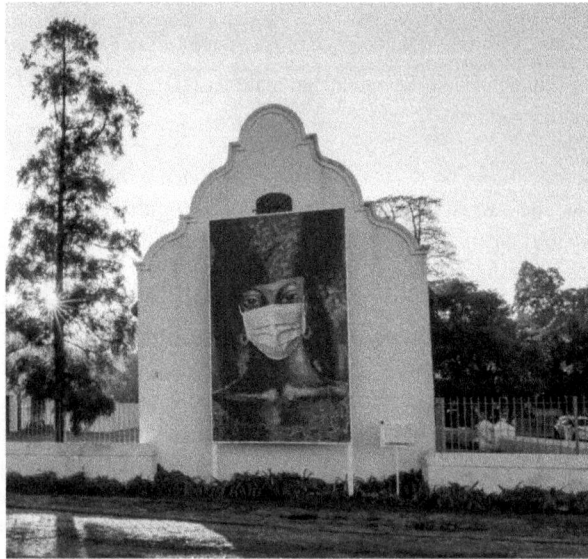

Figure 2.   'The Senegal Woman', photo SU campaign material.

about Sekoto's signature style; his variously elegant and eroticized idealizations of Black female beauty; Africa conceived as voluptuous-cum-nurturing motherland during his exiled displacement in France. I see traces of Negritude's romanticized treatment of the 'dark-skinned female body' (Eyene 430) and consider how this may have been a challenge to Western norms of beauty, even though major South African writers like Keorapetse Kgositsile and Es'kia Mphahlele disagreed.

I drive by the other installation artworks, thoughts following asymmetrical creases of affirmation and unease. Maggie Laubser's 'The Coloured Girl,' a face caught in half side view, as if about to move. Laubser as a female artist from the rural Swartland who, despite time abroad in Britain and Europe, was an outsider to a patriarchal and patronizing South African art establishment. Laubser's bold, distinctive use of form and colour inspired by German Expressionism. Her affinity for local subject matters, *subjects*. Her eventual celebration by the cultural brokers of early Afrikaner nationalism, who valued her depiction of a nostalgic, timeless pastoral farming idyll of 'stable and harmonious feudal relations,' labour presented not as 'determined by social and economic relations,' but 'as an heroic activity' governed by 'the repetitive cycles of nature' (Delmont 7), 'an order … unchanging and natural' (13).

≡

In making one troublesome fold, it's possible I am being difficult. It has been said before. But I cannot escape the queasy apprehension that, from a certain sidewise angle, the *Masked Masterpieces* installation bears bizarre inflections of blackface, and/or racial profiling. The portraits of women/a womxn of colour by various (mostly dead, white) artists are used to perform subordinated raced and gendered identity in a spectacle mounted by a powerful nexus of whiteness in a declarative commitment to transformative justice. A tortuously tautological masking. The selected portraits are tasked to represent the collective institutional goodwill of white privilege towards disadvantaged students (mostly people of colour), at the same time as they serve as the synecdochic, figurative burden of authenticity in representing, standing for, standing in for, sitting still as … the figuring of a predominantly black and coloured missing middle. 'Ethnic' 'femaleness' is accorded the social duty to mediate and 'explain' the figuring of a subordinate group to a dominant group so as to 'bridge cultures' in such a way that would also supposedly benefit the subordinate group (Mary Dearborn qtd. in White-Parks 17). While the *Masked Masterpieces* project hopes to offer innovative intervention, some might argue it takes custody of the (missing) bodies in the artworks, effecting an incongruous, proxy custodial authority for such bodies via the very absence of 'the missing middle'. The visual-conceptual strategizing contributes to an uneasy voiding and avoiding, a disturbingly incongruous fold of agency that collides with the express hope of enabling presence and academic participation.

≡

I first learnt of the *Masked Masterpieces* initiative by email in early August 2020, under Alert Level 3 lockdown. Colleagues in the Visual Arts Programme (VAP) conveyed their critical distance from a university-led public art campaign that was about to launch, a campaign that was conceived without considered consultation with SU experts in disciplines that teach visual studies and interpretative textualities. Colleagues were dismayed. The campaign seemed a top-down *fait accompli*, implemented without sufficient care for ethical caution or critical sensitivity to the decolonial imperative of South African higher education in the global context of Black Lives Matter. They conceded, yes, that the project's consultation team included influential artworld curatorial and critical names beyond SU, and that the external funders had signed off in approval. However, this did not, for the VAP colleagues, alter the perception that *Masked Masterpieces* was a recidivist mis-take, rife with exoticizing and othering, re-popularizing debased 'corporeal schemas' of disease and surveillance that had long been characteristic of the dehumanizing regulation of (in particular) black female bodies under powerful intersections of colonial, Apartheid, patriarchal and capitalist systems (Settler and Engh 144).[1] One academic urged that even with the installation of the artworks underway, University management should be pressed to extend the project to include white masked faces, especially white masked *male* faces: 'Imagine a poster of the Danie Craven statue wearing a mask, for instance, or JS Marais?' Just imagine. (See the paper by Van Robbroeck et al.)

≡

'Consistent with studies in the prior coronavirus pandemic (SARS-CoV) on gender and the likelihood of adopting preventative measures, a recent study revealed that males are less likely than females to wear masks, as wearing a mask is "not manly"' (Zagury-Orly 2020).

≡

Among Stern's works are 'Portrait of a Zulu woman,' 'Malay Girl,' 'Young Xhosa Woman' and 'Zanzibar Lady,' while Tretchikoff paints a Swazi Girl, a Zulu Girl, and an Ndebele Girl, with his world-renowned 'Chinese Girl' portrait felt by the painter perhaps to have 'caught the essence of Chinese womanhood' (Evans 2013). Granted, we cannot anachronistically rebuke artists for using the textual, visual and ideological languages of their day. But is it asking too much of the *Masked Masterpieces*' campaign's 21st-century initiators that they acknowledge such orientalizing categories as expressions of dominant belief and not inherent truth? In the context of Stellenbosch and the difficulties of transformation, the campaign's inability to address the obvious gives a forceful bent to a remark (uneasily ambiguous, I now think), made by Virginia Woolf (1929): 'For masterpieces are not single and solitary births; they are the outcome of many years of thinking in common, of thinking by the body of the people' (55). Which way are these folds made, I mull; to whom inclined and/or against? For the campaign organizers, Chandra Mohanty's 1988 argument shouldn't be news: even under emancipatory suasions, a dominant Western point of view historically tends to relegate so-called 'Third World Women' to homogenized non-speaking subjects who are spoken for, or about: 'they never rise above the debilitating generality of their "object" status' (80). Female sitters. Sitting for 'their' portraits. No wonder then (the beautiful wonder) of the performative slantwise takes on self/portraiture made by Muholi.

≡

It matters, how you label things. 'Masterpieces'. His. Her master's pieces. The term subordinates; others. It implies a reverential attitude to self-evidently Great Art as expressive of High Culture; is associated with (debunked) assumptions of intrinsic worth and transcendent value; it strips away key contextual nuance. Yet, in response to the over-simplifications of *Masked Masterpieces*, I do not wish to over-simplify in return. So, I think of thinkers through whose ideas I might think, in trying to re-think the problematics that are bothering me. Mieke Bal's 'thought-fold' (87) gathers up along the ideas of others, re-folding Gilles Deleuze's argument (1993) for the indeterminacies of a 'Baroque' point of view not as superfluous embellishment but as a generative, *relational* way of thinking that can move understanding beyond linearity, overcoming fixed perspective and complacent aesthetic certainty. In such a thought-fold, there is a co-dependent connection created between thinkers, between object and subject, artwork and viewer. This co-implication unseats easy assumptions of mastery and supremacy. Had such thoughtful disturbance been folded into the planning process of *Masked Masterpieces*, the initiative could have materialized more reflexively as visual-conceptual intervention, rather than cultural complicity.

≡

Stellenbosch, September 2020. Driving again, against being driven crazy, I turn into what used to be tourist central, now vacated. Shuttered shops, restaurants, galleries. The spartan streets in their austere angularity, an animus that belies lives, livelihoods, living here. People are missing. (What are people missing? From bare necessities to home comforts.) I miss people. Drive on towards Jonkershoek, head lost in the atlas of clouds, the changeable sky following, foiling the light, the shadowy folds of a mountainous horizon. The faint scent of fynbos. I have no destination in mind but I had to get out of the house. At the end of the road is the entrance to the nature reserve, which under COVID-19 means Locked. Turn Around. I do. Delay. Stop to check the river. The Eerste Rivier is hurtling; a fierce, oddly late flow has burst the channel and the banks are overcome. Longing for drama, anything to mark and re-route the drawn-out daze of the stalled COVID narrative, I pick a wet way down to the public braai site. The river is everywhere, no longer a burbling stream but a turbulent inland sea, a violent gathering that engulfs wretched fire pits, concrete benches, gargantuan boulders, discarded bottles, plastic bags, masks. Every swirling water rock and heaving reed bend is at once a threat and an exit. Despite the devastation I feel vulnerably alive. I laugh, thinking of a woman as almost unmanned. Sometimes, I wish.

≡

With the pandemic – a series of curfews, lockdowns, prohibitions, deprivations, curtailments – the town streets seem stopped, unhomed, their usually busy time and rhythm slowed to a shallowed pace of barely breathing. Catastrophic, collapsed angles. And home: claustrophobic. Suffocating. A mutual precarity. At the suburban edge of town, I see a familiar homeless woman and her dog. She is masked. Also much thinner than before, in that lost life-world when we ('people'? 'people like us'? 'she and I', 'she', 'I'?) routinely visited the Hospice Bookshop and bumped into local strangers. There, no questions asked, she was free to borrow books, as in a library. Well, one book at a time. Today, the book she has in hand is William Dalrymple's travelogue retracing the journeys of Marco Polo, *In Xanadu: a Quest*. Once, she'd told me about the bad place she was living back then. The noise. Mess. Drugs. Too many people in one small place. But that was life, she said. What else could she do? She is said to be *woes*, very fierce, but I haven't (yet) seen that side of her. In the shady verge, the tawny dog dozes, wet snout on her legs. The woman praises the Woolworths roast chicken. Cries a bit. Says to her dog, Yes, you see, weren't we just now-now praying? I told you! That in His Time, prayers are always answered. I have nothing to offer in reply, my mind egg-dancing in disbelief. Unbelief. Mulling a moment over the likelihood, she asks for a favour: a lift to the top of the long road. I say No, I can't. Not with COVID-19. My husband is over sixty. My elderly mother. The woman lifts both hands to stay my anxious flood; says No problem. Graciously forgives my refusal. Later, she and the dog will make their slow way up Blaauwklippen Road and left into Wildebosch. They will cut through the margins of the wetland, past the half-hearted wall of the abandoned lot, and into the distance of the quivering trees along the watercourse, once a dense poplar grove now cut down to size in the drought for thirst. Since the derelict house in the forest has been demolished to prevent further squatting, that's where she lives these days, as we have seen beyond our boundary wall. When M walks the mutts, he must avoid her and her dog, guiding our pack against the direction of their frenzy, their barking bodies an unleashed mayhem let joyously loose.

≡

The tag line of the Builders catalogue, during Covid: 'Here's to keeping us connected and secure. #HeresToHome. Prices valid at all Builders stores.'

≡

A recurrent thought-fold: *Masked Masterpieces*, as public art, turns from a traditional gallery environment to enact a more dispersed, democratic art experience, outdoors. Could it not, then, have made more of 'the street' as public space? True, 'the street' can be more fraught than friendly, especially for women, women of colour, and queer people, who are more subject than most to scrutiny, harassment and violence in public. So any potential recognition of 'the street' in *Masked Masterpieces* could not have enjoined facile celebration, but only admitted difficult individuation and community: 'the street' imagined as an unstable civic space with the potential to prompt tentative folds of experiential encounter. However fragile the connections, this is an attempt I'd like to have seen, in *Masked Masterpieces*. If you're going for public art, venturing outside the gallery, then go for broke.

Amy Chillag (2020) reports on an artist-driven COVID-19 public awareness campaign in Atlanta, USA, in areas where people of colour have been disproportionately the victims of the virus. Here, existing street mural portraits of figures such as Martin Luther King, Jr, or a black female boxer, have been appended with huge vinyl mask stickers. I envisage this intervention on the mural of a funky, young female face surrounded by king proteas that materialized in Stellenbosch in 2020, a gorgeous painted work grown across an entire wall in the populous, streetwise downtown opposite Tekkie Town. A similar take, adapted to masking, could have carried an element of the SU fundraising vector while also delivering an innovative public health message, displacing the worn idea of 'masterpieces,' risking engagement with the difficultly peopled contemporary streets. An SU campaign using such murals might also have worked to foster an understanding, in the town's somewhat narrow-minded streets, of urban art as a skilled aesthetic practice, a socially critical mode not synonymous with the vandalism of tagging.[2]

But 'the street' was never an integral conceptual element of *Masked Masterpieces*, despite some media commentators invoking comparisons with COVID-produced and COVID-adapted murals in England, such as graffiti artist Banksy's Vermeer parody, 'Girl with a Pierced Eardrum' (2014), which in April 2020 was given an anonymous update with a face mask similar to those worn by key medical workers when treating patients with COVID-19. Instead, the *Masked Masterpieces* portraits seem forms of mask stuck on 'the street,' not holistically part of mobile contemporary thinking about urban design, inherited spatial injustice, geographies of unequal movement, and the demands of human *being*, especially in African cities under COVID. *Masked Masterpieces* does not open up folds from elites to streets, likely a function of the campaign's institutional-ideological underwriting. I notice how the interpretive information board accompanying each portrait refers viewers away from the re-purposed masked portraits to the original artworks, housed in notable venues associated with 'Stellen-bosch' as a 'picturesque' Western Cape visitor destination and desirable residential node.³ Altruistic intervention is subsumed within a self-enclosed, circular economy, so that *Masked Masterpieces* 'excludes from … discussion the power relations that underline philanthropic activities,' presenting 'the often highly racialized, gendered and class-structured practice of neo-liberal philanthropy as an ideal of citizenship' (Rajabi Paak 36). This 'may have the unintended effect of also ratifying an economic culture that creates the need for such benevolence in the first place' (36). Given this masked nexus of cultural, symbolic and material geographies, it becomes difficult for the *Masked Masterpieces* campaign to acknowledge 'the street' and 'street art' as permutably ungovernable cultural formations that valuably intersect with official public com-mentary around art, precisely because they are not subject to editorial control or campaign man-agement (Mitman 2020).

≡

In town I see a rough sleeper, bush-hatted and masked. With his dog, Butchy. The young man's name I do not know, though I know he is a tik addict. Well, is said to be. Is known to be a regular at the tik house in Kayamandi. I don't even know if he is young, his face and body emaciated, though in his constant walking there can sometimes appear to be the trace of a youthful step, so young is what he seems. Once, the man had a bicycle with a homemade wooden seat upfront for the dog. You'd see them here and there around town. Be amazed at the dog's agile obedience. Here boy! And whups, up on the narrow plank, as if life were an easy circus. Then the bike dis-appeared, went who-knows-where, and once again, they walked. You'd see them resting outside the Engen, on the treed verge near the little local Spar. After another while, out on my own bur-dened stroll, I saw him putter by on a beat-up Vespa scooter, the dog perched on the running board between his knees. I looked twice. Felt for a moment oddly uplifted. Then the scooter went too. Sold? Stolen? I don't know the story. These days, the man looks much older. More gaunt. Weather leathered. But the dog seems patiently the same. Patently unchanged. Unmoved in its wandering along the rutted verge, its sun-patched snoozing. The man and his dog are always to be seen outside, sheltering in some chance place. The man gives me the slight-est nod in passing, though I have stopped giving him money. My neighbour from an NGO says he has been offered help – coupons to a shelter; even a temporary flat, apparently. But these are not options, for Butch would have to go to animal welfare. With some other homeless people, this pair lives rough in the forest above Paradyskloof. It's not a forest, really. Just a pine planta-tion. Which is what's left. What people have made of things. Some, more than others, in this Paradise Valley.

≡

      … sadness exhaustion fear frustration mask all with busyness and business.
Make bagels. Cushion. Deckle-edged paper from pond slime. Quick pickles. Administer
and edit. Supervise. Watch Netflix. Cook. Cut, slip, plant. Struggle to read. Read. Desire
                a lively poiesis though/through trapped/released/
                    trappedreleasedtrappedreleasedtra

Some days nights fires floods wars corruption violence extinctions losses suicides excess
                    deaths despairing of bad

thoughts ... I'd do better to scroll clear
of The News. Screened endings plastic shields no family filters all gets the better

of me and worse I
fold, leak, badly.

Then afterwards, because must,
she gathers herself
turns inwards. Holds. Steady.
Ruks roughly reg
and ever ready unfolds
a fresh mask

≡

Lynne Steger Strong adapts Rob Nixon's concept of slow violence to the multiple, pervasive stressors of women's work and the work associated with being women, intensified under the pandemic 'The way we are worked over, run down, reminded again and again to shut up and sit back down.'

> The way the news of eight hundred thousand women dropping out of the work force seems hardly to register. The way that, eight months in, there are no real solutions for most women to get help with our kids ... In thinking about the idea of slow violence, I've been thinking about ... explaining what it has been like, what it is like, to have the world act upon our specific female bodies. What it is like to spend so much time holding tight to feelings no one wants to hear or see. Violence is a word associated with the body, associated with the loud, the immediate, and the concrete. But it is also ... that rickety beat-up feeling we've had our whole lives. What's happening right now to so many female bodies isn't visible. It isn't loud or immediate. It's unrelenting, an accumulation ... it is happening mostly silently. (2020)

≡

A woman folds inwards to create an impassive face, turning away. What was it Levinas said, something about the skin of the face being that which stays most naked, most destitute? The woman must seem unmoved, though with the passage of time (cruel? inevitable?) her companionable old face becomes vividly pinched and tucked with tears (teeyas/tairs) of self-evident emotion. Everything she can no longer hide. In a staff meeting, a colleague once cautioned her kindly against this dangerous transparency. Then how she was disarmed of herself. Unmasked. Before that, she'd imagined she was shielded. What with a little concealer, an uplifting lipstick, the basics would help her pull it off. But apparently: no. Her masking fails. So in some ways the mandatory Covid mask is a safe space, despite the trouble breathing and the misted specs. A convenient guise behind which she can (pretend to) hide her failures, her growing knowledge of inevitable imperfection. The Covid mask is an odd comfort behind which she can escape the constant demands of presenting herself to others, whether as pleasant femaleness or necessary bad cop. The mask is a relief in kind from masking. Dutifully masked, she becomes more difficult to read and can believe herself unreadable; virtually invisible, almost. The pure pleasure of anonymity. Being, without giving anything away.

≡

Aggrieved, aggressive badgering. *Masks masks* masks. Masking? Think *you* fuckn suffering? Fuckkkk ha. Masking is what autistic people have to do every fuckn day, the way you people force us to keep it together. Always beating on us. We never allowed to *be*. Oh no, no, we must follow your fucked up normal standards that fuck up the world. Another new fuckn *normal*. You can't stop me *being*. I am here. I can live. You die! I am so fuckn *tired* of fuckkk, everything. Stupid. Maaaaasks. No! Now your turn. *You* wear. *You* suffer. *You* see how shit it feels. Like how I can't ever breathe myself every day.

≡

For various reasons (aesthetic and ethical pleats that play/ploy/ply/plead), a writer may adopt a mask: a persona (perhaps), a voice, a point of view, a creative crease that tucks the line, and allows her to say what otherwise she c/w/should not. The mask is a paradoxical guise, offering both comfort and licence. On the face of it, first-person is often considered intimate, confessional, authentic, while third-person is assumed to deflect and distance. Yet experienced readers know (readers know from experience) that truth is always difficult to gauge. Who is to determine what is appropriate, and if someone appropriates? Representation is tricky to read.

≡

A woman is mother to a teen on the autistic spectrum. She (meaning 'the woman') has over time become less recognizable to herself, although she is also manifestly herself, being unable to be or become anyone else. Over time, she has gathered what she must do, and she single-mindedly folds and unfolds into a many-faceted support system, a moebius transformer of advocacy, intervention, damage control and care; cooking, cleaning, comforting, coaching, chastising, trying to create ways. Much work of many kinds. To no effect. There is no change to a neurotypical world, closed to difference and disability and neurodiversity. And the change from childhood melt-downs to explosive teenage rage is scarcely change at all. So nothing the woman does changes anything, but if she did nothing, then nothing could ever change. Under COVID-19 this disabling situation grips even tighter.

≡

I wear a mask and keep my distance because I care about the lives of other people.

≡

Masking fold 1: autism spectrum disorders are significantly under-diagnosed in female populations due to an historically male clinical bias, based on studies using young male subjects. Autism has been entrenched in the Diagnostic and Statistical Manual of Mental Disorders as a male neurological disorder.

    Masking fold 2: more recently, researchers of neurodiversity have established that autism in girls and women presents differently than the classic autism profile. Studies now show that behaviours widely modelled as female – politeness, neatness, respect … can mask a girl's autism, precluding diagnosis and access to therapies and educational accommodations.

    Masking fold 3: if a girl exhibits socially non-compliant, risky or disruptive behaviours (more tolerated in young male populations, since 'boys will be boys') she may be misdiagnosed as oppositional defiant or borderline personality (or or or). Again, her special needs may remain unaddressed: significant autistic impairments in areas such as social communication skills, executive function, sensory hyperacuity, impulse control, volatile moods, emotional-cognitive processing …

Masking fold 4: the neurodivergent routinely expend extensive energy on masking in public, mirroring society's preferred behaviours. This is not necessarily to maintain the pretence of 'normal,' but to cope in stressful everyday situations. Under pandemic lockdowns (remote schooling, WFH) autistic masking may diminish as the autistic person might feel less stressed, less compelled to cover compromised competence via exhausting adaptive behaviours.

Masking fold 5: contrarily, lockdowns may mean broken routines, increased anxiety and an escalation in stimming. Perseverative self-regulatory behaviours may include explosive sounding; repetitive singing; flapping; jigging; skin cutting; obsessive cleaning; wound picking; hair pulling; binge eating. Stimming is a crucial form of self-soothing. It can also veer towards the (self-)destructive.

≡

Folds being convoluted, in some lives contiguous, a woman is also mother to a queer young adult. This teen has made it clear: *you* have to learn. *You* think it's difficult? If you think it's difficult to live *with* queer, try asking queer people whether it's easy to live queer, *being* queer. With queer principles.

Under COVID-19, the hard-won supportive networks of 'queer socialities' and 'alternative kin-making' (Trott 88) for young queers in this small part of the world are foreclosed. No more Queer Us. No more Teen Pride. No more clubs. Yet, thrown back into closeted isolation under lockdown, with eight in ten LGBTQ+ young people (in the UK) reporting that their mental health has significantly deteriorated since the pandemic began (De la Cretaz 2021), queer finds connections. WhatsApp groups and video calls; blogs; the wild release of one, two, maybe three out and open-minded out-there friends, who share virtually everything, making life under Covid something remotely possible. This is how a current plague is made bearable.

≡

The portrait that's amiss in *Masked Masterpieces* – a misfit out of place among modernists, for one – is the Zanele Muholi. And yet the project is also reliant on Muholi and their transgressive queer re-figuring. In presenting 'fictionalized versions of a female sitter' in her photographs, 'Muholi invents titles and names, alluding to the places, histories, people, or conditions referenced in the works. In this way choosing to suppress the "sitter's" identity is empowering' (Corrigall 2020). It aims to 'challenge the kind of exoticism that Stern and Tretchikoff sought to summon through their paintings' and offers a 'fitting counterpoint to the other portraits' in *Masked Masterpieces* (Corrigall 2020). Perhaps. But the meanings are more mutable than incontrovertible, more inter-folded than separate (Figure 3).

For example, 'Aphelile IV, Durban, 2020' is first published in *The New York Times*' interactive digital magazine in a COVID-19 photo essay on the question of 'what artists are creating under quarantine' (Anon 2020). The essay features notable contemporary international artists such as Titus Kaphar and Kara Walker. In the brief biotext, Muholi is credited as a photographer and visual artist 'known for documenting black lesbian, gay, bisexual, transgender and intersex people's lives in various townships in South Africa' (Anon 2020). Here, in claiming a photojournalistic, witnessing value for 'Aphelile IV, Durban, 2020,' the understanding of the portrait as a COVID-contextual performative expression of dispersed, seried, manifold staging of selves is

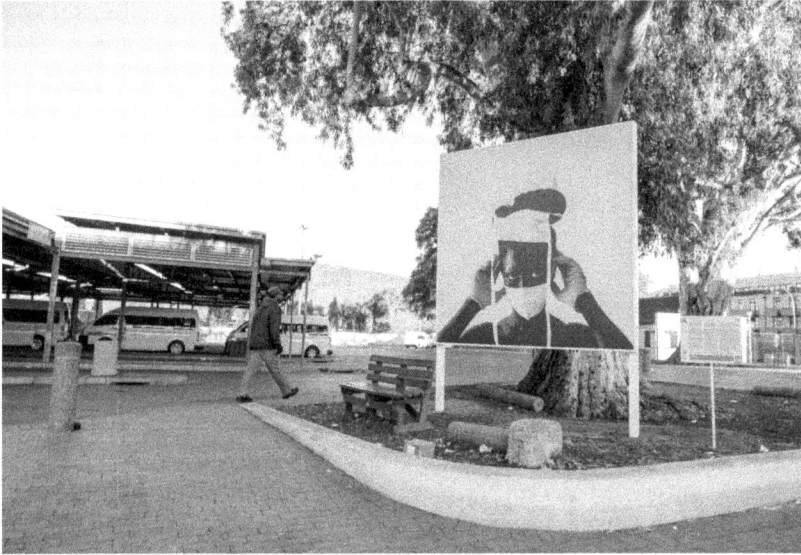

Figure 3.   Muholi's 'Aphelile IV, Durban, 2020', photo SU campaign material.

quelled. Muholi's emphatic visual-conceptual repetition in using *two* masks also escapes notice, whether as a prescient notion of medical double-masking, a comment on the joint burdens of race and orientation, or as an aesthetic gesture to innovative artistic process, especially in uncertain times. The text block alongside the photograph gives the artist's explanation that the 'image was taken on April 11, in South Africa, in response to the emergency and the use of gloves and masks as essentials ... to keep one safe and protected'. Acknowledging strangely folded timelines, Muholi continues: 'I am under lockdown with limited movements and resources to continue production at my usual pace. I have to make use of what is at my disposal' (Anon 2020). This last sentence (in which I at first mistakenly read and typed 'place,' not 'pace') is used to title the whole photo feature. Muholi's phrasing implies a sensitivity to the contradictions of personal protective equipment as (no guarantee of) safety, and yet, in being disposable, endangering the environment. The phrasing also carries an awareness of the hardships caused to creative livelihoods by lockdown, as well as the systemic violence wrought by heteronormativity against the possibilities of queer people's safety and flourishing.

When 'Aphelile IV, Durban, 2020' is re-installed in *Masked Masterpieces*, re-purposed in the ill-fitting company of portraits by Laubser, Sekoto, Stern and Tretchikoff, the performative agency that Corrigall attributes to Muholi is not unequivocally enabling. Given the historical and representational attenuation of the *Masked Masterpieces*' concept and curation, as well as its emphasis on traditional fine art picturing in media such as paint, in the SU initiative 'Muholi' must effect extensive invisible labour, both to be part of the campaign, and on the part of the campaign. (Fold. Re-fold.) The organizers are quick to deflect criticism of the initiative by accentuating that Zanele Muholi expressly asked to participate. Yet this itself is a masked admission of omission, of a neglect to solicit Muholi's participation (perhaps because they and their work were not perceived to meet the campaign's prescriptive criteria of traditional masterwork). The organizers' statement also obliquely speaks of the unspoken anxiety that the criteria of 'currency' and 'critique,' which could be found wanting in the conceptualizing of *Masked Masterpieces*, might be rectified by Muholi as an add-on, added-value contributor. The duty to correct a dearth of insight and lack of thought – a glaring absence – somehow becomes Muholi's responsibility. The Muholi photograph, as well as Muholi's reputation as an artist who stages experimentally performative versions of gender-diverse black subjectivity and, arguably, Muholi themselves as a publicly genderqueer black person who no longer identifies as female, must carry the alternative or radical or transgressively otherwise cultural signatures of the contemporary zeitgeist that *Masked Masterpieces* cannot. This hidden obligation is the cost of Muholi being permitted to participate; an assumed aesthetic-ideological service (even servitude) that Muholi must provide, while the norms of the self-satisfied normative remain blithely unbending. What we have, here, is an instance of the wearying and timeworn workings of the marginalized being burdened with triple loads and multiple shifts, while systemic transformations of thought, practice and behaviour are yet again a dream deferred.

When I visited the site of the Muholi installation in February 2021, the portrait had been gouged in one eye and on the subject's chest, and the information plaque was gone. Such wounding defacement intimates that this artist's queer matter, reputation and/or person are considered by some to require censure, even elimination. I cannot know who vandalized the Muholi at the taxi rank, or why, though my remarks about the challenges of including Muholi's disruptive art and artistic signature in the constricted ambit of *Masked Masterpieces* hint at the perceived unbelonging, for some Stellenbosch publics, of queer black art/ists, whether among local communities, or in the company of supposed artistic masters/masterpieces. I'd hoped that as part of *Masked Masterpieces* 'Aphelile IV, Durban, 2020' would create an imaginative fold in Stellenbosch's social fabric for the 'performance of counterpublicity' (Muñoz 147), unsettling the 'exclusionary and discriminatory' (149) discourses, behaviours and indeed reproducibility of a heteronormative, majoritarian public sphere. But I was never certain of anything. Nothing has changed.

≡

Sometime in early April 2021, with a significant percentage of students back on campus for some form of in-person teaching and learning, the Sekoto, Tretchikoff, and Stern are treated to an anonymous culture jamming, the word COMPLICIT stencilled in black caps across the masked portrait figures (Figure 4). The Muholi is not subject to this intervention. Nor is the Laubser, tucked away in an easy-to-miss alley.

≡

Hoping in difficult times to sustain and console myself by making something otherwise of *Masked Masterpieces*, I work towards a final fold in my material along the lines of an Oulipian potential art.

Imagine this, in your mind's eye.

In the spirit of generative constraint, I work *with* the portraits chosen for *Masked Masterpieces*, making do with givens, yet also asking, 'What if?'

In my re-working of the campaign, my key initial crease is away from the conventionalized, flat portrait surface that can too easily be accorded received status and assumed legibility. Alternatively, I propose a series of visual interruptions that stage uneasy, relational viewing.

Instead of a single flat surface —, think angled panels ^^^^^

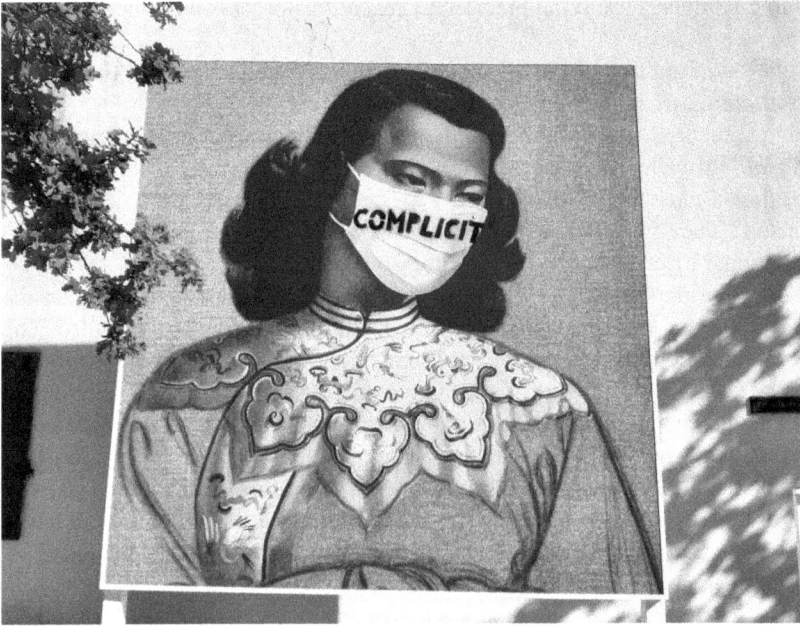

Figure 4.   Anonymous culture jamming of Tretchikoff's 'Chinese Girl', photo S Murray.

In both idea and realization, this allows me to pair *two* images at each installation site (let the wheres be a complication for another day). I set out by taking my reproductions of the five *Masked Masterpieces* portraits and, determining not to be reverential, I tear strips off them; partly slash and burn. (Most of the reproductions will be none the worse and probably all the better for this constructively deconstructive de-facing). When I am done, I re-configure the holed wholes in assemblages, approximations that tangentially reference, but also *skew*, any hagiographic original.

I then source five *additional* portraits, arresting images with a glancing local relevance, *contemporary* pieces that I set in dissonant contrapuntal pairing with *Masked Masterpieces*' time-honoured treasures. Again, it will be the Muholi that blurs neat boundaries. When it comes to who? which? why? when choosing My Five, I will aim for a widely expanded range given to question, over admiration. (Lady Skollie? Mary Sibande? Or?) I will risk innovative styles. I will discuss possibilities and limits with others. I will collaboratively fold and re-fold ideas until their creased complexity is faced head-on and then turned to critical-creative re-purposing.

Once I have the ten portrait pairs, all reproduced to the same scale, as required for application to the ^^^^^ panelled armature, I will apply the masks. (A collaged cut and paste? Digital re-mastering? Neatly? Masking areas other than the mouth? TBC).

Then (a process to be repeated ten times), I take a portrait from a conceptual pair and cut it carefully into five vertical strips of the same dimensions. Each strip I number sequentially so that sections, when assembled 1, 2, 3, 4, 5, will retain the visual integrity of the portrait face. Thinking in kind, this much comfort I will allow my audience. (On the panels, of course, I pencil the corresponding numbers). Working precisely, I repeat this process with the other portrait in the pair.

After this, working from the left, I apply the five numbered strips of a contemporary portrait to each of the similarly numbered (*rising*) hill folds of the ^^^^

The five numbered strips of the related, deconstructed 'masterpiece' portrait I attach to the numbered (*falling*) valley folds of the ^^^^

(Thereafter, I must repeat this process with the four remaining portrait pairs.)

The result? The ^^^^ format situates two portraits together in a single space, a pointed plane of relational meeting at once conjugate, yet separate.

How each portrait appears – whole, emergent, disaggregated – depends on the angle of view. Sometimes, for a flash – longer if you deliberately manage the folded length of the pause – you could apprehend each face almost entire and resolved. More often, you will be challenged to find coherence slantwise in associative processing, your visual sense directed by discontinuity and disorientation that require thought and effort, to establish a reading of 'the face'.

Such a method – however simplistic or imperfect – could 're-sight' the portraits as enfolded cultural re-citations in various Stellenbosch sites. The de-formations, the visual violence, the hard work of making sense ... such features could deflect habit and, even if in passing, reflect other takes on notions of mastery and the picturesque often too easily imagined as *the* Cape Winelands aesthetic.

The ^^^^ design creates a situation where a portrait needs to be materialized in process as a 'conceptually dense text that must be made intelligible, yet remains, in its foreignness, informative as well as provocative, that is, *performative*' (Venuti qtd. in Bal 94). Seeing the faces requires a perplexing effort to 'both dissipate and release the text's otherness'. The ^^^^ structure pointedly reminds a viewer that a culture of mastery 'must be able to estrange itself from its own assumptions, so that the automatic othering of what comes at it ... can be replaced with negotiation' (94). The ^^^^ installation concept aims for 'ethical disturbance' (Serpell, *Seven* 14) and 'uncertainty of agency' (7), 'a shifting, variable mode' (9) of 'heady uncertain mix' where agencies and intentions 'collude and collide' (8) between 'knowing and not knowing' (20).

^^^^ is an invitation to viewers of 'Masked Masterpieces' (Mark II) to open up to the need for a 'transformative participatory process' in art-making and meaning-making; the possibility of different ways of understanding or doing things, of 'becoming otherwise' (Sitas and Pieterse 331). This 'otherwise' 'draws deeply on layer upon layer of experience, thought, feeling, all folding into itself, creating' a rich reservoir that holds the 'potentiality for becoming something or someone else, even if the transition is microscopic' (331). In the traditionalist, still highly unequal Stellenbosch environment, ^^^^ asks you to accept the challenge of mediating 'between the imperatives of sameness (connection, empathy, likeness) and difference (distance, alterity, opposition)' (Serpell, *Seven* 28). Or, as C. Namwali Serpell muses with and against Levinas in her essay collection *Stranger Faces* (2020): looking at a face that both resembles our own and yet is its own distinctive self, how willing are we, limning the lined folds of legibility, to acknowledge what we owe each other? Might we welcome, rather than turn away from 'explored responses to the familiar' that 'surprise us at every turn, seep into the corners of our perception, and make gradual, delicate, enduring shifts in our attitudes. Changes that suddenly highlight all those masked faces we see around us now' (Ciabattari 2021)?

≡

In early March 2020 BC – just Before COVID – a recent SU Visual Arts Honours graduate leads zine-making workshops for creative writing students in the English Department. In the process of preparing portfolios for submission, these emergent writers thrill to experiment with unusual forms of material presentation, learning retro techniques of pamphlet folding and handmade chapbooking. Just maybe, beyond the online presence of personal websites, these tactile, inexpensive modes of making and distribution might enable an alternative audiencing. We intend to hold An Exhibition, in collective celebration. But by mid-March, these cultural ambitions are dead, since COVID-19 curtails all forms of face-to-face university interaction.

≡

Trying to imagine a creative life post-coronial, I wonder: 'what will the arts economy look like once the pandemic is over? Indications so far are not good'. While galleries, venues, acts, artists 'may seem to be holding on … collapse happens slower than you think,' as those in the arts economy 'gradually exhaust their lifelines – savings, loans, emergency purchases from friendly collectors. The crash arrives when no one's looking' (Deresiewicz, 2021).

≡

The zine artist is an accomplished paper folder. Online (@maialehrsacks), I find images of the intricate tessellations she creates, impossibly multi-layered 3-D forms, all painstakingly shaped from the same initial flat surface, a page on which I would need to write and rewrite, both carefully and welcoming chaos, so as to create the illusion of depth. She makes ethereal nautili too, which conjure oceanic environments on the brink of loss – paper creased and angled and curled in on itself to form exquisite shell-like whorls. For the love of nothing more than beauty and skill, I commission nautili in three sizes, each shape the result of a different combination of folds. The paper is off-white Fabriano Ingres. For origami, among this paper's properties are good memory, forgiveness and tensile strength. I will come to know these as a valuable coalescence of characteristics.

The nautili arrive compressed in individually-crafted envelopes. (Surprise: triangular). Each translucent, infolded pod comes with a long, sheer thread tied to an ordinary paper clip that you unbend, making a serviceable hanger. I expand the flatpack forms, unfolding the models in order, biggest to smallest. A, B, C]). I bend the pliable wire and balance precariously to hang the sculptures at different heights from the ugly fluorescent bulkhead in my office. Installed, the shapes slowly find their expanded form, gyring slightly. Twirling thread. Infinitesimal calculus. I switch off the office light, and see the spectral eidolon of ghostly husks, dangling.

Outside my office, the corridors of power form an empty stretch, a long passage that glows clinically white except near the double doors. These are lit by an EXIT sign, burning red. I leave for the day without really noticing all the old familiars – recalcitrant photocopier, posters (new, and faded), course noticeboards, info about reading groups, colleagues' doors with nameplates, pinned clippings ('The Scream'; a Larsson cartoon; a tribute to Toni Morrison).

When push comes to shoving, the departmental doors fold open, and then almost closed. (Always the perennial problem with closure; the unfixable swing-arm at fault). Little do I know, at the time, that virtually overnight the suspended nautili will be left hanging for numerous gathering, successive waves of a global pandemic, an up-in-the-air where days, weeks and months seem slowly to fold into a falter of years.

Notes

1   SU is no stranger to controversy around race and gender, *vide* the mid-2019 scandal around an article by SU researchers on the reputedly compromised cognitive skills of coloured women in the peer-reviewed journal *Aging, Neuropsychology and Cognition*, a study now retracted.

2   I recall the photocopied wheatpaste murals of Scott Eric Williams, a 2019 Mellon 30th Anniversary Artist in Residence in the SU VAP. He deliberately used 'poor' methods and materials, accessible and relatively inexpensive, in a collaborative process easy for students and communities to initiate in their own projects. Williams installed large-scale, haunting images of marginalized people and erased lives around Stellenbosch and adjacent historical worker towns like Pniel. The walls, pasted with anonymous figures from a *lived* past that escapes the archival impulse, were turned into thoughtful portals, openings that asked viewers to look anew into history, present amnesia, and hoped-for futures.

3   The original artworks featured in the campaign are on view as follows: the Tretchikoff at Delaire Graff wine estate; the Sekoto on loan to Stellenbosch University Museum from the Fort Hare collection; the Laubser at the La Motte wine estate museum; the Stern at the Steenberg's Tryn Restaurant; while the Muholi is on show in 2020 at an exhibition at the Norval Foundation, Cape Town.

Works Cited

Anon. '"I Have to Make Use of What is at My Disposal.' What Zanele Muholi, Titus Kaphar, Kara Walters and Other Artists are Creating Under Quarantine'. https://www.nytimes.com/interactive. Accessed on 23 Sept. 2020.

Bal, Mieke. *Travelling Concepts in the Humanities: A Rough Guide*. Toronto: University of Toronto Press, 2002.

Chillag, Amy. 'Black Artists Put Face Masks on Street Murals Because "We're Not Seeing Visual Cues of a Pandemic"'. *CNN*. 1 Sept. 2020. https://edition.cnn.com/2020/07/09/us/black-mural-artists-covid-mask-coverup-iyw-trnd/index.html. Accessed on 20 Sept. 2020.

Ciabattari, Jane. 'This Year's NBCC Award Finalists: *Stranger Faces* by Namwali Serpell'. 4 Mar. 2021. https://lithub.com/this-years-nbcc-award-finalists-stranger-faces-by-namwali-serpell/. Accessed on 21 Mar. 2021.

Corrigall, Mary. 'Masked Portraits Highlight Markers of SA's "Masters"'. 19 Aug. 2020. https://www.investec.com/en_za/focus/beyond-wealth/masked-portraits-highlight-markers-of-sa-masters.html. Accessed on 21 Aug. 2020.

De la Cretaz, Britni. 'COVID-19 is Sparking a Mental Health Crisis Among LGBTQ+ Youth'. *them*. 18 Feb. 2021. https://www.them.us/story/covid-19-lgbtq-youth-mental-health-crisis. Accessed on 25 Feb. 2021.

Deleuze, Gilles. *The Fold: Leibniz and the Baroque*. Translated by Tom Conley. London: Athlone Press, 1993.

Delmont, Elizabeth. 'Laubser, Land and Labour: Image-making and Afrikaner Nationalism in the Late 1920s and Early 1930s.' *De Arte* 36(64), 2001: 5–34.

Deresiewicz, William. 'Stages of Grief: What The Pandemic Has Done to The Arts'. *Harpers Magazine*. June 2021. https://harpers.org/archive/2021/06/stages-of-grief-what-the-pandemic-has-done-to-the-arts/. Accessed on 2 May 2021.

Evans, Becky. "'I Haven't Made a Penny From Being in One of World's Most Famous Artworks": Revelation of the Woman Behind the Green "Chinese Girl" Painting'. *The Daily Mail*, 10 Feb. 2013. https://www.dailymail.co.uk/news/article-2276500/I-havent-penny-worlds-famous-artworks-Revelation-woman-green-Chinese-Girl-painting.html. Accessed on 3 Dec. 2020.

Eyene, Christine. 'Sekoto and Négritude: The Ante-room of French Culture.' *Third Text* 24(4), 2010: 423–35.

Friedman, Michael and Wolfgang Schäffner (Eds.). *On Folding: Towards a New Field of Interdisciplinary Research*. Bielefeld: transcript Verlag, 2016.

Mawere, Tinashe. '(Un)masking Other Dangerous Pandemics Within the Covid-19 Lockdown'. *CSAG*. 17 Aug. 2020. https://www.csagup.org/2020/08/17/unmasking-other-dangerous-pandemics-within-the-covid-19-lockdown/. Accessed 8 Jan. 2021.

Mitman, Tyson. 'Coronavirus Murals: Inside the World of Pandemic-inspired Street Art'. *The Conversation*. 18 May 2020. https://theconversation.com/coronavirus-murals-inside-the-world-of-pandemic-inspired-street-art-138487. Accessed on 25 July 2020.

Mohanty, Chandra Talpade. 'Under Western Eyes: Feminist Scholarship and Colonial Discourses'. *Feminist Review* 30, 1988: 61–88.

Muñoz, José Esteban. *Disidentifications: Queers of Color and the Performance of Politics*. Minneapolis, MN: University of Minnesota Press, 2009.

Rajabi Paak, Mina. "The Epidemic of Spectacles: The HIV/AIDS Pandemic, Visual Culture and the Philanthropic Documentary Archive of the Global South". Diss. University of British Columbia, 2014.

Serpell, C. Namwali. *Seven Modes of Uncertainty*. Cambridge: Harvard University Press, 2014.

Serpell, C. Namwali. *Stranger Faces: Undelivered Lectures*. Oakland, CA: Transit Books, 2020.

Settler, Frederico and Mari Haugaa Engh. 'The Black Body in Colonial and Postcolonial Public Discourse in South Africa'. *Alternation* 14, 2015: 126–48.

Sitas, Rike and Edgar Pieterse. 'Democratic Renovations and Affective Political Imaginaries'. *Third Text* 27(3), 2013: 327–42.

Strong, Lynne Steger. 'Slow Violence'. *The Paris Review*. 14 Oct. 2020. https://www.theparisreview.org/blog/2020/10/14/slow-violence/. Accessed on 16 Oct. 2020.

Trott, Ben. 'Queer Berlin and the Covid-19 Crisis: a Politics of Contact and Ethics of Care'. *Interface* 12(1), 2020: 88–108.

Van Robbroeck, Lize et al. 'On Masked Masterpieces'. In *Covid Diaries: Women's Experience of the Pandemic*. Edited by Amanda Gouws and Olivia Ezeobi. Cape Town: Imbali, 2021. 66–71.

Vyzoviti, Sophia and Joanna Sotiriou. 'Descriptive and Generative Models of Crumpled Sheets'. In *What's the Matter: Materiality and Materialism at the Age of Computation*. Edited by Maria Voyatzaki. Thessaloniki: European Network of Heads of Schools of Architecture, 2015. 521–32.

White-Parks, Annette. 'A Reversal of American Concepts of "Other-ness" in the Fiction of Sui Sin Far'. *Melus* 20(1), 1995: 17–34.

Woolf, Virginia. 'A Room of One's Own'. In *A Room of One's Own and Three Guinees*. London: Vintage, 2001. 1–98.

Zagury-Orly, Ivry. 'Unmasking Reasons for Face Mask Resistance'. *Global Biosecurity* 2(1), 2020. http://doi.org/10.31646/gbio.80.

'As others feel pain in their lungs': Albert Camus's *The Plague*

Hedley Twidle

for D.B. (1981-2020)

This is an account of reading Albert Camus's *The Plague* in the wake of various real-world epidemics, and from a place, South Africa, that emerges as a kind of mirror image of the north Africa in which the novel is set. It suggests that what seems at first like a simple story is in fact a deeply complex, even contradictory work: one that that absorbs and reflects back as much history and difficulty as the reader is willing to bring to it. While giving postcolonial critiques of the work their due, I explore how and why *The Plague* still holds energy and meaning for a 21st-century audience.

1.

In 1947, Albert Camus published *La peste*, the story of a town struck by bubonic plague. He judged the book a failure, but *The Plague* is probably his most successful and widely read work.

In one sense it is a simple story. Rats come out of cellars and sewers, spitting blood, and begin to die in the streets. Then people begin to die. The town is sealed off and we follow the experiences of a small band of characters as they battle the epidemic. Like a classical tragedy, the book is divided into five acts. In parts one and two, the death toll is rising; in part three it is at its height: 'the plague had covered everything' (239).[1] In parts four and five, the disease slowly retreats, and the town is liberated again. Amid the celebrations, the narrator strikes a note of foreboding: 'He knew that this happy crowd was unaware of something that one can read in books, which is that the plague bacillus never dies or vanishes entirely' (237).

The opening lines stress the ordinariness of the setting, the French Algerian port of Oran where Camus arrived in 1941 for tuberculosis treatment, and where he began gathering material for the book:

> The peculiar events that are the subject of this history occurred in 194–, in Oran. The general opinion was that they were misplaced there, since they deviated somewhat from the ordinary. At first sight, indeed, Oran is an ordinary town, nothing more than a French Prefecture on the coast of Algeria. (5)

This short prelude introduces what is in one sense an allegorical 'everytown'. The daily routines of money and love-making, sea-bathing and newspaper reading are charted in a coolly objective, transparent style: 'the style of absence which is,' as Roland Barthes remarked of Camus's prose, 'almost an ideal absence of style' (*Writing Degree Zero* 77). Further down the page are the most quotable lines, which demonstrate his way with an aphorism: 'A convenient way of getting to know a town is to find out how people work there, how they love and how they die' (5).

The opening section of *The Plague* might touch off various moments of recognition, depending from where you read it. I find some answering echoes in the city where I live. Cape Town mirrors the latitude of Oran and was also once a colonial port. It is also a business-minded, tourism-driven place, at least in the oversold city centre, which is 'ringed with luminous hills' but 'so disposed that it turns its back on the bay, with the result that it's impossible to see the sea, you always have to go and look for it' (trans. Gilbert 3–4).

Camus's narrator suggests that there still exist towns and countries where people have now and again an inkling, or an intimation, of something different: *le soupçon d'autre chose*. A hint, a dash, a suspicion or smidgeon. On the whole, he goes on, it might not change their lives, but at least 'they had an intimation, and that's so much to the good' (6) Oran, on the other hand, appears to be *une ville sans soupçons, c'est-à-dire une ville tout à fait moderne*: 'a town without inklings, that is to say, an entirely modern town' (6).

Like so much else in the book, the confident simplicity of the writing is deceptive. The words let on more, betray more and perhaps know more than their author ever intended. The 'peculiar events' of the novel are indeed 'not in their place'. They are misplaced in a complicated and painful sense, with major consequences for how one interprets the book, and whether the great humanist credo that it arrives at can be believed in: 'to say simply what it is that one learns in the midst of such tribulations, namely that there is more in men to admire than to despise' (237).

The opening lines of *The Plague* contain, in embryo, the whole problem of a literary work that tempts you to read it as a kind of universal fable, an allegory of human suffering, stoicism and resistance – but also stubbornly refuses to give up its allegiance to, and imaginative posses-sion of, an actual place. Today the port of وهران (Oran or Wahran) is the second-largest city in Algeria, with a population of around a million people. In nineteen forty-something, it was the town with the biggest population of French Algerians, or *pieds noirs* (of which Camus, born 1913 in Algiers, was one). The pejorative term, 'black feet,' was possibly derived from the boots of the French army that began the conquest of this vast North African territory in 1830: a brutal imperial venture notorious for the military strategy of *razzia* and *ratissages* – punitive raids on Algerian villages.

And why the blank in '194–'? The convention is more common for proper names, signifying someone or somewhere familiar to the author but lightly or partially disguised for the reader. It is really Oran itself that the opening lines should have rendered as 'O–'. That might have avoided some difficulties. Because when you try to place the book – to properly situate it in its historical moment, and in North Africa – *The Plague* becomes a deeply complex, even contradictory work: one that absorbs and reflects back as much history and difficulty as the reader is willing to bring to it.

2.

'On the morning of April 16, Dr Bernard Rieux emerged from his consulting-room and came across a dead rat in the middle of the landing.' This sentence at the start of chapter two could also be a workable first line. *The Plague* has a double beginning in this sense. We move from the distant, generalized register of the first chapter into the mesh of individual human lives and destinies. It begins once as moral fable, and then again as medical thriller.

The five movements of *The Plague* generally follow this structure: first a brief prelude in the voice of collective opinion (*de l'avis général*), then the dive into plot. Like the overture to an opera (and the book does contain one: Gluck's *Orfeo ed Euridice*), the preludes introduce general thematic ideas that will then play out in actual human lives and bodies. The exception is the third movement, when the plague is at its height, which is narrated entirely in the voice of generalized experience.

As soon as we leave Rieux's consulting-room, we meet the old concierge, M. Michel, who is convinced that the dead rats are some kind of practical joke – this is Patient Zero. Dr Rieux is the main character; in fact he is also the narrator, but we only learn that towards the end of the book. For now (if we stay within the realist frame), he is narrating his experience in the third person, while also explaining how it is that he has the authority to tell the story:

> Of course a historian, even if he is an amateur, always has his documents. The narrator of this history has his documents: first of all, his own testimony, then that of others since, by virtue of his role in this story, he came to collect the confidences of all the characters in it; and, finally, he had written texts which he happened to acquire. He intends to borrow from them when he sees fit and to use them as he wishes. He intends ... But perhaps it is time to have done with preliminaries and caveats, and turn to the story itself. The narrative of the early days must be given in some detail. (8)

Here is the punctilious, sometimes pedantic tone of *The Plague*, giving us fiction packaged as documentary (a device that goes right back to the origin of the European novel as a kind of false document). After this briefing on the factual basis of what we are about to read, the rest of part one records the 'troubling signs' of the approaching epidemic, while also introducing us to the five main characters. The narrator is like a midfielder moving the ball quickly and accurately around the football pitch – perhaps in the Spanish style of swift, accurate passing that replaces individual showboating for a dogged collective effort. (Camus was a keen player and there is some football chat in the book.)[2]

First we meet the journalist Raymond Rambert. He is stranded in Oran while on assignment and missing his lover back in Paris. Camus, who obviously split off portions of himself into his ensemble cast, was similarly stuck when he went to central France to recuperate from TB in 1942. With the Allied landings in North Africa in November of that year, the German army occupied the south of France to secure the Mediterranean coastline. Camus was sealed off from his wife and from Algiers.

In letters, Camus described *The Plague* as emerging from a struggle for breath; it was also, he said, a response to a world without women. It is certainly a very male book (but not, I think, a masculinist one) and largely sexless. Dr Rieux's wife (unnamed) leaves Oran just as the story begins. She is going to a sanatorium out of town for treatment; they bid farewell at the train station, promising to make a fresh start on her return. Her place is taken by Rieux's mother, a watchful, largely silent presence who helps take care of her son and his apartment during the epidemic.

Madame Rieux's stoic silence must hold something of Camus's own mother, Catherine Hélène Sintés, who lost her husband in the First World War and during Albert's childhood cleaned houses in the working-class district of Belcourt. Catherine Camus was illiterate, partially deaf, with a speech impediment that meant she hardly spoke. When her son died in a car accident in 1960, at age 46, a briefcase containing a manuscript titled *Le premier homme* was retrieved from the wreck. Only brought into print in 1994 (by Camus's daughter Catherine), *The First Man* evokes a colonial, French Algerian childhood in all the historical texture, social detail and depth of field that seems so absent from *The Plague*. Camus had dedicated his unfinished manuscript to his mother: *To you who will never be able to read this book.*

There is a curious moment just as Rambert is introduced. He tells Rieux that he is '"doing an investigation for a large Parisian newspaper about the living conditions of the Arabs"' and wants information on their health situation (11). Rieux asks the journalist if he can tell the whole truth, by which he means '"an unqualified indictment"' (*condamnation totale*): '"I can only countenance a report without reservations, so I shall not be giving you any information to contribute to yours"' (11–12).

Next we meet Jean Tarrou, a newcomer to Oran, living in a hotel in the city centre and a great lover of swimming. He keeps a notebook, and this is one of the documentary sources that the narrator employs. In counterpoint to the growing tension of the plague plot, Tarrou's notebooks, with their 'deliberate policy of insignificance' (21), work to lighten the atmosphere. With an eye for the absurdity of everyday life, they record chance details and snippets of overheard talk.

Tarrou records how each day an old man comes out onto the opposite balcony, tears up bits of paper and scatters them over the edge, while calling to the cats in the side-street. When they come out and lift their paws towards this shower of white butterflies, he spits on the cats, 'firmly and accurately': 'When one of his gobs of saliva hit the target he would laugh' (22). Elsewhere, Tarrou proposes a kind of mock serious urban fieldwork reminiscent of Georges Perec and the Situationists:

> 'Question: how can one manage not to lose time? Answer: experience it at full length. Means: spend days in the dentist's waiting room on an uncomfortable chair; live on one's balcony on a Sunday afternoon; listen to lectures in a language that one does not understand, choose the most roundabout and least convenient routes on the railway (and, naturally, travel standing up); queue at the box-office for theatres and so on and not take one's seat; etc.' (22)

Camus's prose, wrote one early reviewer, was like Kafka written by Hemingway.[3] Tarrou's vignettes help to activate a Kafkan strain of absurdity and dark comedy in *The Plague*. We watch as city authorities fuss over what to call the epidemic and attempt to deal with it in laughably managerial, bureaucratic ways.

We also get a reverse-angle portrait of the doctor-narrator when we read a quoted description of Rieux: '"He is absent-minded when driving and often leaves his car's indicators up even after he has taken a bend. Never wears a hat. Looks as if he knows what's going on"' (25). This is like the mirror in a van Eyck portrait: we catch a glimpse of the artist, reflected back in the course of depicting his main subjects: 'As far as the narrator can judge, it is quite accurate' (25).

The diaries are also performing another, as yet undisclosed, role in the book. Tarrou, who becomes a close friend of Rieux, will die of the plague, taken cruelly just as the epidemic is ebbing. So the passages that the doctor copies into his chronicle are also a kind of memorial and elegy for a lost comrade. This wry anthology of insignificant acts is edged by unspoken loss and grief.

The three other main characters are Father Paneloux (a Jesuit priest), Cottard (a shady character, probably a criminal, a man with something on his conscience) and Joseph Grand, an ironic name for a small, mild-mannered municipal clerk who tends to speak in clichés. We gradually learn (even though he is very secretive about it) that Grand has been at work on a novel for years, but never managed to get past the first line: 'On a fine morning in the month of May, an elegant woman was riding a magnificent sorrel mare through the flowered avenues of the Bois de Boulogne' (80).

'"What do you think of it?"' he asks Rieux after divulging his secret and reading it aloud, while the sounds of curfew and civil unrest reach them through the windows (81). Rieux says diplomatically that the beginning makes him curious to know what will follow. Grand slaps the manuscript with exasperation:

> 'That's only a rough idea. When I have managed to describe precisely the picture that I have in my imagination, when my sentence has the very same movement as the trotting horse, one-two-three, one-two-three, then the rest will be easy and above all the illusion will be such from the very start that it will be possible to say: "Hats off, gentlemen!"' (81)

A desire for a total and perfect mirroring, or mimesis, of the world in language: the very worst way to set about writing anything. The stuckness and stasis of Grand's manuscript is literary microcosm for the suspended animation of the town: the same films are shown on a loop; the same blues records spin round in the cafes (*I went down to Saint James Infirmary / Saw my baby there ...*). The stranded opera company puts on the same Gluck tragedy each evening (at least until Orpheus falls down on stage, struck down by the plague in the middle of an aria).

Nonetheless, Grand will emerge as the unlikely hero of the book: the person who takes a major role in organizing the health teams that fight the epidemic. When he falls ill in part four and tells Rieux to burn his manuscript (which is just page after page of crossed-out first lines), we finally break out of the frustrated plotting and narrative cul-de-sacs that detain us so long in the middle of Camus's novel. Grand unexpectedly recovers and begins a letter to his estranged wife. The plague graph begins to fall and we move towards a denouement: the 'unknotting' of the destinies of five solitary men – Rieux, Rambert, Tarrou, Grand, Paneloux – who all come to a greater understanding of human solidarity.

So: a novel within a novel, a diary within a diary, a tragedy within a tragedy – *The Plague*, which starts out by claiming to be an objective chronicle, is actually a hall of mirrors.

3.

A man is sitting in his car at an intersection when suddenly his field of vision goes white. The doctor who treats him also goes blind, and before long the 'white sickness' goes global. So begins José Saramago's 1995 novel *Ensaio sobre a cegueira* (published as *Blindness* in English). When reluctantly selling the film rights, Saramago insisted that the city remain unidentified (in the movie it becomes a digital composite of Toronto, Tokyo and São Paulo) and the characters nameless: 'The girl with the dark glasses,' 'The boy with the squint' and so on.

Directed by Fernando Meirelles, the 2008 adaptation is not an easy watch. The sufferers are quarantined in a derelict asylum where all human decency soon breaks down into violence, intimidation, rape and the rule of the strong. Unsure about the blurry placelessness and heavy seriousness of the film, *New York Times* reviewer A.O. Scott wrote that in *Blindness* 'human civilisation is threatened by a sudden and virulent outbreak of metaphor' (2008).

It's tempting to use the same quip about Camus's work. On publication, *La peste* was immediately read as an allegory for the 'brown plague' of Fascism in Europe, as well as the questions of resistance, collaboration and genocide that consumed post-war France. For a friend who had been in the concentration camps, Camus inscribed a copy: 'To a survivor of the plague'. In his notebooks he suggested that the book 'may be read in three different ways':

> It is at the same time a tale about an epidemic; a symbol of Nazi occupation (and incidentally the prefiguration of any totalitarian regime, no matter where), and thirdly, the concrete illustration of a metaphysical problem, that of evil. (qtd. in Todd 168)

This symbolic response to historical events has always had its detractors. 'Camus's world is one of friends, not of fighters,' wrote Roland Barthes, who found its 'ahistorical ethic' troubling ('La peste' 544). Simone de Beauvoir felt that to equate the occupation with a natural scourge was 'a way to escape History and real problems,' and as a result, 'everyone agreed too easily with the disembodied moral emerging from that parable [*cet apologue*]' (144). As Tony Judt points out in his 2001 introduction, this accusation still surfaces in academic treatments of Camus: 'he lets Fascism and Vichy off the hook, they charge, by deploying the metaphor of a "nonideological and nonhuman plague"' (qtd. in Dunn 150: xiv).

If it's wrong to transmute historical events and agents into a metaphorical plague, one can also level the criticism from the other direction: it's wrong to make the very real suffering of disease serve as a symbol for anything other than itself. 'My point is that illness is *not* a metaphor' wrote Susan Sontag in her 1978 discussion of TB and cancer, 'and that the most truthful way of regarding illness – and the healthiest way of being ill – is one most purified of, most resistant to, metaphoric thinking' ('Illness as Metaphor' 1978). The work had emerged, in part, from her regret over describing Western imperialism as a 'cancer'. Ten years later, she extended the argument to HIV/AIDS: 'The age-old, seemingly inexorable, process whereby diseases acquire meanings (by coming to stand for people's deepest fears) and inflict stigma is always worth challenging . . . . With this illness, one that elicits so much guilt and shame, the effort to detach it from loaded meanings and misleading metaphors seems particularly liberating, even consoling' ('AIDS and its Metaphors' 1988).

For me, none of the above charges really stick when applied to a work as subtle and self-aware as *The Plague*. If imagining the Nazi occupation as a seething bacterial epidemic blurs the question of accountability, then perhaps this is because (as Judt points out) Camus's work is suspicious of identifying and blaming too quickly. Or of allowing blame to dominate other, more diffuse questions about everyday accommodations to suffering and tyranny that do not resolve into the easy binaries of victim and perpetrator. In his reflections on 'Paris Under the Occupation,' Jean-Paul Sartre remembered the 'instinctive humanitarian helpfulness' that French citizens would find themselves showing to German soldiers, even while opposing Nazism:

> We remembered the command we had given ourselves once and for all: don't ever speak to them. But, at the same time, faced by these lost soldiers, an old humanitarian willingness to help awoke in us, and another command that went back to our childhood and which enjoined us to not ever leave a person in difficulty. Then, according to one's

> mood and the occasion, one decided to say: 'I don't know' or 'Take the second street on
> the left' and in both cases, one left unhappy with oneself. (3)

Granted, it is odd to read Camus's response to France's wartime experience and find no outright villains. Even Cottard, the shady criminal type who thrives under the plague, is treated with a kind of tenderness. But in the closing moments of the book, as we see him go down under the fists of the police, one senses Camus's scepticism about a post-war climate where individuals were being shamed as collaborators, becoming scapegoats whose publicly advertised crimes might have worked to draw attention away from more subtle and widespread forms of complicity.

As for the question of using disease as metaphor: on one plane the work does full naturalistic justice to the horrors of bubonic plague itself, and the long history of the bacillus *Yersinia pestis* in human affairs (so long that the word 'plague' is, of course, inescapably metaphorical). In the book-length version of *Illness as Metaphor*, Sontag actually exempts *The Plague* from her critique. The work, she says, is not really a political allegory:

> Camus is not protesting anything, not corruption or tyranny, not even mortality. The
> plague is no more or less than an exemplary event, the irruption of death that gives
> life its seriousness. His use of plague, more epitome than metaphor, is detached, stoic,
> aware – it is not about bringing judgment. (147–8)

The sober narrator is all too aware of the rush to judgment that the plague brings, most obviously in the sermon by Father Paneloux. The Jesuit priest interprets the pestilence (in time-honoured religious fashion) as the language of God's displeasure: '"Calamity has come on you, my brethren,"' he begins, '"and, my brethren, you deserved it"' (73). In the book's even-handedness, though, Paneloux is also a sympathetic character; or, at least, not a caricature (still no easy villains). Paneloux has made a study of Augustine (like Camus himself, who wrote a thesis on this African saint). And the second sermon he gives is a much more complex and compelling justification of religious faith. It is a chapter in which one can sense Camus wanting to give full weight to the spiritual counter-argument to his own secular vision. A much fuller weight than that given, for example, to the priest in *The Outsider*, none of whose certainties, says Meursault, 'was worth one strand of a woman's hair' (118).

The Plague, in other words, does not take the easy way out by imagining the worst. It does not scapegoat, nor does it tend towards the complete breakdown of social order that we see in *Blindness* and the many stories of apocalypse that modern human societies like to feed themselves: stories in which civilization is revealed to be (as the aspiring but cliché-ridden novelist Joseph Grand might have said) 'just a thin veneer'.

In an early chapter, Rieux stands at the window looking out at the town, both indulging and resisting the aura surrounding the word 'plague'. 'A word that conjured up in the doctor's mind not only what science chose to put into it, but a whole series of fantastic possibilities utterly out of keeping with that grey-and-yellow town under his eyes' (trans. Gilbert 37):

> A tranquillity so casual and thoughtless seemed almost effortlessly to give the lie to those
> old pictures of the plague: Athens, a charnel-house reeking to heaven and deserted even
> by the birds; Chinese towns cluttered up with victims silent in their agony; the convicts at
> Marseille piling rotting corpses into pits; the building of the Great Wall in Provence to
> fend off the furious plague-wind; the damp, putrefying pallets stuck to the mud floor at

the Constantinople lazar-house, where the patients were hauled up from their beds with hooks; the carnival of masked doctors at the Black Death; men and women copulating in the streets of Milan; cartloads of dead bodies rumbling through London's ghoul-haunted darkness – nights and days filled always, everywhere, with the eternal cry of human pain. No, all those horrors were not near enough as yet even to ruffle the equanimity of that spring afternoon. The clang of an unseen tram came through the window, briskly refuting cruelty and pain. Only the sea, murmurous behind the dingy chequer-board of houses, told of the unrest, the precariousness of all things in this world. (trans. Gilbert 38)

Occasionally the restrained, even pedantic, narrative voice gives way to rhetorical set pieces like this. One can sense Camus the lyrical essayist seizing the controls from his alter ego Dr Rieux. But the passage conjures up these nightmarish images – climaxing with the plague-fires described by Lucretius, where Athenians fight each other with torches on the seashore to secure a space for the funeral pyres of their loved ones – only to set such visions aside.

Most of the time, *La peste* offers something much less sensational, much more humdrum: a lockdown, sometimes terrifying, but often just boring and frustrating, that we all have to get through after our own fashion: 'The trouble is, there is nothing less spectacular than a pestilence and, if only because they last so long, great misfortunes are monotonous' (138).

4.

In March 1900, a ship called the SS Kilburn arrived in Cape Town from the grain-exporting port of Rosario, Argentina. It was carrying fodder for the horses of the British army, then fighting against the Boer republics in the South African War.

Five crew members were ill and the captain had died a day before docking. A quarantine camp was set up in Saldanha Bay and the crew taken there under armed guard. But by September 1900, large numbers of rats were dying in the Cape Town docks. 'The stench was unendurable,' an officer reported to the Plague Advisory Board: 'they had to have the floors up to remove the dead rats. He himself had seen numbers of sick rats coming out to the open in daylight, in a dazed state so that you could catch them with your hand' (qtd. in Phillips 42–43).

In early 1901, a number of cases were reported among dockworkers who had been unloading the grain and fodder that harboured rats (and their fleas carrying the plague bacillus). Tented camps were set up: first on the beach, then at Uitvlugt Forest Station, a few kilometres away from the city centre. Using a Public Health Act introduced in 1883 after a smallpox epidemic, the city's Medical Officer ordered that over 6 000 black Africans living in the city centre were to be forcibly removed from their homes and marched there.

Untouched by the sixth-century Plague of Justinian and medieval Europe's Black Death, southern Africa was now part of the so-called Third Pandemic. It began in Chinese ports in 1894 and encircled the globe for the next decade, a seaborne epidemic carried along the global shipping routes established by European colonialism.

The southern African story, as told by Howard Phillips in *Plague, Pox and Pandemics*, makes for grim (and grimly predictable) reading. The outbreak provided authorities with an 'unchallengeable opportunity' to effect rapid, large-scale social engineering (60). At a time when the germ theory was radically changing ideas of disease transmission (but had not yet vanquished more nebulous ideas of plague being transmitted through miasmas and bad sanitation), authorities could draw on the 'richest genealogy of fear in the Western psyche' as a tool of political expediency (Cradock qtd. in Phillips 40: 124). All of which was now further infected by the most harmful elements of colonial ideology: racial pathology, prejudice, scapegoating, stigma and paternalism.

In Cape Town, the tented camp at Uitvlugt became Ndabeni, the first 'native location' in the city. Special legislation was rushed through, preventing those detained there from living any-where else. This was met with widespread protest, including rent and train boycotts. Slum dwell-ers in the city centre tried to prevent the removal of bodies; Cape Town's Islamic community opposed the isolation of patients, and especially the handling of their dead by non-Muslims. Mounted police were called in to break up mass meetings against forced removals. 'By what legal process or right of law or equity have you acted?' asked community leader Alfred Mangena in 1901: 'Let us assume a *vice versa* position and what would the white man feel and say?' (qtd. in Phillips 60).

In retrospect, the arrival of plague in Cape Town can be seen as a catalyst and trial run for the political project – continuing throughout the 20th century via different methods and in different guises – which sought to unscramble a creolized port city into fixed racial blocs and then lock these down spatially. Responding to this prototype of apartheid's Group Areas legislation, the *Cape Argus* specu-lated that the outbreak might have been 'a blessing in disguise' (qtd. in Phillips 61).

To tell the story of a deadly bacillus, parasite or virus – whether *Yersinia pestis*, malaria, HIV/AIDS, Ebola or COVID-19 – is to reveal, unerringly, the fault lines and psychopathologies of human societies. The question of disease is always political, and hardly a flight into disem-bodied allegory or apolitical moral fable. This is why *The Plague*, when read in the time of cor-onavirus, 'doesn't need the lens of metaphor to maintain its resonance' (Williams 8). It is a work that has been re-literalized by global events and comes across, in one sense, as an all-too-plaus-ible account of life under lockdown: 'a malevolent holiday' in which 'a jittery simulacrum of normal life persists' (Williams 8).

And yet for all its verisimilitude, Camus's book retains a great and puzzling silence about its Algerian setting, and about the way that an epidemic would actually have played out in a colonial city like Oran: who would have been treated, and treated humanely, and who not.

5.

Why does Rieux refuse to help Rambert with his investigations into 'the Arab quarter'? Why is the matter raised – and in the context of an insistence on the whole truth – only to be dropped?

For Conor Cruise O'Brien, writing in his 1970 Fontana Modern Masters series on Camus, the answer is simple. To include the Muslim, Arab and African inhabitants of Oran (and so to frankly acknowledge the colonial setting) would cause the allegory of resistance and oppression to break down. O'Brien suggests that it came naturally to Camus, because of his background and education, to think of Oran primarily as a French town, 'and of its relation to the plague as that of a French town to the Occupation':

> But just below the surface of his consciousness, as with all other Europeans in Africa, there must have lurked the possibility of another way of looking at things – an extremely distasteful one. There were Arabs for whom 'French Algeria' was a fiction quite as repugnant as the fiction of Hitler's new European order was for Camus and his friends. For such Arabs, the French were in Algeria in virtue of the same right by which the Germans were in France: the right of conquest. The fact that the conquest

had lasted considerably longer in Algeria than it was to last in France changed nothing in the essential resemblance of the relations between conqueror and conquered. From this point of view, Rieux, Tarrou and Grand were not devoted fighters against the plague, they were the plague itself. (47–48)

O'Brien's short book lands a tremendous polemical blow. It did much to dislodge the Western idea of Camus as a kind secular saint, and to reveal how his works – most often read as universal, existential parables – are actually riven by the paradoxes of the colony. In *Culture and Imperialism*, Edward Said extends this idea of Camus as a late imperial writer who, in assuming the ordinariness of a place like Oran, comes to naturalize what was really a vast geographical and ideological fiction: that Algeria was part of France, even down to its French postcodes. For Said, Camus is someone who could never quite face the historical reality of Algerian nationalism, and whose work is profoundly marked by this imaginative failure. His writings, Said concludes, 'express a waste and a sadness we still have not completely understood or recovered from' (224).

In one sense, such charges are unanswerable. Oran does become a 'partly unreal' place, a 'never was' city in which the stuckness of quarantine might be figuring another kind of paralysis (O'Brien 49, 47). In the decade after the Second World War, Algeria entered a political interregnum in which the old order was dying and the new had not yet been born. This was a context in which, as Antonio Gramsci wrote in his prison notebooks, 'a great variety of morbid symptoms appear' (a line often applied to South Africa in the dying days of apartheid).

Yet it is not true that Camus was disengaged from the reality of a dying colonialism, and the question of what would come after it. He started his career as an investigative journalist for *Alger républicain*, writing exposés about how French policy had caused poverty and famine in Kabylia. And the analogy between Nazi occupation and French colonialism was not (as O'Brien claims) beyond the horizon of his awareness: he had made the point himself in an editorial of the journal *Combat*. In a piece of 10 May 1947, Camus denounced the 'methods of collective repression' used by the government in Algeria in the wake of anti-colonial protests, along with torture and all forms of racism:

> Three years after having experienced the effects of a politics of terror, the French received this news with the indifference of people who had seen too much. Yet the fact is there, clear and hideous as the truth: we are doing in these cases what we reproached the Germans for doing. (*Actuelles I* 28).

The editorial, appearing in the same year as *La peste,* was titled 'La contagion'.

So one can adduce evidence to refute the charges levelled by O'Brien and Said, and to defend Camus's honour – but that is not really the point. The real quandary that *The Plague* presents is its ethic of non-violence amid the morbid symptoms of the late colony. In the wake of the French empire and the terrible conflict that brought it to an end, is Camus's vision of human fellowship credible? And how does his steadfast refusal to justify 'the necessary murder,' or glorify any form of killing, read today, at a greater historical distance, and from a different part of the world?

6.

In 1961, Nelson Mandela, the 'Black Pimpernel' who was banned and in hiding from the apartheid regime, travelled to Morocco. In Oujda, just over the border from Algeria, he received his first military training from the armed wing of the *Front de Liberation Nationale* (FLN). As with the massacres at Sétif in 1945 that had radicalized Algerian nationalists, the killings at Sharpeville in 1960 had made the African National Congress abandon its strategy of non-violent resistance: they were one of the last liberation movements in the world to do so. In *Long Walk to Freedom* (1994), Mandela wrote that the situation in Algeria 'was the closest model to our own in that the rebels faced a large white settler community that ruled the indigenous majority' (298). After his release in 1990, Algeria was the first country that Mandela visited; he never forgot the support that the FLN offered to the South African liberation struggle.

In this photograph from 1962, one sees the future icon of peace and reconciliation receiving guerrilla training from the revolutionary movement that had sworn to erase utterly the French Algerian culture into which Camus was born – such was the cruelty, bitterness and ideological polarization of the Algerian War of 1954 to 1962.

This was a political climate – structurally violent, highly militarized – in which Camus's call for a civilian truce (delivered as hardliner *pieds noirs* shouted for his death outside the venue in Algiers) was regarded by many on the Paris left as hopelessly naïve. Camus's language 'had never sounded hollower than when he demanded pity for the civilians,' wrote de Beauvoir: 'The conflict was one between two civilian communities' (qtd. in Horne 125). When she heard Camus's statement after he won the Nobel Prize in 1957 – 'I believe in justice, but I will defend my mother before justice' – de Beauvoir was 'revolted' (qtd. in Horne 235). 'Between justice and my mother, I choose my mother': this was what Camus's words were soon reduced to in the press, a formulation for which he was roundly mocked and condemned.

What he actually said was different from either of the two versions above:

> I have always condemned terror. I must also condemn the blind terrorism that can be seen in the streets of Algiers. People are now planting bombs in the tramways of Algiers. My mother might be on one of those tramways. If that is justice, then I prefer my mother. (*Algerian Chronicles* 216)

The whole meaning of the statement was held in the conditional premise ('If that is justice'), but this did not survive the press paraphrases and subsequent polemics. 'He was not sentimentally exalting his mother above justice,' writes George Scialabba in a review of Camus's *Algerian Chronicles*, 'he was rejecting the equation of justice with revolutionary terrorism' (2013).

After the failure of his 1955–1956 campaign for a civilian truce, and holding steadfast to his position – that no values can remain after a justification of torture or terror – Camus lapsed into public silence on Algeria, a silence seen as culpable by his detractors on the left. In private, he campaigned against the death sentence for Algerian freedom fighters, intervening in over 150 cases (Todd 399). But he could never accept the FLN's version of nationalism, or the idea of Algeria as an essentially Arab nation. He viewed his native land as a polgyglot society – partly Arab, African, Mediterranean, Jewish, indubitably French – and argued for a federation that would recognize and reconcile these elements. He believed (contra O'Brien) that 130 years of French settlement in Algeria had rendered the society like the one he grew up in 'an indigenous population in the full sense of the word' (*Algerian Chronicles* 3) – a comparable but more plausible claim lies at the heart of the white Afrikaans experience in South Africa. And finally, the poverty of Camus's upbringing in Belcourt meant that he could not easily imagine himself or his family as colonial elites or oppressors. In Algiers, the telegram bringing news of his Nobel had to be read aloud to his illiterate mother.

'Yes, there is beauty and there are the humiliated,' he wrote in the essay 'Return to Tipasa': 'Whatever difficulties the enterprise may present, I should like never to be unfaithful either to the second or the first' (*Selected Essays* 153). It is one of several gnomic formulations in which one senses, even in the syntax, the impossibility of the undertaking – it can only be broached negatively, conditionally, hypothetically. After these lines, the essay continues: 'But this still sounds like ethics, and we live for something that goes beyond them. If we could name it, what silence …' (153).

In his 2016 biography, Robert Zaretsky suggests that Camus's silence over the war ravaging his native Algeria 'did not transcend ethics. Instead, it flowed from his recognition that the humiliated were on both sides in this conflict: the great majority of *pieds noirs* as well as Arabs' (86). This is, perhaps, something like the understanding that Nelson Mandela evolved during his long incarceration: of white Afrikaner nationalism as emerging from British colonialism and the humiliation of the South African War. This late imperial catastrophe would incubate apartheid thinking across the 20th century, with black South Africans becoming (as Edward Said claimed of the Palestinians) the victims of the victims.

For the exiled Algerian writer Assia Djebar, Camus was a Mandela-like figure: she read his campaign for a civilian truce as a moment in which Algerian history might have gone differently, a last chance for reconciliation instead of bitter violence. This is very different to Said's idea of Camus as a late imperial writer unable to imagine a postcolonial future. In *Fantasia: An Algerian Cavalcade* (1985), Djebar classes him (with Frantz Fanon) as an annunciator of a history that never came to be, a herald of a lost possibility that he died too young to see so utterly lost. In *Algerian White* (1995), she keeps circling back to the unfinished manuscript of *Le premier homme* found in the car wreck that killed him, wondering what the book might have become.

7.

At the back of my mind when reading *The Plague* is always the sense that the histories of Algeria and southern Africa mirror each other in some ways, even as their paths out of colonialism and white minority rule are in another sense diametrically opposite.

In one case a suspended revolution and negotiated settlement; in another an eight-year war of liberation, one of the most violent and brutal of all the decolonial conflicts, in which between 400 000 and 1,5 million people lost their lives. In South Africa, a project of national reconciliation, based on the assumption that erstwhile victims and beneficiaries of apartheid were 'condemned to live together': a phrase from Camus's 1955 'Letter to an Algerian Militant,' his friend Aziz Kessous (*Algerian Chronicles* 114). In North Africa, the expulsion of virtually the entire population of French Algerians (and Algerian Jews) after the FLN government took power in 1962 (and warned the *pieds noirs* that they could leave either via *la valise ou le cercueil*: with a suitcase or in a coffin). The torture, atrocity, spiralling violence, reprisals and the targeting of civilians on both sides of the conflict had by that time made any negotiation or reconciliation unthinkable.

In a 1996 preface to his book on the Algerian conflict, *A Savage War of Peace* (1977), Alistair Horne begins at Tipasa, the site of the Roman ruins where Camus had asserted the 'invincible' or 'unconquerable' summer that lay at the heart of his being. Horne points out how the beauty of the place 'casts a deceptive cloak over a much more ferocious past,' as the violence of the Algerian Revolution spills, retroactively, into Camus's lyrical essay:

For it was on a sunny beach close to Tipasa that French women and children, as well as men, were machine gunned as they bathed by freedom-fighters of the Algerian FLN. At Zeralda, just a few miles to the east, Algerian suspects died in a French torture camp; and it was from the barracks of Zeralda that rebel units of the elite French paras launched a nearly successful coup against President de Gaulle's Fifth Republic in April 1961. (12)

In the same year, 1961, that *la guerre d'Algérie* almost precipitated a right-wing coup on French soil, Frantz Fanon's *The Wretched of the Earth* appeared with a preface by Sartre. The preface seems partly addressed to his old adversary; though one wonders if Sartre would have published it in this form, had Camus still been alive:

In Algeria and Angola, Europeans are massacred at sight. It is the moment of the boomerang; it is the third phase of violence; it comes back on us, it strikes us, and we do not realize any more than we did the other times that it's we that have launched it. The 'liberals' are stupefied; they admit that we were not polite enough to the natives, that it would have been wiser and fairer to allow them certain rights in so far as this was possible; they ask nothing better than to admit them in batches and without sponsors to that very exclusive club, our species; and now this barbarous, mad outburst doesn't spare them any more than the bad settlers. (17–18)

How different this is to Sartre's earlier reflections on occupied Paris, and the 'instinctive humanitarian helpfulness' that Parisians found themselves offering, despite themselves, to German soldiers. In writing about what he had lived through, Sartre's language is measured, reflective, humane, alert to moral complexity, ambiguity and failure. But in addressing violence far removed from his own experience, Sartre's prose has taken on another tone:

They would do well to read Fanon; for he shows clearly that this irrepressible violence is neither sound and fury, nor the resurrection of savage instincts, nor even the effect of resentment: it is man re-creating himself. I think we understood this truth at one time, but we have forgotten it – that no gentleness can efface the marks of violence; only violence itself can destroy them. The native cures himself of colonial neurosis by thrusting out the settler through force of arms. (18)

Sartre's preface is torrential, passionate, scornful. It brought Fanon's work to a wider European audience, but perhaps also traduced it. Fanon wrote from the experience of a psychiatrist treating those damaged by the violence of the colony, both as victims and perpetrators, and on both sides of the conflict. Nothing in his writing approaches the kind of relish Sartre shows here: a glee in violence seen and celebrated from afar. Out of a self-appointed sense of historical necessity, it is working – polemically but also with a sense of unmistakeable rhetorical self-satisfaction, even pleasure – to justify the indiscriminate killing of men, women and children. In other words, it is infected with the plague bacillus.

Contrast this with the preface that Camus wrote to his 1958 collection *Algerian Chronicles*, his last published statement on his native land. The book was met with deafening silence at the time. The author's embattled humanism seemed impotent and irrelevant in the wake of revelations of widespread torture by the French army. But how does it read today?

The truth, unfortunately, is that one segment of French public opinion vaguely believes that the Arabs have somehow acquired the right to kill and mutilate, while another side is prepared to justify every excess. Each side thus justifies its own actions by pointing to the crimes of its adversaries. This is a casuistry of blood with which intellectuals should, I think, have nothing to do unless they are prepared to take up arms themselves. When violence answers violence in a mounting spiral, undermining the simple language of reason, the role of the intellectual cannot be to excuse the violence of one side and condemn that of the other, yet this is what we read every day. ... Metropolitan France has apparently been unable to come up with any political solution other than to say to the French of Algeria, 'Die, you have it coming to you!' or 'Kill them all, they've asked for it.' Which makes for two different policies but one single surrender, because the real question is not how to die separately but how to live together. (*Algerian Chronicles* 28–29)

Sartre, de Beauvoir and their followers 'won' the battle with Camus at the time. Only violence, writes Sartre, never gentleness, can efface the marks of violence. The diagnosis, the whole tonality, of *The Plague* could not be more different. It carries the sense not of rhetorical victory but incipient moral failure. Written out of a personal reckoning with disease, Camus's work is not a triumphal diagnosis; it reads instead as a record of what it means to live through the pain and contradiction of French Algerian history. Many times in his letters and diaries, Camus runs together the metaphors of his native land and his illness: 'Sometimes I think of health as a great land full of sun and cicadas which I have lost through no fault of my own' (qtd. in Todd 153). The blurring of private body and body politic reaches towards something not quite coherent or articulable, but deeply felt and deeply embodied: 'Believe me when I tell you,' Camus wrote to his radicalized friend Kessous as the conflict escalated, 'that Algeria is where I hurt at this moment, as others feel pain in their lungs' (*Algerian Chronicles* 113).

Ultimately, *The Plague* is a pacifist text (and unexpectedly, given that it emerges from the French Resistance). Whatever violence there is occurs in the background: heard as distant gunshots through the window as Rieux and Grand discuss the endlessly trotting horsewoman, or listen to Louis Armstrong sing 'St James Infirmary' one more time. This makes the work partly unreal, but also unfinished, in the sense that it is never finished saying what it has to say. Today, it stands as prescient of the painful historical irony borne out in so many postcolonial and post-conflict societies: when no limits are placed on the means being used to resist injustice, then the form of resistance to one form of the plague can become the carrier for the next outbreak.[4]

8.

'A literature of failure is not a failure of literature,' wrote Albert Memmi, reflecting on the French literature of the Maghreb.[5] *The Plague* fails to resolve its internal contradictions or the noise within its allegorical schema. But Camus's failings can seem preferable to the success of those intellectuals who cheered on murders and massacres from afar. He himself judged *La peste* a failure; but perhaps the ability to perceive this, and then to write from within it, is what carries the book's wisdom.

'"I was already suffering from the plague long before I knew this town and this epidemic"' (189). In Tarrou's confession to Rieux, just before they take a night swim together, the idea of a 'healthy carrier' is broached by the work (one of several moments when the text seems to half-acknowledge the unspoken, colonial occupation that flickers on the edge of its awareness). Within the story, Tarrou is talking about living in a society that condones the death penalty. But his words reach further than that, and continue to reach out in a world where so much of what passes for politics rests on the desire to construct a simplified, less-than-human other – and then to argue for their removal, expulsion, cancellation, disappearance or death. '"And this is why,"' Tarrou concludes, '"I have decided to reject everything that, directly or indirectly, makes people die or justifies others in making them die"' (195).

When we hear, in the final section of *The Plague*, about the death of Tarrou, Rieux reflects that his friend '"had lost the game"': 'But if so, what has the narrator of his history won?' In his measured way (and how difficult to have brought off a novel with such a restrained narrator), Rieux answers:

> All he had gained was to have known the plague and to remember it, to have known friendship and to remember it, to have known affection to have one day to remember it. All that a man could win in the game of plague and life was knowledge and memory. (224)

The work moves to close with a double ending (much as it had a double beginning). There is the hopeful motto about there being more in men to admire than to despise. And then the foreboding cadence of the bacillus never disappearing or vanishing entirely – a kind of suspended sentence hanging over the whole work. The famous last lines loop back into the work we have finished, inviting rereading: 'He knew that this happy crowd was unaware of something that one can read in books … ' (237).

But much of the book's life is actually held in the smaller, less quotable moments. '"Next thing they'll be wanting a medal,"' says the old man who Rieux has been treating, watching the townsfolk celebrating, '"But what does it mean, the plague? It's life, that's all"' (236):

> 'Tell me doctor, is it true that they're going to put up a monument to the victims of the plague?'
> 'So the papers say. A pillar or a plaque.'
> 'I knew it! And there'll be speeches.'
> The old man gave a strangled laugh.
> 'I can hear them already: "Our dead … "' (236)

January 2019 – March 2021

Notes

1 All quotations are from the 2001 Penguin Modern Classics translation by Robin Buss, unless otherwise stated.

2 At one point we hear that 'there is no finer place in the team than a midfielder': 'the centre-half is the one who positions the game and that's what football is about' (113). Though Camus himself took on the greater moral anguish of being goalie.

3 See Todd 155.

4 This formulation is adapted from Carroll (*Camus the Algerian* 55–6).

5   Memmi's line from *Anthologie des écrivains français du Maghreb* (1969) is used by Carroll as an epigraph ('Camus's Algeria' 517).

My thanks to Jan Steyn for his help with translation.

Works Cited

Barthes, Roland. 'La peste: Annales d'une épidémie ou roman de la solitude'. In *Oeuvres complètes*. Edited by Eric Marty. Vol. 1. Paris: Seuil, 1993.

Barthes, Roland. *Writing Degree Zero*. 1953. New York: Hill and Wang, 1968.

Camus, Albert. *Actuelles I (Chroniques 1944–1948)*. Paris: Gallimard, 1950.

Camus, Albert. *Algerian Chronicles*. 1958. Translated by Arthur Goldhammer. Cambridge: Harvard University Press, 2013.

Camus, Albert. *The Outsider*. 1942. Translated by Stuart Gilbert. London: Hamish Hamilton, 1946.

Camus, Albert. *The Plague*. 1947. Translated by Robin Buss. London: Penguin, 2001.

Camus, Albert. *The Plague*. 1947. Translated by Stuart Gilbert. 1948. London: Penguin, 2010.

Camus, Albert. *Selected Essays and Notebooks*. Translated by Philip Thody. London: Penguin, 1970.

Carroll, David. *Albert Camus the Algerian: Colonialism, Terrorism, Justice*. New York: Columbia University Press, 2007.

Carroll, David. 'Camus's Algeria: Birthrights, Colonial Injustice, and the Fiction of a French-Algerian People.' *MLN* 112(4), 1997: 517–49.

Craddock, Susan. *City of Plagues: Disease, Poverty and Deviance in San Francisco*. Minneapolis: University of Minnesota Press, 2000.

de Beauvoir, Simone. *La Force des choses*. Paris: Gallimard, 1963.

Djebar, Assia. *Fantasia: An Algerian Cavalcade*, London: Heinemann, 1985.

Dunn, Susan. *The Death of Louis XVI: Regicide and the French Political Imagination*. Princeton University Press, 1994.

Fanon, Frantz. *The Wretched of the Earth*. 1961. Preface by Jean-Paul Sartre. Translated by Constance Farrington. London: Penguin, 2001.

Horne, Alistair. *A Savage War of Peace: Algeria 1954–1962*. 1977. *New York Review of Books*, 2006.

Judt, Tony (Introd.). *The Plague*. Translated by Robin Buss. London: Penguin, 2002. vii–xvii.

Mandela, Nelson. *Long Walk to Freedom*. Boston: Little Brown, 1994.

O'Brien, Conor Cruise. *Camus*. London: Fontana, 1970.

Phillips, Howard. *Plague, Pox and Pandemics: A Jacana Pocket History of Epidemics in South Africa*. Auckland Park: Jacana Media, 2012.

Sartre, Jean-Paul. 'Paris Under the Occupation'. *Sartre Studies International* 4(2), 1998: 1–15.

Scialabba, George. 'Resistance, Rebellion and Writing'. *Bookforum*. April/May 2013. www. bookforum.com. Accessed on 1 May 2020.

Scott, A.O. 'Film Review: "*Blindness*"'. Rev. of *Blindness*, dir. Fernando Meirelles. *New York Times* 2 Oct. 2008. www.nytimes.com. Accessed on 1 May 2020.

Sontag, Susan. 'AIDS and its Metaphors'. *New York Review of Books*. 27 October 1988. www. nybooks.com. Accessed on 1 May 2020.

Sontag, Susan. 'Illness as Metaphor'. *New York Review of Books*. 26 January 1978. www. nybooks.com. Accessed on 1 May 2020.

Sontag, Susan. *Illness as Metaphor; and, AIDS and its Metaphors*. New York: Picador/Farrar, Straus and Giroux, 1989.

Todd, Olivier. *Albert Camus: A Life*. London: Chatto & Windus, 1997.

Williams, Thomas Chatterton. 'A Malevolent Holiday'. *Harper's*. June 2020. www.harpers.org. Accessed on 1 May 2020.

Zaretsky, Robert. *A Life Worth Living: Albert Camus and the Quest for Meaning*. Cambridge: Harvard UP, 2016.

SELF/ISOLATION

Dan Wylie

I woke

I woke, sweating in the darkness,
having dreamt that the cat was dead,
and sat up, suddenly sobbing –
for her life, and for mine,
for my long-departed dad,
and my mother fading
like a banknote crumpled in the rain,
for the whole green world wrecked
by my beautiful, reckless kind
with its greedy machines,
its recurrent plagues.

I went out into the night
looking to regain myself,
shining my torch
into all those haunted corners
and upwards into the sky
as if I might somehow
brighten the stars.

The cat of course was there all along
at my feet, licking a silvery paw,
and, like a supplicant
clutching the promise of a goddess,
to my stricken chest
I held her,

furiously purring
and very much alive.

In her small self

In her small self
the cat can occupy large tracts of space.
You wake to find yourself
buckled along the edge of the double bed,
the cat a triumphant nugget of stripes in the middle,
or stretched in a clever diagonal
excluding all other configurations.

A small fear can be like this;
or a single consuming pleasure.
For one, you can grow static and obese;
for another, so thin you might vanish from sight.

All causes are unconscious of their stature.
A plate dropped in the sink might dominate history.
A bat trapped in a tiny cage
might infect the world.

This autumn day

This autumn day
can scarcely believe its luck.

Somebody else's pandemic has stilled
the moil of commerce and machines.
The earth can hear itself breathe again.

The pine stands calmly beside the rhus;
the leafless erythrina alongside grass.
A breeze coaxes the moon across a sanded sky.

Humans, longing for roots, can't achieve this.
Their furies and financials, their nasdaqs and vaccines,
plunge and rear like horses in a storm.

This autumn day is a hummingbird, an emerald.
Soft doubloons of sun bank up in the porch.
The cat basks in a corner, a vault of gold.

The jasmine is freshly lathered
with its good fortune, the season
uncurling. Still, don't the erythrinas long
for the burden of leaves, grass
to converse once more with rain?

I know

I know, I know
the situation is appalling:

the streets are emptied of life
the hospitals have turned into cripples
our leaders stumble into the traps of their own bombast
the corrupt seethe in the acids of their wealth
the ribs of the poor become racks of need
fears balloon behind every unsmiling mask

But what's locked down exactly?

Not the weather, blustering along the escarpment
not these caterpillars climbing the walls of their days
not the coppery wasps hunting the caterpillars
not even the wasps' larvae self-isolating
in their voracious silos beneath the eaves
not the polished drongos hunting the wasps
not the caterpillars surviving to be charaxes
nursing the pollen in the boerboen flowers
and spreading it like words across pages of wind
not the mind that leafs through the words
through storms and the pools between the storms

I could go on
and on tracing the lines of the uncontrolled
uncontrollable beauty
uncontrollable cruelties
the lines that escape delineation
the spaces spilling over their rims
dimensions unfurling within and around
in fractals of fragrant regress

everything, despite everything
more alive than ever

As they grow older

As they grow older, the hills
become more sentimental, angers
and desires worn down at the brows.

They begin to don drab colours,
only on special occasions affect
a splash of red aloe in a shy lapel,

or a yellow scarf of sunlight
on a scarp, pretending they might tempt
that green young valley closer.

They are more inclined to weep,
quietly into the elbow of a kloof,
stricken by something perfectly mundane:

the echo of a bar from Schubert,
or the violet eyes on a butterfly's wing,
or the scent of crushed horsewood

reminding them of something primordial,
brave, once loved, and lost. For what
has it all been about, they ask themselves:

all the upheavals of granite and schist,
the politics, plagues, volcanoes, and floods,
the paintings, the churches, the disastrous mines?

On these coppery, autumn days
blue with smoke, they hunker down alongside
their own forebodings and bones,

complaining, We've been on lockdown
forever, when will it all end? And observe
a man scrambling up a scree, also weeping,
but for what they cannot discern.

If the self

If the self is an illusion,
what is there to isolate?

Search where you will, it melts away:
in cupboards, only thread, elastic, colour
in fridges, only chlorophyll, sinew, oils

on bookshelves, only motile mythologies
already chewed by moths and other mouths
chemical legends owned by no one

already and always am I all
liquid drawn from aquifers, all viral,
bacterial, parasitic on parasites

the lungs are a wet delta almost reaching the sea
the brain a tangle of rope spooling towards the stars
the heart pumping its Mississippi, Orinoco, Nile

Atlantic saline structures the blood
calcium scoured from mountains scaffold the bones
tears condense and evaporate across nations

Why then does this poem feel so alone?
Why does the cry that is torn from me
want only to find a home?

What am I

What am I becoming, in my solitude,
the plague tapping in the porch, itinerant and blind,
like a wind rattling at an unlatched sky?

Am I becoming

just a procession of redundant ideas,
like elephants on a pelmet,
one of porcelain, one of glass;
one of mukwa, one of wire;
one of horror, one of hope;

a shiver of self-reflections
in panes framing those fading tales:
the sepia smile of an uncle dead before I was born;

the cracked map of a land
growing stranger by the day;

just the bones of a futuristic book
whose predictions of destruction and dust
find themselves already written
in the lymph and the lungs;

or an urn that burns with thoughts
already corroding their host from the inside,
hunting for another warm place to live?

Plague and Cultural Panic: Edgar Allan Poe's 'The Masque of the Red Death'

Laurence Wright

Abstract

Poe's 'The Masque of the Red Death' turns on the paradox of a privileged elite succumbing to a plague that is ravaging society at large, and from which they believe themselves completely protected. The horror of the story consists not in the devastation of external society – that is taken for granted – but in the abject failure of the elite's supposedly impregnable defences, their faith in which is exposed by the 'Red Death' as utterly delusory. 'Put not your trust in Princes' (Ps. 146.3) takes on an entirely new meaning.

> I built my soul a lordly pleasure-house,
>> Wherein at ease for aye to dwell.
> I said, 'O Soul, make merry and carouse,
>> Dear soul, for all is well.' (Tennyson, 1832: 'The Palace of Art' 1–4)

Poe's short story of 1842 has been the 'go-to' candidate for many journalists and commentators seeking to hallow the worldwide COVID-19 pandemic with a literary referent. As recently as 1989, Hubert Zapf called the tale 'a strangely contemporary text' (217). How much more is this so in the aftermath of 2020.[1]

A Prince, 'happy and dauntless and sagacious,' whose dominions have been so ravaged by a pestilence called the 'Red Death' that the population has halved, chooses a thousand 'hale and light-hearted friends from among the knights and dames of his court' and retreats to one of his 'castellated abbeys' surrounded by 'a strong and lofty wall' (670). Once inside, the iron gates are welded shut, leaving the chosen few means 'neither of ingress nor egress' (671). After five or six weeks of enjoying 'the appliances of pleasure,' they give themselves up to decadent revelry in a masquerade ball, hosted by the Prince. We are made to understand that beyond this privileged enclave, devastation and death ensue unabated. All detail of the circumambient horror is occluded from the story, unremarked and unreferenced, left wholly to the imagination. 'The external world could take care of itself' (671). Protected by secluding walls, the Prince's elite company is meant to be safe. Except they are not: they all die.

The relevance of the tale today seems patent if puzzling. COVID-19 has been no respecter of elites despite the advantages wealth and privilege can buy. The literary *topos* is well worn. Consider this stanza from Thomas Nash's haunting 'A Litany in Time of Plague' (1600) (as it is titled by modern anthologizers), another obvious literary bellwether in these trying times:

> Rich men, trust not in wealth,
> Gold cannot buy you health;
> Physic himself must fade.
> All things to end are made,
> The plague full swift goes by;
> I am sick, I must die.
> Lord, have mercy on us! (8–14)

Similar instances could be multiplied. The puzzle is that the text of 'Masque of the Red Death' offers no explicit indictment of wealth. Poe's tale certainly impugns elitism, but on what grounds? Poe's editor, Thomas Mabbott, confidently sees in the tale 'a clear moral that one cannot run away from responsibility' (667). Obviously, elites can and do abdicate responsibility – as Poe's tale suggests. In any case, as with much of Poe's writing, ethical judgment is left to his readers. The charge might be one of arrogant confidence in privileged hierarchy, or culpable neglect of others' welfare, or careless epidemiological bravado or just breathtaking social insouciance. Or perhaps something else – a different kind of panic?

A striking feature of the tale is its total avoidance of any close-up treatment of the Red Death's ravages being inflicted on the general populace. Instead, in the opening paragraph, the reader is given a succinct account of the plague's physical manifestations:

> There were sharp pains, and sudden dizziness, and then profuse bleeding at the pores, with dissolution. The scarlet stains upon the body and especially upon the face of the victim, were the pest ban which shut him out from the aid and sympathy of his fellow-men. And the whole seizure, progress and termination of the disease, were the incidents of half an hour. (670)

This is magnificently grim and portentous, and readers might consequently anticipate a tale embellished with agonizing accounts of suffering, individual and collective. This never materializes. The story pretext insists that the tell-tale scarlet stains on the body and face of victims isolate them from human sympathy; society shuns plague victims because of public fear of contagion. On the contrary, what really excludes them from the reader's sympathy or empathy is the author's brutal determination to excise them from the story's imaginative universe. Their suffering is determinedly 'offstage'. This is both odd and puzzling. Equally intriguing is the prognosis that from start to finish, inception to death, the progress of the Red Death takes 'half an hour,' almost exactly the time it takes to read Poe's story carefully. It would seem that 'Masque of the Red Death' may be a plague of a different kind, a literary *thanatos*, a metonym for the reader's own imagined death as a reader. Poe leaves his audience in a world wherein 'Darkness and Decay and the Red Death held illimitable dominion over all' (677).

Poe has his readers accompany the 'happy and sagacious and dauntless' Prince to a castellated abbey, remote from suffering society, where they imaginatively indulge in a decadent and extravagant 'lockdown' party, believing themselves wholly immune to the plague thanks to elaborate physical quarantine measures (670). Of course, they are not safe, as the story's denouement makes plain. 'Put not your trust in Princes' (Ps. 146.3). But why not? The physical barriers are robust. There is no hint of a possible route by which plague might enter the abbey. In that era there could be no recognition of viral transmission, a mechanism only discovered at the end of the century, and even if there were, the abbey is locked down, secluded, amply provisioned and self-sufficient. In terms of the realized constitution of Poe's fictional world, the reader would be 'cheating' were he or she to imagine some means of secret ingress for the plague, physical or metaphysical, that the authorial voice somehow forgot to mention. The supposition would be completely impermissible according to the tale's narrative logic.

Yet the uninvited masquer does arrive, wholly unexpectedly, to disrupt the Prince's revelry. He is clad in lineaments that gruesomely portray the plague those present have striven to escape and from which they believe themselves completely shielded. When directly confronted and attacked by the Prince, the intruder is literally disrobed and, as his garments drop to the floor, inside is found ... absolutely nothing. Not only do the Prince and his company die, one after the other, presumably according to the aetiology of the plague (this is left tantalizingly unclear), but the fictional universe itself succumbs, leaving only the plague and decay. The half-hour read is up. 'Masque of the Red Death' seduces its readers into experiencing, or at least contemplating, what death might mean. The narrative arc of the story subsides into imaginative nullity, its conclusion offering us no escape route. The whole suffering world is notionally there, beyond the isolated abbey and outside the story, but we as readers are deemed to know nothing of it. We have 'died'.

The question arises as to why Poe created this elaborate phantasy of escape only to insist, paradoxically, that there is in fact no possibility of escape. The Prince and his guests suffer the fate of the populace. To put it another way, would not a realist account of the progress of the plague among the suffering populace serve his purpose just as well? Why satirize the self-indulgent escapism of an elite locked away in a castellated abbey, especially if their escape attempt proves unsuccessful?

Poe is an enormously conscious and deliberate artist. In the second of his two 1842 reviews of Hawthorne's *Twice-Told Tales*, he was theoretically insistent that 'there should be no word written, of which the tendency, direct or indirect, is not to the one pre-established design' (299). The issue of *Graham's Magazine* where this review appeared is the very one that ran 'The Mask of the Red Death. A Fantasy'. Poe later changed 'Mask' to 'Masque' and dropped the subtitle. This ambivalence over his title goes to the heart of the story. The masque sets out to mask the plague but fails abjectly. Poe's irony is directed not at the plague itself, but at the presumptuous human culture that seeks to ignore and evade it.

(To bring the story for a moment into our own 21st-century pandemic crisis, consider the 'illegal' house parties that violate COVID-19 lockdown rules, those gormless crowds milling about unprotected on the beaches of Florida during Spring Break, mindless sun-bathers in the parks of Europe, all social distancing forgotten in the bliss of 'normal' freedoms, and we begin to understand how a Poe-like virus, uninvited, may already be attending the human 'party'. The virus is invisible.)

But 'Masque of the Red Death' offers a more profound challenge than these contemporary instances might suggest. Poe's strictures are directed, not at trivial human behaviours such as those that drive today's evasion of simple protocols introduced to curb COVID-19 – partying from habit or to forget – but at the more fundamental way the whole fabric of human culture loses its significance, buckles and collapses, in response to plague because it has no cogent means of understanding or acknowledging the insurgence. Poe tells his readers that the external world can take care of itself. The implication must be that the threat that interests him is to the internal world.

This is a horror story, but the horror does not consist in the ravages of the plague visited offstage on the helpless populace. The elite revellers die from this inscrutable pestilence, an imperceptible nothingness, as readily as ordinary people. Poe's tale is an elaborate parable indicting the nescience of human art and culture measured against the malignant will of the plague – something COVID-19 has emphasized emphatically for our own generation. The real horror is the inexplicable ease with which the plague infiltrates and undermines what has been (for better or worse) formally established as an irrefragable elite enclave, namely the rich defensive legacy of human culture – a castellated abbey of the mind. This high culture is humanity's 'home,' our collective refuge, a richly endowed resource and legacy inherited from countless earlier generations, something the privileged treasure and wallow in, while the disadvantaged populace sleep-walks unregarding through this (to them) invisible heritage. Unmasking the intruding masquer – disguised as the 'Red Death' – reveals his nothingness, and this 'nothingness' in turn unmasks the masque, exposing its nullity. What then does the decadent masque symbolize and how is its significance realized in Poe's story?

Various 'Poes' are discernible in today's literary criticism. Take your pick: the sickly Southern outcast, the self-conscious craftsman, the Freudian exemplum, the proto-deconstructionist, the hack writing for money, the aesthetic theoretician, the not-so-covert racist, the literary rebel. Of special importance is Poe's catalytic role in the evolution of French Symbolism. *Fin de siècle* England scarcely knew what to make of his influence on French art and letters, leading T.S. Eliot to observe of writers such as Baudelaire, Mallarmé and Valéry that 'we should be prepared to entertain the possibility that these Frenchmen have seen something in Poe that English-speaking readers have missed' (Eliot 328). That seminal 'something' was canvassed, deliberated over and disseminated during leisurely Tuesday receptions hosted by Mallarmé in his small fourth-floor apartment in Paris's Rue de Rome, attended variously by the cream of contemporary experimental writers, French and English, including Huysmans, Laforgue, Valéry, Remy de Gourmont, André Gide, Arthur Symons, W.B. Yeats, George Moore, Oscar Wilde and others, not excluding 'modernizing' painters such as Manet, Gauguin and Whistler, each of whom made off in a different direction with the fruits of this discourse. The core message was Poe's disconcerting swerve away from naturalism towards *la poésie pure*: the work of art as an end in itself (Eliot 338) – as *symbolic*. Significant distinctions between the meanings of 'symbol' and 'allegory' emerged only at the end of the eighteenth century. Gadamer points out that earlier, across Europe, the two terms were virtually synonymous (72). Symbolism traded the earlier notion of symbol as conventionally understood – as a one-for-one sign standing in for publicly available knowledge – for the deliberate deployment of idiosyncratic figures evoking obscure ambiences, feelings and notions unique to the artist. In his *Maxims and Reflections* (1809–1836), Goethe explained that with symbolism 'the more particular represents the more general, not as a dream or shade, but as a vivid, instantaneous revelation of the Inscrutable' ('Maxim 202' 1906). Texts and images must operate by suggestion and indirect evocation, avoiding direct statement. It was a risky strategy. Communication might fail (Balakian; Pach; Wilson).

Critics have vigorously indulged various forms of allegory and allegoresis in their efforts to interpret 'Masque of the Red Death'. The starting point must be to ask whether anything in the text absolutely demands such treatment. What happens if the allegorising impulse is resisted? For instance, were we to posit a naïvely vacuous ideal reader, one with no literary or artistic experience at all, merely a literal command of the English language, there is no compelling reason why 'Masque of the Red Death' should not be received as a simple univocal horror story devoid of allegorical potential. Several critics have insisted that this is indeed how it should be taken, notably Julian Symons (1978) and Nicholas Ruddick (1985). Typical of the approach is Stuart Levine's remark that 'One can best convey the nature of "Red Death" by saying that it is really not about a moral issue at all, but is really "about" the thrill of horror it hopes to produce in the reader' (200). On this view, the tale is best construed as if it were a monological horror film, lacking anything demanding further reflection or interrogation. The story's superficial impact adequately exhausts the text.

For readers of this persuasion resisting allegoresis is barely a decision. More complex choices are cognitively unavailable or resisted on principle as, inherently, these readers hew to a version of Occam's razor, prioritizing simplicity of response. Such an attitude gains analytical support by regarding the Prince's retreat to the sealed confines of a 'castellated abbey' as a technical device to invoke the claustrophobic atmosphere of horror, a mere writerly mechanism. Poe himself admitted, 'It has always appeared to me that a close circumscription of space is absolutely necessary to the effect of insulated incident: it has the force of a frame to a picture' ('Composition' 166). This point of view is valid if, and only if, we accept the assumption of a sentient but vacuous reader, a decoder of text whose reflective capabilities and literary experience have been so limited that the tale is experienced solely at the level of 'This is what happened'. Achieve this imaginative nullity and our putative reader is appropriately equipped to conclude, as Donald Trump did of COVID-19, that '"it is what it is"' (Cole and Subramanium 2020).

Better informed readers would probably note that retreat from the exigencies of the world to a secluded castle is a staple of the symbolist imagination, celebrated in many extravagant romantic and aesthetic detours from the mundane world. They might think of Horace Walpole (1717–1797) reconceptualizing his mansion, Strawberry Hill, on the banks of the Thames at Twickenham, in line with neo-Gothic prescripts. Dozing off, Sir Horace dreams of a 'gigantic hand in armour' floating down the banister of a great staircase. This odd fusion of mediaeval fantasy and his amateur architectural obsessions produced *The Castle of Otranto* (1764), the strange work that inaugurated the Gothic novel, an undoubted precursor to 'Masque of the Red Death'. The example of an eccentric aristocrat retreating from hum-drum modernity to a world of private fantasy embodied in antique architecture is certainly congruent with aspects of Poe's fabulation.

An equally cogent instance of aesthetic retreat from the contemporary world, stemming directly from the symbolist reaction to naturalism that Poe (via Baudelaire and Mallarmé) had in large measure inspired, would be J-K. Huysmans' *Á Rebours* (1884), often translated as *Against Nature*, the French decadent novel that became an important influence on Oscar Wilde's *The Picture of Dorian Gray* (1890). Baron Jean des Esseintes, sole survivor of a once powerful aristocratic dynasty, having wrecked his physique with riotous living in the flesh-pots of Paris, conceives of a restorative aesthetic retreat. He buys a villa high above the village of

Fontenay on the outskirts of the City, alters it to his own demanding architectural specifications and fills it with objects designed to satisfy his obsessive sensory connoisseurship – paintings, literature, furnishings, lighting, liqueurs, aromas, music and so forth. Urban modernity, the industrial *demos*, is to be kept at bay. He rejoices that 'the height on which [his home] was perched and its isolation insulated him from the hubbub of the vile hordes which the vicinity of a railway station invariably attracts on a Sunday afternoon' (Huysmans 35). In the end this insupportable decadent/aesthetic project collapses, implying that Des Esseintes's approach to life is indeed *À Rebours*, 'Against Nature' or 'the wrong way'.

Then there is Villiers de l'Isle-Adam's play *Axël*, published serially in *La Jeune France* between November 1885 and June 1886, a work that had little success on stage but is regarded as perhaps the archetypal symbolist drama. Villiers was a friend of Baudelaire's and adored both Poe and Wagner. His story evokes the retreat of a handsome young Count, Axël d'Auersperg, to a remote castle in Germany's Black Forest where he immerses himself in hermetic philosophy under the direction of a Rosicrucian adept, preparing himself for some final revelation of alchemical mysteries. He is joined by a beautiful young French noblewoman, Sara de Maupers, also a Rosicrucian, who has escaped from her convent prior to taking the veil and brings with her knowledge of the whereabouts of unimaginable riches hidden in Axël's castle. Sara finds the treasure, and the two, Axël and Sara, abandoning their cherished hermetic austerity, fall in love. In principle, everything the world has to offer now lies open to them. Long pages are devoted to description of imaginary romantic ecstasies available in places round the world that they could freely sample. But no, having wallowed in these enticing possibilities, Axël rejects them, and proposes suicide as the only apt culmination. When Sara suggests a night of passion beforehand, he demurs, arguing that being in thrall to her body would fatally jeopardize his spiritual harmony. Preferring his private carapace of abstract contemplation, Axël eventually persuades Sara of death's supposed superior freedom, they drink a goblet of poison, and perish in ecstasy.

The instances of escapist aesthetic fantasy described above suggest the idiosyncratic temperament of the symbolist 'hero,' typified in much European literature of the era, and summed up marvellously by Walter Pater in his *Marius the Epicurean* (1885), where he writes of Marius: 'He was become aware of the possibility of a large dissidence between an inward and somewhat exclusive world of vivid personal apprehension, and the unimproved, unheightened reality of the life of those about him' (133) – exactly the predicament Poe sets up in 'Masque of the Red Death'. These stories uncover connections between aesthetic and sensual aspiration as the mainspring of personal desire, and embody an inherent elitism symbolized by architectural retreat and spatial remove from the quotidian populace. Almost as if he were generalizing from the predicament explored in 'Masque of the Red Death,' the philosopher Schopenhauer has this to say about art and elitism in his magnum opus, *The World as Will and Representation*:

> the most excellent works of any art, the noblest productions of genius, must eternally remain sealed books to the dull majority of men, and are inaccessible to them. They are separated from them by a wide gulf, just as the society of princes is inaccessible to the common people. (234)

Readers who can readily place Poe's 'Masque of the Red Death' in the rarefied aesthetic company briefly explored above are clearly marked off from 'the dull majority of men'. They belong in 'the society of princes'. From this realization, a disturbing reflexive critique flames back at Poe's readers: 'If it is my own reservoirs of literary meaning which inform and sustain my response to the tale, may I not, by analogy, be complicit with Poe's noxious elite roistering away in a castellated "literary" abbey, exuding callous neglect of quotidian humanity?' Robert Regan puts it this way: 'Finding the right clue occasions a smile, a murmur, a glow of self-esteem; it delights us because it raises us above less perceptive readers – in other words because it debases the easily deluded mass of mankind' (298). Readers have been seduced into entering an aesthetic retreat, a fictive Strawberry Hill or Axël's castle, of their own making. Superior literary percipience – if this is what it is – separates them from naïve readers in much the way that the Prince's chosen few are hived off from the mass for incarceration (or 'protection') in his luxurious abbey. But their separation cannot save them from horror. Indeed, this is the horror.

In search of Regan's 'right clue,' consider the Prince's name, Prospero. The symbolic cue is highly attenuated in its vehicle, a mere fragment, yet open to huge indeterminate vistas in its tenor. The literary minded will immediately think of Shakespeare's Duke in his elegiac play, *The Tempest* (1610–1611). A salutary check to such presumption results from consulting Professor Google: no such correlation emerges in the first page of search results. Not one mention of Shakespeare. Indeed, nothing in Poe's text insists on Shakespeare. *We* must make the connection and nail our literariness to the masthead as we do so. Both Prosperos, Poe's and Shakespeare's, put on masques, each of which is radically disrupted. Poe's Prospero has his masque invaded by a figure in the guise of the Red Death, whose unmasking actualizes instant mortality for everyone; Shakespeare's Prospero has his masque disrupted by a belated memory of the slave Caliban's hapless insurrection:

> I had forgot that foul conspiracy
> Of the beast Caliban and his confederates
> Against my life. (4.1.139–40)

… a mental irruption that precipitates Prospero's apocalyptic vision of annihilation in which the 'cloud-capped towers, the gorgeous palaces, / The solemn temples' and, finally, 'the great globe itself' dissolve, leaving 'not a rack behind' (4.1.152–53). This is horror on a grand scale. The world is as illusory as art, as the theatre itself. Moreover, if we recognize in Shakespeare's 'cloud-capped towers' speech a deft moralizing re-write of Virgil, we will recall that Aeneas's elegiac meditation on the destruction of his home city of Troy takes place in Juno's temple at Carthage, with the walls of Dido's new city rising around him, the emerging heart of a fresh trading empire. In telling parallel, Prospero's meditation hymning the anticipated demise of human civilization is enacted in the Globe Theatre on the banks of the River Thames, with some impressive towers, palaces and temples rising on the opposite bank, heralding an incipient British Empire (Pitcher; Wright). Early Modern London was regularly troped as *Troy Novant*, an important staging post in the grand arc of the *translatio imperii*, that sprawling mediaeval myth whereby political legitimacy, knowledge and prestige, stemming from ancient Babylon and going back to the Biblical Eden, were supposedly transferred from ancient Greece westward across time, following the trajectory of the sun (as happens in miniature in Poe's story) in history's longer purview – first to Rome and from thence to Paris and London and, eventually, to the New World and Edgar Allan Poe (see Curtius).

In these rhetorically parallel moments from the *Aeneid* and *The Tempest*, history is paused, hanging in the balance. Prospero's masque celebrating dynastic triumph and political restitution is emblematically disrupted by Caliban, Aeneas's reverie by the arrival of Queen Dido; for Dido is the temptress whose affair with Aeneas could potentially derail his destiny to become the future founder of Rome, as told in W.F. Jackson Knight's prose translation: 'As Aeneas the Dardan looked in wonder at these pictures of Troy, rapt and intent in concentration, for he had eyes only for them, the queen herself, Dido, in all her beauty, walked to the temple in state ... ' (*Aeneid* 42–43). The two mythicized moments of crisis (both narrative crises and historical-cultural crises) enact threats to the continuity of human (Western) civilization. Fortunately, according to the Virgilian mythos, Aeneas's *Romanitas* holds firm, and he deserts Dido to successfully found what becomes the imperial city of Virgil's literary patron, the Emperor Augustus. Prospero's vertiginous glance into the void, provoked by his sudden memory of the rebarbative Caliban, proves equally ephemeral. Instead of dissolving like 'the baseless fabric of this vision' (4.1.151), the real-world towers, palaces and temples of London grow and thrive to sustain the largest and richest empire the world has known. Prospero's private nightmare premonition of all-encompassing *vanitas* is seemingly forgotten. He stills his 'beating mind' and returns to Milan in dynastic triumph, leaving Caliban to his fate.

In both cases the vision is double-sided: the comedic 'happy ending' that transpires historically (the rise of Rome, Prospero's return to Milan, the development of what will become the British Empire) is shadowed by two incipient disturbances, unregarded at the time, but increasingly acknowledged today. The parallel disasters, which shadow allied civilizational developments in this historical vortex, announce themselves in two famous literary curses: Dido's curse on the faithless Aeneas; and that which the slave Caliban pronounces on his master, Prospero. Abandoning Dido provokes the Punic Wars, perhaps presaging, emblematically and fancifully – why should we not make such leaps? – the struggles of the Women's Movement across the long 20th century. Abandoning Caliban speaks eloquently to the future history of slavery and thence to Black Lives Matter in our own century. The burgeoning British Empire is doomed from its inception. Civilizations and their constitutive visions rise and fall, synchronically and diachronically, both sequentially and in historical parallel: Virgil, Shakespeare and Poe. Contrarian potentialities are ever present. The effect is not far from Herakleitos's famous aphorism: the way up is the way down (DK B60).

Which brings us to the climax of 'Masque of the Red Death,' a third significant moment when, narratologically speaking, history holds its breath. The intertextual allegoresis functions with (seemingly) only the slightest nudges from author to reader. There is nothing in Poe's text granting cogency let alone legitimacy to the giant cultural riff we have been following, no necessary pointer to *The Tempest* and therefore none to Virgil. The only explicit handhold on this otherwise smooth referential cliff-face would be Caliban's curse in *The Tempest*, 'The red plague rid you [kill you] / For learning me your language!' (1.2.363–64). Surely not! – Poe's whole literary structure premised on one slight and arcane referent? What superlative literary cheek. Allow that possibility, and readers have admitted themselves *a fortiori* as paid-up citizens in what Jacques Barzun once called *The House of Intellect*. They have deliberately entered an arcane bastion of literary *jouissance* and artistic experience (like the Prince's 'castellated abbey,' Axël's castle, Des Esseintes's Fontenay retreat, their own 'Strawberry Hill') that alienates them, marks them off, from the concerns of quotidian humanity. Perhaps the intent of 'Masque of the Red Death' is indeed to help us reassess such language, especially to re-evaluate cultured literariness, by alerting us to its equivocal nature. These pretensions are no defence against plague.

The uninvited masquer wearing the mask of the Red Death (we remember Poe's equivocation over 'mask' and 'masque' in naming his tale) makes his way gravely through the seven chambers in which the revels are taking place until, at the climax of his stately progress, he is challenged by the Prince, greatly incensed by the gross tactlessness of this unwanted guest's presence and attire. Two things happen. The Prince chases after the intruder and attacks him 'with dagger born aloft,' until the latter turns on him, a 'sharp cry' is uttered (by whom remains unclear), following which, using Poe's characteristically estranging syntax, 'instantly afterwards, fell prostrate in death the Prince Prospero' (676).[2] The revellers seize the intruder, but gasp 'in unutterable horror at finding the grave cerements and corpse-like mask, which they handled with so violent a rudeness, untenanted by any tangible form' (676). There is nothing inside. They all die, one by one, at which point time stops: 'the life of the ebony clock went out with that of the last of the gay' (677). 'And now was acknowledged the presence of the Red Death. He had come like a thief in the night' (677). The story concludes with sombre finality, 'And Darkness and Decay and the Red Death held illimitable dominion over all' (677).

The tale's conclusion invokes two venerable motifs: the tragically misguided attempt to thwart death by assaulting the allegorical figure of Death, and then the ungraspable, incomprehensible vacuity of death itself. To illustrate the first, we might recall Chaucer's 'Pardoner's Tale' in which three young drunks, deeply affronted on hearing that a friend has died, swear they will seek out Death and kill him:

> 'Herkneth, felawes, we thre been al ones;
>   Lat ech of us holde up his hand til oother,
>   And ech of us bicomen otheres brother,
>   And we wol sleen this false traytour Deeth.
>   He shal be slayn, which that so manye sleeth,
>   By Goddes dignitee, er it be nyght!' (410–415)

Through their own cupidity, treachery and stupidity, all three end up dead. They kill each other, enlarging death's dominion, while Death itself evades their attentions. The second motif is magnificently illustrated in Epicurus's *Letter to Menoeceus*:

> So death, the most terrifying of ills, is nothing to us, since so long as we exist, death is not with us; but when death comes, then we do not exist. It does not then concern either the living or the dead, since for the former it is not, and the latter are no more. (85)

Poe collapses the two motifs into one. The Prince attacks the Red Death and dies, after which the masquers unmask the 'Red Death' and find 'nothing' – and they also die. Only after the allegorical figure of death has been 'slain,' his disguise fatally punctured, can the presence of the Red Death be acknowledged, and this happens when no-one in the tale is alive to do any acknowledging. The one surviving process is decay, pointing towards final entropic dissolution and a plenum of nothingness.

The entire superstructure of Western art and culture has been symptomatically invoked, its diachronic rise and fall, systole and diastole, and has proven wholly incapable of resisting the Red Death; as incapable, indeed, as those people unacquainted with any of its pretensions.

The plague unmasks the masque of Western cultural afflatus, exposing its nescience in the face of a malignancy it cannot apprehend.

Except, of course, for the surveillant consciousness of the reader responding to Poe's narratorial voice. This is the paradox on which the meaning of Poe's tale finally turns, the symbolist's *redux*. The Red Death comes 'like a thief in the night'. In the Bible, that which comes 'as a thief in the night' is 'the day of the Lord,' the much longed-for salvation where 'the heavens shall pass away with a great noise, and the elements shall melt with fervent heat, the earth also and the works that are therein shall be burned up' (2 Pet. 3.10). Poe's apocalypse is quieter. The narrating voice simply stops. We are left palpably on our own. But we are there. The reader's irrefragable conscious aliveness is the symbolists' nirvana, the untapped arena in which fresh, unsullied apprehension and even appreciation become possible. This is what the tale's symbolism has delivered. The Red Death emancipates the reader by rehearsing and then symbolically ridding the would-be creator of moribund artistic-intellectual tradition – flattening the whole inflated construct with more than Platonic zeal. Having survived this 'death,' the *avant garde* are once more on a par with quotidian humanity and can begin to create from a position of egalitarian clarity and alertness.

As readers, we are left attempting to adjudicate between 'Masque of the Red Death' as a monological horror story that exhausts its meaning in the mere telling, horror for the sake of horror, and the tale as a seductive, reader-driven narrative springboard for scuppering cultural allegoresis, delivering visions that melt 'into air, into thin air' until, 'like this insubstantial pageant faded,' they 'Leave not a wrack behind' (*The Tempest* 4.1.150, 155–56).

Poe designedly caters for both modes of narrative apprehension. The choice is there – sheer horror or cultural fabulation – but, ironically, the choice exists only for readers properly equipped to sojourn fruitfully in what Tennyson in 1832 called 'The Palace of Art'.[3]

Notes

1   For example, *The Boston Globe*: 'These days, the short story strikes me as a metaphor of a kind Poe never intended but which is applicable to this crisis: Who among us is akin to the ghastly, ghostly figure who wanders through the party spreading disease?' (Lehigh 2020); *Medium*: '"The external world could take care of itself". For Donald Trump, it wasn't just the rest of the world, but even parts of America itself that were to be left on their own' (Carlson 2020); *Livewire*:

  The central character ... decides that barring a thousand-odd friends among the nobility and the rich, his castle would be closed off to those who contract the illness. In short, those with resources would be protected from the disease, but those stranded outside would be left to possibly die. (Chakraborty 2020)

  Psychology Today: 'The palace had been sealed, as it turns out, to no avail. The deadly disease was already inside. The ruler and his revellers had quarantined themselves with death' (Fileva 2020); *The Prospector Daily*: '"Masque of the Red Death" serves as a parallel not only to the tragic deaths it can foresee, but in the lack of morality in human behavior' (Martinez 2020).

2   Poe is a hugely conscious stylist. Controversy over the effectiveness, sophistication and felicity of his prose and poetry has been fierce. The debate is summarised in Zimmerman (3–27). Sadly, despite the brilliance of his literary constructions, I incline to the view

mordantly expressed by Harold Bloom: 'Poe is inescapable though a vicious stylist in all his works' ('Editor's Note' vii). However, in mitigation, Bloom has also contributed one of the finest summative insights into his work: 'Poe dwells, with the rest of us, in Plato's Cave but wants, more desperately than most do, to find his way out into the disembodied light' ('Introduction' xi).

3 See the epigraph to this essay.

Works Cited

Balakian, Anna. *The Symbolist Movement*. New York: Random House, 1967.

Barzun, Jacques. *The House of Intellect*. 1959. New York: Harper Torchbooks, 1961.

Bloom, Harold. 'Editor's Note'. In *Edgar Allan Poe's 'The Tell-Tale Heart' and Other Stories*. Edited by Harold Bloom. New York: Bloom's Literary Criticism, 2009. vii. Bloom's Modern Critical Interpretations.

Bloom, Harold. 'Introduction'. In *Edgar Allan Poe*. Edited by Harold Bloom. New York: Bloom's Literary Criticism, 2008. xi–xii. Bloom's Classic Critical Views.

Carlson, Michael. 'COVID-19: Our Modern Masque of the Red Death'. *Medium*. 20 March 2020. https://carlsonsports.medium.com/covid-19-america-britain-and-poes-masque-of-the-red-death-c58dfe06cef6. Accessed on 10 July 2020.

Chakraborty, Abhinav. 'Edgar Allan Poe's 'Red Death' in the Times of Coronavirus'. *Livewire*. 19 March 2020. https://livewire.thewire.in/out-and-about/books/edgar-allan-poes-red-death-in-the-times-of-coronavirus/. Accessed on 11 July 2020.

Chaucer, Geoffrey. 'The Pardoner's Tale.' *The Canterbury Tales*. Edited by Sinan Kökbugur. http://www.librarius.com/cantales.htm. Accessed on 2 January 2021.

Cole, Devan and Tara Subramanium. 'Trump on Death Toll: "It is what it is"'. *CNN Politics*. 3 Sept. 2020. https://edition.cnn.com. Accessed on 2 January 2021.

Curtius, Ernst Robert. *European Literature and the Latin Middle Ages*. 1948. Translated by W.R. Trask. London: Routledge & Kegan Paul, 1953.

Eliot, T.S. 'From Poe to Valéry'. *The Hudson Review* 2(3), Autumn 1949: 327–42.

Epicurus. 'The Letter to Menoeceus'. *Epicurus: The Extant Remains – Text, Translation and Notes*. Edited and translated by Cyril Bailey. Oxford: Oxford University Press, 1926. 83–92.

Fileva, Iskra, 'Dancing with Death'. *Psychology Today*. 1 April 2020. https://www.psychologytoday.com/za/blog/the-philosophers-diaries/202004/dancing-death. Accessed on 11 June 2020.

Gadamer, Hans-Georg. *Truth and Method*. Translated by J. Weinsheimer and D.G. Marshall. London: Sheed and Ward, 1993.

Goethe, Johann Wolfgang von. *The Maxims and Reflections of Goethe*. 1809–1836. Translated by Bailey Saunders. New York: The Macmillan Company, 1906. http://www.gutenberg.org/files/33670/33670-h/33670-h.htm. Accessed on 16 January 2021.

Herakleitos. *The Fragments of Heraclitus*. DK (Diels-Kranz) B60, from Hippolytus, *Refutation of All Heresies* 9.10.4. http://www.ou.edu/logos/heraclitus. Accessed on 2 January 2021.

Huysmans, J.-K. *Against Nature*. Translated by Theo Cuffe. 1884. London: riverrun, 2018.

Lehigh, Scot. 'A Question from Poe: Are you Spreading the Coronavirus?' *Boston Globe*. 19 Mar. 2020. https://www.bostonglobe.com/2020/03/19/opinion/question-poe-are-you-spreading-coronavirus/. Accessed on 10 July 2020.

Levine, Stuart. *Edgar Poe: Seer and Craftsman*. Deland, FL: Everett/Edwards, 1972.

Martinez, Jacqueline. 'The Relevance of Edgar Allan Poe's "Masque of the Red Death" in the Era of COVID-19'. 31 Mar. 2020. *The Prospector*. https://www.theprospectordaily.com/2020/03/31/in-review-the-relevance-of-edgar-allan-poes-masque-of-the-red-death-in-the-era-of-covid-19/. Accessed on 11 June 2020.

Nashe, Thomas. 'A Litany in Time of Plague'. *The Works of Thomas Nashe*. Edited by Ronald B. McKerrow. Vol. 3. Oxford: Basil Blackwell, 1958. 283.

Pach, Rémi. 'Symbolism in French Literature'. *Literator* 11(1), April 1990: 67–76.

Pater, Walter. *Marius the Epicurean*. London: Macmillan, 1910.

Pitcher, John. 'A Theatre of the Future: *The Aeneid* and *The Tempest*'. *Essays in Criticism* 34(3) 1984: 193–215.

Poe, Edgar Allan. 'The Masque of the Red Death'. *Tales and Sketches: 1831–1842*. Edited by Thomas Ollive Mabbott. Vol. 2. Cambridge, MA: The Belknap Press, 1978. 667–78. The Collected Works of Edgar Allan Poe.

Poe, Edgar Allan. 'The Philosophy of Composition'. *Graham's Magazine* 28(4), April 1846:163–67.

Poe, Edgar Allan. 'Review of Twice-Told Tales. By Nathaniel Hawthorne'. *Graham's Magazine* 20, May 1842. *The Collected Works of Edgar Allan Poe*. Edited by Thomas Ollive Mabbott. Cambridge, MA: The Belknap Press, 1978: 298–300.

Regan, Robert. 'Hawthorne's "Plagiary"; Poe's Duplicity'. *Nineteenth-Century Fiction* 25(3), 1970: 281–98.

Ruddick, Nicholas. 'The Hoax of the Red Death: Poe as Allegorist'. *Sphinx* 4, 1985: 268–76.

Schopenhauer, Arthur. *The World as Will and Representation*. Translated by E.F.J. Payne. Vol. 1. New York: Dover Publications, 1969.

Shakespeare, William. *The Tempest*. Edited by Stephen Orgel. Oxford: Oxford UP, 1987.

Symons, Julian. *The Tell-Tale Heart: The Life and Works of Edgar Allan Poe*. 1978. New York: Penguin 1981.

Tennyson, Alfred. 'The Palace of Art'. In *Alfred Tennyson: The Major Woks*. Edited by Adam Roberts. Oxford: Oxford University Press, 2009. 35–43.

Villiers de L'Isle-Adam, Auguste, comte de. *Axël*. 1885–1886. Translated by Marilyn Gaddis Rose. Dublin: The Dolmen Press, 1970.

Wilde, Oscar. *The Picture of Dorian Gray*. 1890. London: Oxford UP, 1974.

Wilson, Edmund. *Axel's Castle: A Study in Imaginative Literature of 1870–1930*. 1931. Collins: The Fontana Library, 1961.

Virgil. *The Aeneid*. Translated by W.F. Jackson Knight. London: Penguin, 1956.

Wright, Laurence. 'Epic into Romance: *The Tempest* 4.1 and Virgil's *Aeneid*'. *Shakespeare in Southern Africa* 9, 1996: 49–65.

Zapf, Hubert. 'Entropic Imagination in Poe's "The Masque of the Red Death"'. *College English* 16(3), 1989: 211–18.

Zimmerman, Brett. *Edgar Allan Poe: Rhetoric and Style*. Montreal & Kingston: McGill-Queen's University Press, 2005.

Two Paintings

Ingrid Winterbach

'Running the Gauntlet'

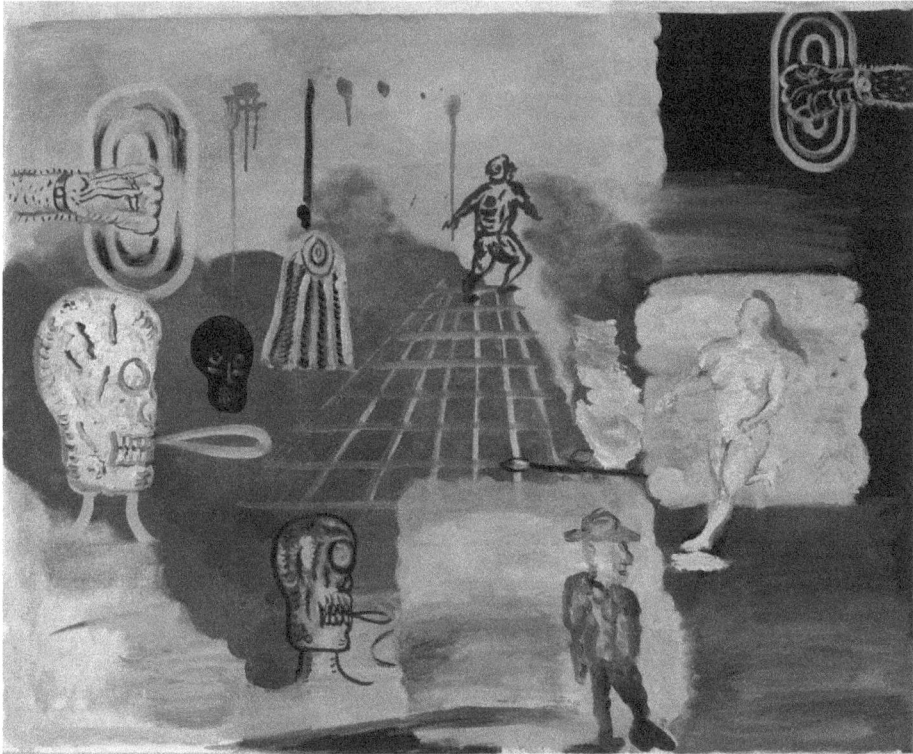

'Wat/What'

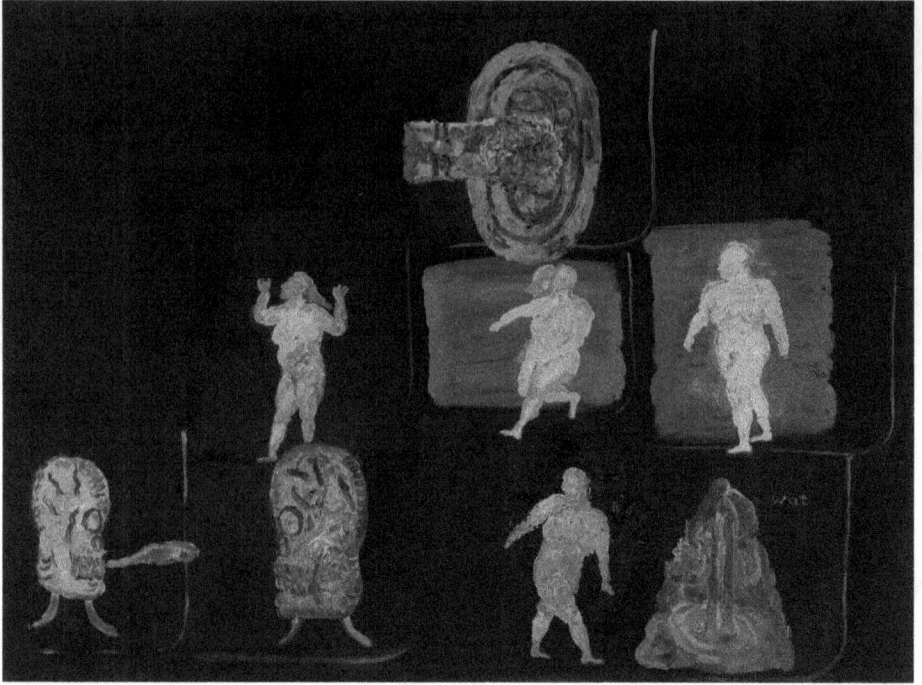

Towards a Poetics of Disaster: Chinese Poetry in Combatting COVID-19

Yanbin Kang

Abstract

China's campaign against the COVID-19 epidemic has triggered an upsurge in literary creation and animated discussions on writing about disaster. This essay explores the emergence of a disaster poetics in the COVID-19 war which considers poetry as revelatory, ameliorative and cathartic in both personal and national terms. This strand of poetry, which blends humanism, philosophical exploration, and a skeptical impulse, reexamines the isolated state of being, resists glorification, concerns individual lives and redefines heroism as quiet courage, love and compassion in despair among ordinary people, displaying a Chinese forbearance, wisdom and wry humor in facing grim reality. These poetic voices register admirable artistic courage, spiritual depth, self-critical reflection and stylistic ingenuity.

Combatting COVID-19 through poetry

China's nationwide campaign to combat COVID-19 at the onset of 2020 has triggered a poetic outpouring, a 'COVID-19 poetic tide,' as Jiang Hongwei calls it, utilizing various platforms including newspapers, literary magazines, WeChat and websites. (In Mandarin 'COVID-19 poetic tide' is more accurately translated as 'anti-epidemic poetic tide' – 'COVID-19 poetry' implies this throughout this article.) *Guangming Daily*, an influential newspaper in China, published over 200 poems from 28 January–28 February 2020 on its website. In January and February, *Poetry Periodical* on WeChat featured COVID-19 poems by 41 poets who were in shutdown Wuhan or worked on the frontline. 'Chinese Poetry,' which has its own website and circulates on WeChat, published around 200 COVID-19 poems, while the Hubei Writers' Association published over 100 poems on WeChat. Major Chinese poetry journals, such as *Poetry Periodical*, *Journal of Selected Poems*, *Poetry Monthly*, *The Poetic Tide* and *Chinese and*

Western Poetry, have had special columns featuring COVID-19 poems. Further, two anthologies published by Writers' Press and Guizhou People's Press include epidemic poems by around 200 poets.[1]

The surge of COVID-19 poetry has led to discussions about the effectiveness of this type of poetic creation. In an essay published on 7 February 2020, Wang Zheng points out that anti-epidemic literature and art needs to combine immediacy and transcendence to examine people's spirit in disaster. This emphasis on truth is further reinforced by Huo Junming, who maintains that literature needs to 'explore possibilities about reality, truth, human nature and disease'. For them, COVID-19 poetry should abstract the reality of the crisis to reveal a universal vision that is of significance when divorced from the specific context. In a widely circulated article published on 11 February 2020, Li Xiuwen, president of Hubei Writers' Association, proposes that 'the sole ethics of disaster literature is to reflect on disaster,' calling for 'reexamining the national character' and 'protecting individual dignity'. Following Li's principles, Guan Yue observes that the value of literature lies in its aesthetic and revelatory function and that its duty is to question and to reflect. He rejects the prevalent practice of writing 'memorials' that are marked by 'obsequious flattering' and 'insincerity,' suggesting that a writer needs sufficient distance from disaster in order to accommodate a broader vision. A similar idea is proposed by Huang Lihai, who edited a themed issue concerning COVID-19 poetry for *Chinese and Western Poetry* in March 2020. In his editorial, he suggests that 'the role of poetry at this time is not to praise, but to question, to ridicule, to critique and to reflect'.

Guan Yue's resistance to glorification is shared by other writers, who also seek to value the lives of individuals directly affected by the disaster. Xu Zhaozheng observes that disaster writing should be 'anti-lyrical' and must not attempt to condense any 'lofty significance' from the disaster but rather adopt 'a sober, restrained, disciplined, and transparent language which differentiates from the corrupted one' (37). Jiao Dian affirms the therapeutic function of disaster writing and contends that it must avoid 'shouting slogans and singing high-sounding words' lest 'grandiose concepts and big names conceal the small individuals and small emotions' (40–41). Zeng Pan maintains that literature and the arts have a public dimension orientated towards mobilizing people and consoling them, yet it also needs to go beyond 'superficial straightforward slogans,' and 'return to literary form and texture'.

Li Xiuwen's 'reflect upon disaster,' Xu Zhaozheng's 'anti-lyricism,' Jiao Dian's 'not shouting slogans' and Zeng Pan's emphasis on 'literariness' all suggest that successful COVID-19 poetry needs to respond to the disaster, yet must rise above social reality, taking critical thinking, individual lives and aesthetics into consideration. Indeed, as Wu Sijing observes, Chinese COVID-19 poetry, the quality of which is uneven, can be regarded as a collective catharsis, while the best poems display a compassionate, humanistic and reflective spirit (51–54). Taking account of the context of the epidemic poems, I explore the emergence of a *disaster poetics* in combatting the COVID-19 epidemic. These poetics encapsulate a commitment to the notion that poetry is potentially revelatory, ameliorative and cathartic both personally and nationally. The most effective poems blend humanism, philosophical exploration and a skeptical impulse, while also reexamining conditions of living, resisting glorification, turning our attention to individual lives, redefining heroism as quiet courage, love and compassion among ordinary people, and displaying Chinese forbearance, wisdom and wry humor in facing the grim reality. These poetic voices and perspectives reinforce one another, demonstrating the complexity of Chinese psychology in the process of cultivating a resilient, detached and calm way of dealing with the overwhelming disaster. The signal aspect of these poetic voices is that they register great artistic courage, a self-critical reflection and stylistic ingenuity.

Reexamining Isolation, Despair and Cure

How might we think of the COVID-19 epidemic and its impact upon our state of being? When the virus was confirmed to be transmissible among humans, China adopted the strictest and most comprehensive control measures, including locking down the city of Wuhan on 23 January 2020, and restricting movement of the 60 million residents in Hubei province two days later. Isolation became the norm and a dominant theme in COVID-19 discourse. In the face of the virus, which is invisible and omnipresent, human beings are helpless; as Yu Xiaozhong, a Wuhan poet, observes, we became 'cautious and eager to be in armor like a mollusk' (*CW* 76). Huang Lihai evokes the sudden ubiquitous presence of locusts to suggest the way in which the arrival of the virus caught people off guard (*CW* 81). The nondescript, pervasive sense of anxiety and dread is rendered eloquently and heartbreakingly by Zhang Zhihao, a poet who lives in the locked down Wuhan: 'The lights are getting denser and denser like ants in a hot pot / I'm not going anywhere. This is all I have left anyway' (45). Xi Chuan writes in his 'Ode to Facemasks': 'Wuhan people, confined at home, and choked madly, like maggots crawling / and by the window sending wishes' (*CW* 8). The maggot image describes how insignificant people's futile struggles are. The phrase 'maggot crawling' was broadly disseminated during China's lockdown. It typifies, as Matt Jenkins observes, a Chinese self-deprecatory way of 'finding joy amidst sorrow'. The people, who considered themselves prisoners, drifted aimlessly through their days, but nevertheless struggled to make the best of things.

Mo Yaping's 'Sonnets,' which arose in direct response to the COVID-19 pandemic, both place him in English poetic traditions and align him with Feng Zhi (1905–1993), a modern Chinese poet who uses sonnets to undertake philosophical explorations. 'Sonnet: Compatriots in the COVID-19 Period' deftly captures the common psychology of the people walking on desolate streets, wearing masks: 'people hold their breath unconsciously,' 'you fear that others cough up the virus / I fear that there is a virus in birdsongs'. Everyone suffered from a constant sense of fear, which is represented as an inescapable part of daily life. The virus, given its unknown origin, is compared to a bullet shot as if from nowhere: 'God knows where the sniper lies / whether it will give you or me a fatal blow'. Everyone craves human contact, striving to break out of one's isolated shell, and simultaneously distrusts everyone who might be a potential carrier of the virus: 'now I want to hug you more than ever / but instinct keeps me two meters away'. In this unique time, Wang Dandan writes, 'love, becomes a virus' (*JSP* 42–43). Wang is a poet who works on the frontline and here comments on the situation when a returning father rejects his little son's welcoming embrace until he has thoroughly cleansed himself. The tenuous nature of existence in extremity also undergirds Ye Xiubin's 'Survivor,' where even being a somewhat lucky survivor amounts to a misfortune because one is haunted by the pain of losing others and the constant fear of death: 'the rope of birdsongs tightens my throat / Breathing every second / may wake me up from a sleeping dream' (*CW* 95). Comparing the nocturnal birdsong to a rope that threatens one's life, Ye's poem speaks on behalf of the survivors whose lives are damaged beyond repair, questioning the myth that survival can be equated with triumph.

The epidemic triggered a reexamination of history. Poets pondered whether, in comparison with the SARS virus 17 years ago, there has been any improvement in dealing with the new epidemic. Huang Jinhu compares 2020 to a 'wrecked ship in the middle of the sea, losing its way,' upon which 'quarrels and abuses' run rampant. The vision of the historical cycle suggests the poet's indignation and disappointment which is rendered through an ironic rewriting of a Chinese proverb about the Changjiang River's irresistible flow: 'the lesson of history has been forgotten, and it goes on and on, like the old wave beating / new wave'. Like the ebb and flow of the sea, epidemics seem inevitable, repetitive, and even cyclic; trying to hold back the waves is senseless. Finally, the speaker points out that 'the iceberg of the new corona-virus' is all over the sea, and 'to stay away from this reef, we have to let go of pride and ignor-ance' (*CW* 99). In Yi Miyi's 'Wuhan's Closure,' which laments the suffering of Wuhan people, the speaker similarly criticizes the folly of forgetting history: 'I think that's learning from suf-fering / in fact, the pain is followed by forgetting' (*CW* 101). The poets are agonizingly aware that collective forgetfulness results in recurrence. This forgetting begins with the languor follow-ing the heightened tension, a psychology which is adroitly explored by Hu Zibo's 'A Residue of Life'. In Hu's poem, life in the later phases of the epidemic is compared to 'a pot of boiled water' in which 'the water gradually cools,' and 'anxiety and fear' '[condense] into a residue of the past … silent, hard, gray … seen or unseen'. This conveys the exhaustion and indifference experi-enced after a great calamity.

Looking back on the past also involves relating to artists across time and space, attempting to explore the common destiny of people. In Shu Dandan's 'Seclusion,' which can be regarded as an ekphrastic poem, the speaker records the isolated life at home, 'mopping the floor with diluted disinfectant / wiping furniture, sitting on the balcony,' studying Edvard Munch's paint-ing 'Self-Portrait after Spanish Influenza'. The speaker sympathizes with Munch's life which was plagued by illness and anxiety: 'a ship with no rudder,' yet with 'the consolation of creation / the ballast stone of the ship of life' (*CW* 96). These observations can be read as the poet's self-examination and affirmation of art as her life-support. The speaker continues to find the 'hope of life' in details such as 'warm furniture, carpet, and books,' referring to 'a small white spot' at the top of the picture as 'artistic therapy,' which enables one to transcend the limitations of life, rather than sinking into despondency (*CW* 96–97). For many people, poetry functions to sustain the self in quarantined solitude and despair. In 'On Island,' Yu Xiaozhong writes: this winter, 'poetry, as a small patch of ground' 'more resembles a small temple,' 'if self-isolation can be uplifted to self-redemption' (*SCC* 50–51).

Disaster propels people to consider what wise living entails, which is inextricable from a fruitful life. When autonomous breathing becomes a luxury, Xiao Qin writes, people realize the primacy of restraining needs: 'A steady lung is far more important than a desirous stomach' (*SCC* 106–107). In 'If I Can Survive,' Wang Yuewen proposes a humble, authentic and essential way of living: to love intensively, not to dominate others' lives, to eat plainly, to tell plain truth and to return to an original innocence. Wang ascribes survival to the mask, emphasizes its protection, and extends gratitude to ordinary people, including peasants, workers and those involved in the production and delivery of masks (*SCC* 99–100). The most comprehensive and trenchant self-critique is proffered by Zhang Jinfeng's group poems. In 'I have been kneeling, wiping,' the speaker uses the act of wiping to suggest cleaning, a deep reflection, in particular allowing 'hard wounds' to remain discernable when the disaster is over. The poem advocates a humble posture of 'kneeling,' urging people to abandon the desire to dominate; to rather seek repose in nature and enjoy harmony with a myriad of things (*SCC* 19–20). In 'Prayer,' Zhang prays that human beings will prevail over disaster, evoking a sparrow outside the window as an agent of God's punishment of those who are guilty of ignoring the wellbeing of other creatures (*SCC* 20). In 'A Hug,' inspired by a photo-graph of a baby in an isolation ward opening its arms for a hug, the speaker first laments human loss, yet extends compassion to the bat, which is generally viewed as our mortal enemy, and sees a similar vulnerability in the bat and the baby: 'A poor bat with its wings forced spread / how similar their postures are / it has been praying for human beings to embrace it' (*SCC* 21). Recognizing a natural community that shares its future with mankind undergirds Liu Liyun's poem in which the speaker realizes that relatives, the beloved and our enemies, sorrows, joys and grief are an integral part of life, yet 'so are the birds, trees, soil / beasts' (*PM5* 103–104).

Considering various problems which have arisen in this unique time, Cheng Jilong explores the therapeutic concerns and lists masks, the dead, bats, people's hearts, spring and frivolity as infected objects in need of treatment. Masks have been stigmatized. As carriers of the virus, people passed away without the company of relatives and without funerals to ensure speedy cre-mation. Bats were likely the original host of the virus, and their 'imposed crimes' need to be erased. Constant fear breeds distrust and trust needs to be re-established. People 'report neigh-bors,' are 'suspicious when meeting,' and are struggling with estrangement and 'loneliness'. In addition, during lockdown, the shops close, the square is empty, and spring is deprived of its vitality. Alluding to his verbal outpourings, activated by closure and estrangement, significantly he turns to self-reflexivity, to his own act of writing: to 'cancel everything I wrote above,' dis-missing it as mere 'frivolity' (*CW* 98).

Resisting Glorification

Deeply sympathetic towards sufferers, conscientious poets resist any gesture of glorification. They deconstruct the master narrative advocated by mainstream media, which was marked by collectivism, instrumental rationality and the heroism of humanity conquering the virus. In the suffering and grief of the whole society, any singing, laughing and even speaking amount to disrespect of the dead. Death lurks everywhere, casting a sobering pall over even the shiniest act of heroism. Wang Yan points out: 'when a lot of families are in grief, it is not appropriate to sing carnivalesque songs, especially not in public spaces, for they constitute a cruel contrast'.

Such restraint is embodied by the title of Ai Meili's poem 'In Sad Days, I Don't Want to Sing'. The speaker refuses to sing because in the context of disaster eulogizing tends to deceive: 'a voice says don't lie / we have paid the price of lying' (*CW* 104). Resisting glorifica-tion indicates aversion to political slogans as well as to reducing the suffering of others to a pol-itical maneuver. Li Li's 'Elegy of Epidemic' comments on a fictional suicide note left by an infected female doctor at Wuhan University: 'who added feet to a snake and changed a clumsy tragedy into a comedy and slogans! "Be filial to your parents! China will win!"' (*CW* 40). Wang Jiaxin's 'Leap Year' also critiques praise; the 'sweet life' presented on the front page of newspapers when Wuhan people were plagued by endless suffering (*CW* 17). In Yang Xiaobin's 'Newspaper Reading Guide,' the speaker is appalled simultaneously by the number of deaths, confirmed cases and the infection statistics given in the press, and the contra-dictory 'colorful pictures / like peach blossoms on a tree' and the headlines that represented 'life as sweet as honey' (*CW* 48). 'Extinction and Songs' by Liu Jiemin highlights the incompatibility of death and singing; the final lines indicate the preposterousness of extolling victory in the midst of such disaster: 'those in high position will urge gratitude again / whereas every face shows the scar of the mask stripped from the face' (*CW* 102). The final lines in Jin Du's 'Sealed Winter' contextualize the disaster in cyclic history and reject the narrative of victory because of the irrevocable losses:

> The time has repeated a stagger,
> Empty streets, old people, children, lovers
> And adults, are all shaken off.
> There, I believe life goes on
> There will be victory. Memory of paper
> is not exactly so. The pain there is borne by us. (*CW* 105)

Using 'we,' the speaker identifies with the victims, offsetting the claimed 'victory' with 'pain'. Here, writing is an attempt to correct error, reminding readers not to forget all the pain when celebrating victory. For the victims, death is an irretrievable loss that cannot be compensated for by an abstract victory and the survivor needs to bear the exorbitant emotional costs of survival. Such repudiation against triumphalist propaganda, a leitmotif in Chinese epidemic poems, represents the Chinese poets' consciences and critical thinking. They agree with Susanne Hillman, who challenges the myth of heroic survival in Holocaust narratives: 'To emphasize the positive outcomes of their frightful ordeal is as problematic and morally questionable as to downplay or smooth over the lasting wounds they sustained' (216).

Resisting glorification is also reflected in homages to medical workers. In the war against the epidemic, in which medical workers are commonly celebrated as soldiers, a significant portion of poetic articulation reiterates the discourse of revolutionary martyrs in modern Chinese literature which represents the heroes as 'invariably fearless, sexless, selfless, and untiring, ever ready to lay down their lives for the glory of the socialist cause' (Lau and Goldblatt xxiii). For instance, the image of strong, fearless, valiant soldiers can be seen in Wu Ziran's poem, 'The countermarch is moving mountains' (*SCC* 125). Xie Keqiang writes, 'Go forward / without grandiloquence / with only total loyalty / and a doctor's professional ethics' (*SCC* 48). Zhu Youhua and Huang Yazhou position their vignettes depicting volunteering in China's larger revolutionary history and accentuate the volunteers' virtuous sacrifice (*SCC* 37–39; 53–54); volunteers' fearlessness can be also seen in poems by Wang Jiuxin and Shan Ha (*SCC* 10; 31). Ding Xiaowei elaborates the military trope, stating that 'the epidemic means a war without gunpowder,' praising the soldiers' selfless dedication to their country (*SCC* 56). Tian Xiang uses an epithet 'iron policeman' to commemorate Liu Daqing, a 58-year-old martyred police officer, stressing that with an ordinary body, Liu had an ironlike will and character and devoted all his time to, and sacrificed his life for, the cause (*SCC* 64–65). This strand of poems, which are thematically and stylistically very close to journalistic writings, play in tandem an instrumental role in invigorating people and mobilizing them to embrace collective action.

Some poets, such as Long Qiaoling, Li Li and Wang Jianzhao, however, find such uplifting heroism unsatisfactory or insufficient. They portray so-called 'heroes' as ordinary people possessed by fear and other emotions and as experiencing a succession of frustrations. They disrupt the monolithic discourse of heroism in multiple subtle and persuasive ways. Wang Jianzhao's poem 'The Word "Hero" is Still Too Light' reformulates heroism by evoking honesty and duty and, thus, subverting the bravery and victory of heroic martyrdom that marks revolutionary optimism. The speaker undercuts the glory of any victory that entails the hero's death or emotional collapse, while endorsing the primacy of life and suggesting that it is not shameful to surrender and to weep – 'If you can't hold on, do not be ashamed, / Tears can't wash away evils, yet can restrain grief' (135). An underlying logic is that the hero's vulnerability is justified since he is human, rather than an omnipotent god who can keep the forces of evil at bay. Having experienced egregious hardships and irreparable losses, the heroes need cathartic outlets for emotional release and spiritual cleansing. More provocatively, the second part of Wang's poem, a parodic account of the fearless soldier ready for combat, adopts 'I' as the narrative voice, so that the hero can self-disparagingly evoke an image of a beleaguered rat to confess to experiencing cowardice, anxiety and fear, despite his armed exterior. The conventionally unheroic speaker pleads for forgiveness for lacking bravery and downplays the role of sacrifice— 'we are ordinary people, as you are / A self-lit, faint light, occasionally lights the world's limited / darkness' (135). Wang's eschewal of glorification, as Chen Xuguang argues, like Wang Dandan's denial of fearless countermarch, constitutes a new understanding of heroism in a civilian era – 'lives matter to both the saved, and savers, hero is an external title and unnecessary sacrifice should be avoided' (60–61). Similarly, Liu Dawei acknowledges his inability to endorse militarized notions by indicating that medical workers' toils should not be glorified in these terms since such glorification is heartless: 'There was another doctor who was exhausted / I was too ashamed to shout "come on" for him' (*SCC* 117). The tension between the impulse to praise doctors and the impotency of language also confronts Su Rencong, who writes, 'when I cannot write, I show mother a video where doctors fall down, / till her eyes are overbrimmed with tears' (*SCC* 104). For these poets, a hero's greatness does not consist in supernatural strength and determination, but rather in fulfilling their duties despite their ordinariness. This revision, rather than being anti-patriotic, suggests poets' deep respect for a selfless hero and profound humanism.

Li Li's 'Thus Spoke the Young Nurses Who Died of COVID-19' unapologetically deconstructs the grandiose version of heroism by offering a glimpse into a mother's psyche when she is facing imminent death. The speaker wishes to tell her two-year-old daughter the meaning of death plainly by listing all the small things that will be denied to her after her mother's death – her mother can no longer cook for her, send her to kindergarten, tell her bedtime stories at night or accompany her to the park to see blooming flowers. Rather than celebrating a traditionally heroic dying, the poet suggests, we should see that for the little daughter her mother's death means the collapse of life: 'love is gone'. The speaker disavows glorifying phrases such as 'the pride of the motherland' and belittles the overblown concept of martyrdom: 'Tell her about her mother's death / It was nothing more than a stone thrown into the Yangtze River' (*CW* 39). While mainstream media often describe medical staff going to 'the battlefield' as fearless volunteers, such bravery often stems from ignorance about 'the power of the enemy's weapons'. This is an implied indictment of systemic dereliction in providing medical staff with personal protective equipment and needlessly risking their lives. She repudiates the sublimation of her own death, saying that 'the dead, become / a number, are nothing' (*CW* 39). This critique is particularly forceful because it emanates from a much vaunted individual.

The most forceful critique of glorification is made by Long Qiaoling, a poet and nurse from Gansu Province, who volunteered to serve in one of the makeshift *fangcang* hospitals in Wuhan. Two of her widely circulated and critically acclaimed poems undercut the image of an indefatigable hero. In 'Please Do Not Disturb,' the speaker does not conceal her tiredness, rejects praise and acknowledges that 'I am just doing my duty / a healer's conscience / Often one has to join the battle, unarmed,' which suggests that the speaker has no interest in heroism whatsoever but rather aspires simply to go home alive. In 'Little Sister, Tonight I'm Ashamed of the Praise,' the speaker recounts a nurse's hardship when having to work without PPE because of a shortage, 'All songs of praise,' she writes, 'are guilty' (Tao Quoted 16–17). Zhai Yongming ascribes these poems' success to Long's experiences as a medical worker and most importantly to her critique of those poems which are sentimental and declaim victory.

Similarly, Chen Xuguang celebrates poems from the frontline, observing that Long's exorcising grandiose phrases stems from an intense attachment to living and her adherence to duty (55–56). Tao Dongfeng aptly considers Long's poems to be 'Wuhan anti-hero stories written by a hero,' arguing that her poems subvert a recurrent narrative pattern in COVID-19 discourse which inherits the progress narrative from modern and contemporary Chinese literatures, which eagerly invoke images of light, victory and spring, and bombastically transform tragedy into comedy and disaster into an opportunity, by neglecting the voices of sufferers (16). In short, Long's effort to deflate heroism, or at least to avoid referring to it in terms of nobility, indicates a true heroism within oneself, rather than acting in terms of abstract ideals for public rewards. Rather one's conduct should be fashioned from a genuine sense of duty. Her non-glorification is interwoven with valuing individual lives, which links her to the other poets, but her status as a witness endows her voice with greater evocative power in the public domain. In addition, her anti-heroic stance enables her to record in plain language the mutual support of ordinary people, which develops an alternative version of heroism characterized by quiet courage, love and mutual compassion. I will return to this conception.

Re-membering Lives

In conceiving of poetry as a vehicle for comforting and cheering people, especially those who live, suffer or work facing imminent danger, poets recognize that the ethics of writing about disaster needs to centre the lives of individual sufferers or workers situated at the epicenter of disaster. They believe that poetic exploration should focus on the individuals' experiences, especially sufferers' experiences, and describe the struggle of the oft-ignored little people in the whirlpool of time. Poets should also reveal how the most vulnerable members of society are most deeply affected by the epidemic. These poets refuse to allow those who have suffered or those who lost their lives to fall into oblivion. Through depicting the sorrows, despair and death of ordinary people, including medical workers, they urge readers to remember every individual, and to re-member every individual who has been wrongly neglected, excluded or rejected during the perilous and inconceivable epidemic that made the conditions of life bleak for so many.

The suffering of Wuhan's people became a national concern. As indicated by Yi Miyi's 'Wuhan Closure,' Liu Jiemin's 'Extinction and Song' and Jin Du's 'Sealed Winter,' among many others, the people of Wuhan in the locked down city constantly faced the threat of the virus, witnessed the frequent, sudden deaths of their close friends and colleagues, often in close proximity, and experienced anxiety and despair when insufficient hospital beds were available and the infected could not be treated. According to Nan Ou, 'Wuhan is an innocent city / She stood in the middle of the storm and for the world / Bore the bitter fruit of ignorance and greed' (*SCC* 26). Wang Jiaxin's 'Leap Year' foregrounds the suffering and indignation of the Chinese people generally (indicated in the poem by the smog of Beijing) and Wuhan's inhabitants particular (*CW* 17). Appalled by the virus's unidentifiable malevolence and implacable manner, some Wuhan people drifted towards hysteria and tried to flee the stricken city after its lockdown. In 'Run, Rabbit,' Wang extends sympathy towards those who ran away. The association of the

Wuhan people with rabbits underscores their fragile position relative to the virus; the deadly grip of the epidemic is compared to a butcher who inflicts senseless harm (*CW* 17).

Mo Yaping's 'Sonnet: My Country is a Hospital Bed' views the media's carnival from the perspective of a patient who is waiting helplessly for a hospital bed. The speaker first presents the context: 'the COVID-19 war is tense'. The speaker watches a video in which 'fireworks are set off in the area of the Yangtze River Bridge / like a signal bomb for the counterattack launched by Wuhan'. Fireworks wrote anti-epidemic slogans in the sky: 'eliminate the virus,' 'refuel China,' 'eradicate COVID-19' and 'refuel Wuhan'. For the healthy person, these slogans were exciting. However, the speaker is not interested in the gorgeous fireworks display, but is appalled by the 'giant fireworks' which to him resemble a huge virus. These splendid fireworks demonstrate the strength and happiness of the collective yet are only dispiriting for the afflicted. All the abstract praise and encouragement do little to assuage the suffering. As the speaker says finally, 'To me, my country is a hospital bed'.

Several poets commemorate the victims of COVID-19 by emphasizing the connection between the living and the dead. 'The death of a stranger is also / - a part of me,' observes Shi Bin in 'Warning,' because all the pain experienced by the dead 'will reappear in a living person'; 'the living is all survivors / how can survivors feel at ease?'; 'the dead are too weak, and / the living cannot be too noisy' (*CW* 66). Chen Yujia in 'Wuhan's Notes' similarly expresses this view:

> How many people die when one person dies?
> How many people live in one person?
> My friends, Sisyphus in Stonehenge,
> Finally, dropping the stone in hand, bravely
> Break into that hard data. (*CW* 66)

Addressing friends as 'Sisyphus' suggests that, even confronted with a hopeless situation, they chose not to flee from Wuhan, but rather heroically accepted their fate and defied death. Yet, as with Sisyphus, the rock continuously rolls downhill, and their plight is not captured in published data, which does nothing to differentiate and distinguish the dead.

The most profound tributes to COVID-19 heroes who rose above their quotidian limitations, many of whom passed away, adopt a restrained tone. Mo Yaping depicts Dr. Peng Yinhua, from the Respiratory Department of the first hospital in Jiangxia District, Wuhan, as an ordinary hero by articulating Dr. Peng's unrealized wishes. Dr. Peng postponed his wedding ceremony to join the frontline. When he was infected with the virus, lying in bed, he finally allowed himself to think about the postponed wedding. Yet even the imagined wedding could not be completed because he was constantly interrupted by his cough, and his life ended on 20 February 2020. His unfulfilled wish is represented in the last couplet: 'now only unsent invitations are left in his drawer; / the smallest wedding hall in the world'. Depictions such as this render the hero more familiar, and his sacrifice more poignant.

The death of Li Wenliang, a doctor who was criticized by authorities for alerting friends about the coronavirus, triggered a national outpouring of grief. It became a public event which, as Shen Xingpei observes, heightened national sentiment. It also became a 'literary event' in Chinse COVID-19 literature (*CW* 7–8). He is acclaimed a hero before being accorded martyrdom, the highest honorary title awarded by the Chinese government. Li Li proposes that a monument be erected on which his last words be engraved: 'a healthy society should not have only one voice!' (*CW* 38). Qi's poem proclaims Dr. Li's immortality: 'a man with conscience will not die,' and 'every living being is your / dwelling place' (*CW* 79). Lan Lan remorsefully acknowledges her guilt: 'I feel responsible for your death' (*CW* 14). Wang Jiaxin's 'After Many Days when Dr. Li's Gone' concludes: 'Dr. Li is gone, gone forever / the comment area under his microblog is still updated / like a long line every day before the desperate clinic' (*CW* 16). The juxtaposition of Li Wenliang and the people of Wuhan hopelessly waiting for treatment suggests that both the dead and the survivors are shrouded in sadness and despair. The commemoration of a hero functions as a public means for finding consolation and support in a precarious world. 'Impermanence' by Yu Jian introduces the personal, human and everyday dimensions of Li Wenliang's being. The poem portrays Li as a content, loving and life-affirming person, 'Craving eating and dressing … caring about the neighbor's saltshaker, admiring Kobe'. The understated final line conveys a restrained sadness: 'it is only ordinary people who are to be killed' (*CW* 20–21). Yet, these quotidian details are symbolically rich. For instance, comparing Li's playing badminton to a gull dashing at the sea establishes a link with Du Fu, the Chinese poet of the Tang dynasty, who lamented his unrealized ambition to serve the country, and affirms Li's readiness to meet challenges. The Chinese name of Clivia, a plant which Li waters in the poem, combines the images of a noble man and orchid, suggesting Li's integrity.

The discrimination against particular regions, which was triggered by the epidemic, has been the subject of much poetic reflection. The people of Wuhan, as well as of the Hubei province of which it is the capital, were ostracized when the first case was reported there and the epidemic subsequently began to spread. Yet even those from Wuhan and Hubei who did not live there also encountered unprecedented discrimination. Everyone connected to Wuhan and Hubei was considered as a potential carrier of the virus. Fei Ya's 'He was Rejected by a Hotel' records a person who was rejected by nine hotels because he came from 'that central province' and thus was regarded a 'potential patient / and an extremely dangerous element'. Denied accommodation, he ate New Year's dinner in a Kentucky Fried Chicken, 'like a bird drenched by a storm / lonely / stranded without a habitat' (*CW* 107). The speaker does not give him a name to highlight the fact that all people from Hubei were subtly or outrageously labeled, stigmatized and excluded.

Other citizens who were severely affected or lost their lives are also mourned and honoured by the poets. On 13 February 2020, Liu Decheng, a beekeeper from Sichuan Province, committed suicide in an apiary tent. In Wang Jiaxin's 'The Death of a Beekeeper,' the speaker voices a lament, presents Liu's act of suicide as resistance to the devastating situation, accentuates his intense attachment to life, and urges readers to acknowledge social problems. The speaker first lists the much-mourned deaths of several historical figures and the officially mourned deaths of doctors and nurses during the war against the epidemic. Adding the death of a beekeeper to this list suggests the speaker's intention to record, remember and immortalize a life which is at risk of being forgotten. Being a beekeeper meant chasing the seasons, following blooming flowers. Liu Decheng, a diligent and joyous person, did not lack strength of spirit; he could make the most of a nomadic life. The final lines evoke the flower of life, poignantly conveying the pain of elusive happiness: 'he died, in a tent that no one dares to approach / in the quietest spring - / the most flourishing flowering period he has ever seen in this life' (*CW* 16). The poet suggests mournfully that Liu's suffering and death was caused, not by mere misfortune or his personal mistakes, but by stringent measures inappropriately enforced by local officials.

Shortly after his passing, the police investigated the cause of Liu Decheng's death and discovered unsent messages on his mobile phone, among them, 'most bees died from poisoning due to excessive use of bee mites and local oilseed rape flowers'. On 17 February, *Global Times* published an article entitled 'Beekeeper's wife dispels rumors that claimed her husband's suicide was due to epidemic'. The article quotes Liu's wife to the effect that the outbreak of the epidemic did not contribute significantly to Liu's death; that Liu died because he could not bear the death of the bees. But, if there had been no epidemic, things would have continued as normal and there would probably not have been a swathe of bee deaths – and then no last straw that overwhelmed Liu Decheng. The death of the bees emblematizes the loss of honest, meaningful work. Wang Jiaxin's poem invites readers to think about why a man who loved singing and flowers and was in the spring of life lost the will to live. By giving a voice to the powerless and deceased, poems such as 'The Death of a Beekeeper,' supplement journalistic representations of the epidemic. Liu might not have been a direct victim of the epidemic yet the overall effect of the attendant historical, social and economic circumstances, led to his suicidal panic and despair.

Redefining Heroism

With the outbreak of the epidemic in Wuhan, the whole country sent supplies, including protective masks and testing kits, and dispatched doctors. In line with the state's propaganda, the literary outpourings at this moment advocate a heroism based in medical workers' determination to fight; their selfless sacrifice, patriotism, unwaveringly committed to triumph and the conviction that Chinese people's invincible strength is fostered by solidarity. The most distinctive feature of COVID-19 literature and art, as Fu Daobin observes, is heroism that is based on patriotism (30). These invigorating poems commonly have a pronounced, rhythmic pace which seems to subsume individual impulsiveness in collective action. This quest for the heroic, when combined with skepticism towards obsequious glorification, a concern with individual lives and an emphasis on the quotidian, produces a humane heroism which is expressed in a restrained, lowly voice.[2] What makes this alternative version of heroism especially touching is the figure of the ordinary hero, deeply involved in the disaster, who nonetheless remains life-affirming, and fulfils his duties in the face of adversity, remaining capable of love and sympathy. This hero takes care of people in immediate danger and the moribund, cultivates happiness, reciprocity and fulfillment amidst suffering and despair. The ordinary people's mutual support and compassion enables mutually affirming relationships that break down isolation and allow for unironic representations of heroism.

Quiet courage sustains the verse of the Wuhan poet, Zhang Zhihao, who lives 'in the center of darkness' (45) and often feels 'the deafening cries for help' (47). In 'Words in Snow,' he evokes snow falling to emblematize the helplessness of 'living amidst death,' the 'powerlessness and preciousness of the strugglers,' and sufferers' 'dignity' despite their 'humiliation' and 'despair' (47). 'It's Not Poetry' laments the masked, ubiquitous death which is not accompanied by tears, obituaries and memorial services. The final lines urge one to redouble efforts to live since 'in the territory occupied by death / Only living itself can make a poem' (46). Even in his darkest moment, Zhang yearns for poetry and a free, loving, happy life. In 'Poetry Outside,' a family of wild ducks paddles leisurely upon the lake, and the threat of dying is muted by the poet's concord with nature, if not actually cancelled by the fortitude of living. The final lines juxtapose the hospital and the metasequoia trees by the lake the shadows of which are lengthened in turn by the morning and afternoon sunlight (47). 'I come from the

Mountain' features a person lying on the bed, listening to an orchid song; 'I come from the Mountain' is sounded by a sprinkler. Then the sound of the sprinkler is displaced by that of a disinfectant vehicle. The desolation of the empty street is underscored by the memory of the noisy street, when people jumped, laughed and dodged cars. This stark contrast is intensified by the lingering convivial song, which evokes free movement and the orchid's fragrance. But the song, rather than being refreshing, comes to feel suffocating to those confined in lockdown. On the verge of sinking into despondency, the speaker draws attention to the metasequoia trees along the street. They have been pruned down to mere trunks and seem dead, but the speaker knows that, after winter passes, they will 'restore their erstwhile vigor, / be able to climb ranges of mountains' (46). The understated final lines serve as the poet's encouragement in despair, both for himself and more generally for Wuhan, which he is certain will also overcome this great adversity.

Wang Jiaxin's widely circulated 'Wuhan Girl Shanshan' records a mother's note, scrawled in the last moments of her life. It expresses an ethic of loving that incorporates courage, detachment and self-restraint. The speaker tells us in a matter of fact tone that Shanshan has infected her parents and older brother – and her mother dies, leaving the orphaned daughter a note. The mother's last message, devoid of fear, relates tossing out expired cake flour, seemingly trivial examples of domestic prudence and finally an apology to her daughter for her nagging. These mundane details emphasize earnest, diligent living, urging one to accept the transience of life, let go of losses and make the best use of what one owns. These homely injunctions render all the grandiloquent epidemic narratives frivolous and meaningless. This is a measured reexamination of the poet's mission and the ethics of writing. The speaker laments the impotency of writing and the inadequacy of words, 'Words are so heavy that we cannot drag them … . We have written too many' (*CW*17). Particularly, the speaker evokes Du Fu, who climbed the three-story tower overlooking Lake Dongting in late-winter 768 and helplessly lamented a national tragedy and his personal losses. The speaker implies that even the greatest poet, Du Fu, lacks the love, wisdom and fortitude of a dying mother who calmly leaves behind a message urging intense living.

Another important epidemic poet who explores the inner, latent heroism of ordinary people is Long Qiaoling, a nurse-poet who worked in Wuhan. Long's 'Bus Driver' recounts the stories of Dai Yong, who on Valentine's Day, warm-heartedly sends garlands of roses to nurses, then silently leaves. Girls jubilantly wear the garland of roses, as if the spring has arrived, with flowers blossoming in the cold night. When, in a late afternoon, the speaker meets Dai Yong who wears a mark and hazmat suit, she requests him to leave the bus which needs to be sterilized, and shares Lanzhou noodles with him (115). A horrifying effect of the epidemic has been the apathy caused by the dreadful power of death. To win the battle, one needs to be as impregnable as iron, a typical image representing determination and strength. Long's poem suggests that hardship does not deprive Chinese people of tenderness, which is a fundamental aspect of our humanity. To record the warm moment of mutual support and comfort among ordinary people serves to salvage the light of humanity amid desolation and dread.

An intimate and human heroism can also be seen in Long's poem 'The Night Watch,' which portrays the compassion of two ordinary people, a security guard and a nurse on night shift. The night refers metaphorically to the death, darkness and the despair that pervades Wuhan. The speaker addresses the guard as an older brother though she is unsure of his age and dismisses this question as trivial given the virus's undifferentiated destruction of people. There can be no less conventionally heroic figure than this brother who 'Nestles in the sofa, shrinking into a cocoon,' silhouetted against Wuhan's chilling cold. Han Hong's song 'Sky Road' plays repeatedly, suggesting his hankering for a pure place untouched by the virus. This scene indicates man's pitiable smallness in the face of the ravaging sickness, but simultaneously hints that heroism might merely entail persevering in the face of the threat. Whenever he sees the nurse, this humble man, immensely guilty about the disaster, apologizes on behalf of Wuhan, an apology that suggests, really, a gratitude towards medical workers who provide assistance, possibly at the cost of their own lives. The speaker silently disabuses him of self-blame, advocating solidarity and embracing the common destiny of 'Breathing the same air'. Stanza Four depicts how the brother, driven to despair by the cooling weather, 'tightens himself ... retracts into the inner storm, and pretends / Not to hear the bad news' (116). This depiction of the helpless guard renders him more human and admirable. At midnight, the speaker sends some food to him, yet refrains from disturbing his sleep and interrupting his dreams. Her restraint, empathy with his plight and hope, and her proffering food, amount to a profound act of compassion, the most important gift one person can give another. By living and fighting so closely together, the Wuhan brother and the nurse break down their isolation, develop true interpersonal contact and support one another. They replace more nebulous ideas of heroism with less lofty, but perhaps more substantive ideals of friendship and immediate, proximate duty. The compassion shared by common people sustains them in desperate times and provides a light of warmth to those struggling in the dark.

Fortunately, as the virus is rampant, love and compassion are also infectious, passing from one person to another. Liu Chun's 'Two Photos' describes two moments which are deeply affecting for Chinese people. First, a little boy forms a heart shape with his hands to express his love for the nurse who is going to vaccinate him, and who, in response, gives him two thumbs-up for encouragement. The second is when a baby in an isolation ward opens his arms for a hug and a doctor, outside the creche, turns her head and covers her face, crying. The desire for human contact is a powerful need, especially in times of suffering. The boy is loved, and thus capable of loving; the baby spontaneously yearns to love and be loved. Such scenes inspire the speaker's empathy, who, in the third and fourth stanzas, indicates the need to be a patient, to 'Embrace them and replace them,' and a resolve to regard all the medical workers as 'brothers' and 'lovers' (32). Such responses signify a radiant circulation initiated by the loving doctors and nurses. The two photos and Liu Chun's poem indicate that love begets love, and compassion begets compassion.

In March 2020, a photo of two figures watching the setting sun, a seriously ill and bedridden patient, and a doctor in full protective clothing, quickly went viral on the internet. The patient is Wang Yi, an 87-year-old erstwhile violinist, and the doctor is Liu Kai. They had stopped for a moment to watch the sunset on their way back from a CT scan at Renmin Hospital at Wuhan University. Unlike the sentimental journalism and sloganeering poetry inspired by this photo, Sun Xiaoya's 'Sunset Has Love,' a lyric which is sung by Li Shan and was made into a video, subtly explores the nuanced change in the patient triggered by watching sunset with the doctor. The speaker first describes the mundane details of doctors who take care of patients in isolation and console them in their despair. The second stanza alternates between the perspectives of the melancholic patient and the young doctor: 'for me, the sunset is transient' and 'aloof' whereas 'you' are quietly smiling; 'for you, the sunset is so gorgeous' and 'you can see morning in the sunset'. For a dying patient, the resplendent sunset merely intensifies his sense of the transience of living, the ruthless march of time and the sneering of fate. Yet, the doctor's company, vigor and optimistic vision inspire him to see a dawn of hope. Their interaction culminates in both acknowledging the infinite and the possibility of transcending death. The singer's soulful performance, accompanied by plangent and wistful music, and the verbal and visual images of spring thawing the ice and the end of a cold winter, poignantly render the patient's journey from despair to rekindled hope and courage. Listeners and viewers are invited to achieve a similar spiritual catharsis.

Coda: At Least My Shadow Remains

Since June 2020, the COVID-19 epidemic has been largely under control in China. After great pain, China has begun to start over. I would like to conclude this essay by reading Mo Yaping's 'Sonnet: At Least My Shadow Remains,' which adroitly integrates personal losses and social critique with philosophical meditation. On a sunny day, the speaker, after a long time in isolation, comes to the Lijiang River to breathe the fresh air. Reflecting on people's losses and his deceased father, the speaker is not sentimental, nor does he express his yearning for those who have died. Rather he decides to seek consciously for what is left, saying with mingled resignation and congratulation: 'at least my shadow remains / at least, the reflection of tower-hill in Lijiang River remains'. By describing shadow and the reflection of the tower in the flowing river, the speaker appeals to a recognition of interiority, which is often neglected, but which is integral to life, to the natural state of being and the coexistence of things. The third stanza explains:

> If I have no shadow in the sun,
> or tower-hill no reflection in the Lijiang River,
> Or only one sound echoes in the valley,
> What an appalling scene it is!

The absence of shadow and reflection implies the denial of aspects of life which are essential to good living. This disquieting absence is further compared to the situation in which 'there's only one sound in the valley'. This alludes to Dr. Li Wenliang's words: 'a healthy society should not have only one voice'. The speaker quietly pays tribute to birdsong, flowers' fragrances and, particularly, the tower's reflection in the river, which suggests the abundance, freedom and harmony of nature, and corresponds to humankind's inner nature. This is an idealized utopia for Chinese people: a place and approach for achieving peace of mind.

Funding

This work is supported by the National Social Science Fund of China under Grant Number 20&ZD222.

Notes

1   According to Jiang Hongwei's statistics, more than 5 000 Chinese poets published more than 10 000 poems before 31 January 2020. A COVID-19 poem column is featured in *Poetry Periodical* 詩刊 (5,7) which includes 15 poets, *Poetry Monthly* 詩歌月刊 (2,3,4,5) which includes 85 poets, *Journal of Selected Poems* 詩選刊 (3) which includes over 160 poets, *Chinese and Western Poetry* 中西詩歌 (1) which includes 64 poets, *The Poetic Tide* 诗潮 (3,4,5) which includes 35 poets, *The Stars* 星星 (7,10) which includes 21

poets. *Song of Combatting COVID-19* (Xiao Qin, ed. Beijing: Writers' Press) includes 40 poets. This essay refers to the initial journals and anthologies published in 2020.

2   This reformulation of heroism interweaves the contemporary artistic and poetic trend, a 'quotidian turn' if we adapt Tang Xiaobing's phrasing. Tang argues that 'the heroic and the quotidian – two complementary visions of reality … constitute the inner dynamics of Chinese literature in the twentieth century' (6). Contemporary films question 'conventional tales of martyrdom, such as omnipotent heroes, gender rigidity, and patriarchal loyalty to the collective' and 'challenge the exclusively political representations of traditional martyr figures' (Yang 183). Rejecting Misty's poetry's 'grandiloquence and tragic heroism,' Yu Jian, among others, in the early 1980s, began to propound a colloquial poetry, 'a poetics of the everyday, with minimal use of high-modernist metaphor and symbolism, low-key language usage, and much room for humor and irony' (Denton and Fulton 416).

Works Cited

Chen, Xuguang陳旭光. 'COVID-19 Poetry: Bugle, Mirror, and Lamp'(疫情詩:疾馳的號角及鏡與燈). *Poetry Periodical* 詩刊 11, 2020: 54–63.

Denton, Kirk A., Bruce Fulton, and Sharalyn Orbaugh. *The Columbia Companion to Modern East Asian Literature.* New York: Columbia University Press, 2003.

Fu, Daobin 傅道彬. 'Lighten the Lamp of Heroism'(點亮英雄主義的文學之燈). *China Literature and Art Criticism* 中國文藝評論 5, 2020: 28–36.

Guan, Yue 管樂. 'Dream as a Horse: What Kind of COVID-19 Literature Do We Need?' (以夢為馬/我們需要怎樣的抗疫文學?). *Ta Kung Pao* 大公報. 14 February 2020.

Hillman, Susanne. '"Not Living, but Going": Unheroic Survival, Trauma Performance, and Video Testimony'. *Holocaust Studies* 21(4), 2015: 215–235.

Hu, Zibo 鬍子博. 'Hu Zibo's Poems of Combating COVID-19'(鬍子博抗疫詩歌). Unpublished Manuscript.

Huang, Lihai 黃禮孩. (ed.). *Chinese and Western Poetry* (1), 2020.

Huo, Junming 霍俊明. '"There is a Light": A Lyrical Poet in the Disaster' ("要有光":非常時期的抒情詩人). *Journal of Literature and Art* 文藝報, 10 February 2020.

Jenkins, Matt. 'In China, Finding Hope Amid Coronavirus'. https://www.bbc.com/travel/article/20200426-in-china-finding-hope-amid-coronavirus. 27 April 2020. Accessed 14 July 2021.

Jiang, Hongwei 薑紅偉. 'Memorandum on the Outbreak of "COVID-19 Poetry Tide" in Chinese Poetry Circle'(書寫大美大愛 鼓舞信心士氣 謳歌眾志成城——中國詩壇爆發"抗疫詩潮"備忘錄). *Liao River* 遼河 (4), 2020: 113–116.

Jiao, Dian 焦典. 'Literary "Medicine": on the Therapeutic Function of Disaster Literature' (文學的"藥":淺談災難文學的療救作用). *Literary Comment* 創作評譚 (04), 2020: 37–41.

Lau, Joseph SM, and Howard Goldblatt. *The Columbia Anthology of Modern Chinese literature.* New York: Columbia University Press, 2007.

Li, Xiuwen 李修文. 'My Heart is Chaotic, I Can't Write Now' (我的心是亂的 現在沒法寫作). *Xinmin Weekly* 新民週刊. 11 February 2020.

Liu, Chun 劉春. 'Liu Chun's Poems' (劉春的詩). *Journal of Selected Poems* 詩選刊 (7), 2020: 31–34.

Long, Qiaoling 龍巧玲. 'Poems by Wuhan Fangcang Nurse.' (武漢方艙醫院護士的詩). *Liao River* 遼河 3, 2020: 114–116.

Mo, Yaping莫雅萍. '20 Sonnets About Combating COVID-19' (抗疫十四行詩20首). Unpublished Manuscript.

Shen, Xingpei 沈杏培. 'Narrative Ethics and Writing Taboo in Disaster Writings'(災難文學的 敘事倫理與書寫禁忌). *Yalu River* 鴨綠江 10, 2020: 4–12.

Sun, Xiaoya 孫曉婭. 'Sunset Has Love'(夕陽有愛). https://wap.peopleapp.com/video/ rmh12528782/rmh12528782?from=message. Accessed on 20 April 2021.

Tao, Dongfeng陶東風. 'Wuhan Anti-hero Stories Written by a Hero: Long Qiaoling's Poems as Witness Literature' (一個英雄寫的反英雄的武漢故事——从弱水吟的诗说到见证文 学). *GBA Lite* 粤港澳大湾区文学评论 4, 2020: 16–20.

Wang, Jianzhao 汪劍釗. 'The Word Hero is Still Too Light' (英雄這個詞還是太輕). *Southern Literature* 南方文學 2, 2020: 135.

Wang, Yan 王焱. 'Disaster Writing Needs Rational Reflection' (公共災難的文學書寫需理性 反思). *Social Science Weekly* 社會科學報. 20 February 2020.

Wang, Zheng 汪政. 'What Kind of "COVID-19 literature" Do We Need?' (我們需要怎樣的"抗 疫文藝"?). *Journal of Literature and Art* 文藝報. 7 February 2020.

Wu, Sijing 吳思敬. 'COVID-19: Call for Conscience and Test of Humanity '(抗疫詩歌:良知的 呼喚與人性的考量). *Poetry Periodical* 詩刊 1, 2021: 51–54.

Xu, Zhaozheng 徐兆正. 'Refusing Imagination: Guideline of Disaster Literature ' (拒絕想像:災 難文學論綱). *Literary Comment* 創作評譚 4, 2020: 34–37.

Yang, Haosheng. 'Myths of Revolution and Sensual Revisions: New Representation of Martyrs on the Chinese Screen.' *Modern Chinese Literature and Culture* 24(2), 2012: 179–208.

Zeng, Pan 曾攀. 'The Public Nature of a Private Lyricism' (個體抒情的公共性). *China Arts Daily* 中國藝術報. 1 June 2020.

Zhai, Yongming 翟永明. 'Women's Status Does not Change with the Increase of Buying Power' (女性地位,並沒有因消費力增強而改變). Interview by Yu Yaqing. *The Beijing News* 新 京報. 26 April 2020.

Zhang, Zhihao 張執浩. 'Zhang Zhihao's Poems' (張執浩的詩). *Bianjiang Literature* 邊疆文學 4, 2020: 44–47.

Ten Chinese COVID-19 Poets

Translated by Yanbin Kang

1.

The Night Watch
Long Qiaoling

Every nightshift I meet an older brother on duty in the hotel,
Nestled in the hall sofa, shrunk into a cocoon.
I incline to ask, who is older, he or me?
Damn it! Now, why bother to ask?
The virus has gone mad, attacking whomever!

His mobile phone replays Han Hong's 'Sky Road,'
A wish that Wuhan
Be clean as Tibet, a pure land.
Every time he is asked to lock door, he always apologizes:
I am sorry! Wuhan gets you into trouble!
Wuhan, big brother,
The pressing issue is not to blame.
Tied together, we share a pot of rice,
Breathing the same air, facing the same death

The weather forecast says that Wuhan is cooling,
Lightning, gale, hail, and blizzard.
You wrap yourself up in your military coat,
Retract into the inner storm, and pretend
Not to hear the lousy news

At midnight, I bring some food to him.
The body in the sofa is snoring.
I pause for quite a while. Yes,

I shall not disturb a person's sleep.
Let him return to his middle-aged daily life,
Let him enjoy children's presence in his dreams.

Long Qiaoling, from Gansu Province, volunteered to serve as a nurse in Wuhan Shelter Hospital. Her poems about the experiences in Wuhan gained wide popularity.

2.

Wuhan Girl Shanshan
Wang Jiaxin

Shanshan, a girl from Wuhan, her parents and brother also infected.
Mother finally left, leaving only a note:
'Your cake flour is out of date. I've taken it away. Food
has a shelf life.'
'You, living alone, should buy small packages; things
need to be classified in case you forget them.'
'Not to use up things is also a waste.'
'The days need to be carefully arranged.'
'Don't frown upon your mother's nagging, this is the last time … '

After reading this note, I burst into tears, going downstairs.
I think we should not write poems.
Words are so heavy that we can't drag them.
How shall we live after this day: use oil, salt, sauce and vinegar sparingly,
Du Fu on Yueyang Tower did not know either.
We also lack an orphan's ear
To hear instructions from heaven.
All of us have written too much.
To take poetry as last words, leaving every word of love behind,
Only a mother in her last moment
can.

3 March 2020.

Wang Jiaxin is an internationally acclaimed Chinese poet. He has published over forty volumes of poetry, collections of essays, and translations. He is the recipient of a number of poetry prizes, most recently the Li Bai and Du Fu Poetry Award (2018) and the Changyao Poetry Award (2020).

3.

Impermanence
Yu Jian

Never plots against anyone, nor curses fate,
Longs for the coronation of life,
Young man, who dreams about being the king of life.
Craves food and clothing, studies recipes, abides by medical advice.
And when playing badminton, he imitates a gull high above in the sky
stabbing at the sea, waters the Clivia,
Tolerates a homeless ghost, follows grandmother
To feed it, at dawn on the balcony dries a pair of
wet shorts, cares about the neighbour's saltshaker, and admires Kobe.
He doesn't know Nihilism. In the spring
He dies, wearing a mask, as azure as the sky.
That is the spring of 2020, and in this plague
Clearly, it is only ordinary people who are killed.

Yu Jian is one of the most original and influential poets in contemporary China. His recent poetry volumes include *Tattooing the World* (2015), *Move* (2017), *Works of Yu Jian* (5 volumes, 2018), *Notes on Paris* (2019) and *Giant Web* (2019).

4.

The Word 'Hero' is Still Too Light
Wang Jianzhao

Compared to human goodness,
The word hero is still too light,
Honesty and duty are your largest legacy.
What is the victory?
The difference is fiasco or collapse.
Hold on? Precious life is everything,
If you can't hold on, do not be ashamed,
Tears can't wash away evils, yet can restrain grief.
At the moment, I am wearing a mask,
Fully armed, like a soldier joining the war,
Yet, inwardly weaker than a mouse crossing the street,
voicing inarticulate, unclear sounds,
You must forgive us who are ordinary people, as you are.
A self-lit, faint light, occasionally lights the world's limited
darkness.

Wang Jianzhao is a professor at Beijing Foreign Studies University, an important poet and a major translator and critic of Russian literature. He has published volumes of verse: *Crow Age of Poetry*, *One Second More Than Forever*, and *Selected Poems of Wang Jianzhao*.

5.

A Poem of Shame
Liu Dawei

To see the state of epidemics sinks my heart
In addition to tidying bookcases, these days
All I can do is turn on my phone again and again,
Read news from all sides.
Every message compels me to see my smallness
my weakness, my lightness, my emptiness.
I can't write a decent line
I fear it loses balance, is pretentious and meaningless.
I fear it blocks the only hole through which the sun shines
Look, in Moments on WeChat
Another doctor is exhausted, nearly falling.
I am too ashamed to shout 'Come on'.

Liu Dawei is an Associate Professor at Qinghai Normal University who has published several poetry and essay collections, including *Snow Falling upon the Forest*, *Soaring Below* and *Gazing upon Qinghai Road*. He has twice been awarded the Literature and Arts Prize of Qinghai Province (2014, 2019).

6.

'I Come from the Mountains … '
Zhang Zhihao

Every morning the sprinkler sings
Driving into the yard from outside
When it sings around the corridor,
I can smell the fragrance of orchids, while lying in bed.
Now the sprinkler is replaced by a disinfection car.
There is no one on the empty road
And gone are pedestrians who dodge, jump, and laugh.
It still sings:
'I come from the mountains with orchid plants … '
But the song is like a string that gets tighter,
Wrapping around our increasingly flaccid body.
The metasequoia trees by the street have only trunks left
Last year I thought they were going to die

But after winter, they restore their erstwhile vigor,
able to climb ranges of mountains.

Zhang Zhihao is one of the most prominent writers from Wuhan. He is a recipient of several
major literary awards in China including the People's Literature Award, Southern Media Literature Award and the Lu Xun Literature Award.

7.

Survivor
Ye Xiubin

Maybe I'm a survivor
A battle of swords
Might build a vision in a desolate place.

In the late autumn, a rope of birdsongs tightens my throat,
Breathing in every second
might wake me up from a deep sleep.
To dream is good. Why waken from a good dream?

But I still wake up
and see the rope tightening around my throat.
How lucky; the survivors stay alive,
How unlucky; the survivors stay alive.

Ye Xiubin's poems have appeared in Chinese journals such as *Poetry Periodical*, *Poetry
Monthly* and *Poetry Tide*. He has published a collection of poetry, *Gathering Moonlight* (2019).

8.

Two Photos
Liu Chun

A five- or six-year-old boy sitting on a stool
With his hands over his head is facing a nurse injecting him.
He draws a heart shape. The nurse stands him up,
Two thumbs

A baby a few months old, expectant
Reaches out to the doctor opposite
For a hug. The young doctor turns his head,
Covers his face and cries.

At that moment, I would like to be a patient,
Go to them,
Embrace them and replace them.

At that moment, I regard the worldwide
doctors as my brothers,
my lovers

Liu Chun has published collections of poems, essays and literary criticism, including *Happiness Blossoms Like a Flower*, *By the Literary Circle* and *A Poetry History of a Person*.

9.

A Residue of Life
Hu Zibo

Life in the latter phase of the great epidemic
Is a pot of boiled water.
Viruses and bacteria
Hardly make waves.
The water gradually cools,
Anxiety and fear
Gradually subside,
Condensing into a residue of the past.
It is silent, hard and grey,
Attached to the bottom of the pot,
Not affecting the clarity or cleanliness of the boiled water
Nor its potability
Ordinarily
It becomes an acceptable part of the pot,
Visible, yet invisible,
Occasionally
You have an urge to remove it
But it's hard and obstinate.
You think about it for a while
And let it go -

21 February 2020

Hu Zibo is an avant-garde poet who has published two volumes, *A Sleepless Person* and *The Unknown Thing*. He lives in Guilin.

10.

Sonnet: At Least My Shadow Remains
Mo Yaping

The sun finally breaks through the dark clouds, smiling,
Leaving home, I come to the Lijiang River.
Where men and women, old and young, wear masks,
But there is a sweetness in the air, which cannot be masked.

People lost so much during the epidemic,
I even lost my beloved father.
But I say to myself, 'at least my shadow remains,
At least, tower-hill is reflected in the Lijiang River.'

If I have no shadow in the sun,
nor tower-hill a reflection in the Lijiang River,
Or only one sound echoes in the valley,
What an appalling scene it is!

In the birdsongs and flowers' odors by the Lijiang River,
I pay homage to the reflection of tower-hill with my gaze.

24 March 2020

Mo Yaping has published a volume of poetry, *Humor and Sublime*, as well as Chinese translations of *The Devil's Dictionary*, *The Pickwick Papers* and *The Adventures of Tom Sawyer*.

Funding

This work is supported by JNU Collaborative Innovation Center for the Communication of Chinese Culture in Hong Kong, Macao, Taiwan and Overseas under Grant Number JNXT2021016.

Ancient Chinese Poetry and Chinese Calligraphy in Combatting COVID-19

Zhiyong Mo

In the global fight against the COVID-19 pandemic, countries, regions and international organizations dispatched personal protective equipment (PPE) to frontline workers and afflicted people. Lines of ancient Chinese poetry were printed on the side of boxes dispatched by the People's Republic of China both nationally and globally, as well as some sent from Japan to China.[1] Many of these lines invoked shared histories and the long tradition of cross-cultural communication and international friendship between China and other countries. But the printing of poetry was also motivated by a desire to remove people – albeit temporarily – from the context of COVID-19 suffering, to lead them to a more peaceful and harmonious world.

The good will and friendship among people, as well as the common destiny of all humanity, is a recurrent theme. On the boxes of PPE sent to Wuhan, initially the most affected city, by the Chinese language academy (HSK) in Japan, eight Chinese characters read, 'Mountain, River, Different, Areas / Wind, Moon, Same, Sky' (Figure 1). The elemental and ethereal images, wind, moon and sky emblematize a lofty, magnanimous, and capacious mind, able to accommodate 'ten thousand things'. These words were first embroidered on a thousand cassocks – on the orders of Japan's Emperor Tenmu's grandson Prince Nagaya (circa. 684–729) – and were sent to the Tang Dynasty court about 1300 years ago. After receiving them, the high monk Ganjin (Jianzhen 688–763), inspired by the gift, sailed to Japan to propagate Buddhism there. Invoking and rekindling this ancient memory of Japan reaching out – reiterating the gift – the HSK affirmed the long history of solidarity between the two nations.

As the pandemic unfolded, China reciprocated the gift by sending PPE to Japan. China's poem to Japan also affirmed their common heritage despite the distance separating them. The Tiantai Sect was founded during the Tang Dynasty and Japanese monks traveled to Tiantai to study, which led to them establishing the Tiantai Sect in Japan and instigating ongoing exchange. The Buddhist scholar Juzan's lines allude to this history by using the metaphor of a tree's blossom spreading its fragrance to two places (Figure 3). In the lines by Southern Song Dynasty poet, Zhang Xiaoxiang (Figure 7), printed on the PPE

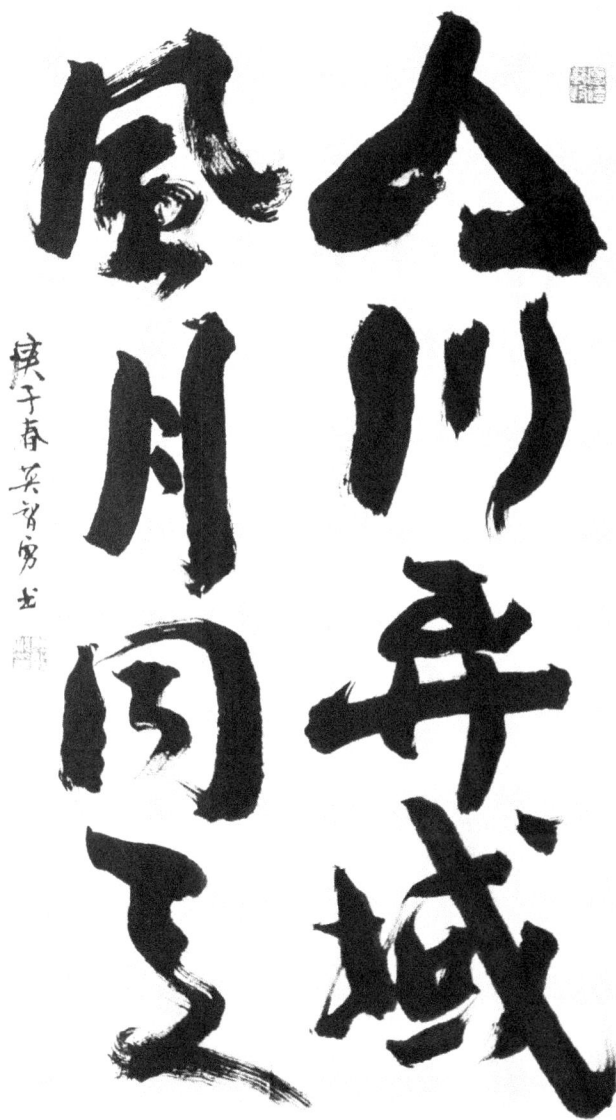

Figure 1: 山川異域, 風月同天 (Mountain, River, Different, Areas / Wind, Moon, Same, Sky). By Prince Nagaya (circa 684–729) to the Tang Dynasty's high monk Jianzhen (688–763), who helped to propagate Buddhism in Japan. The Chinese Proficiency Test (HSK) secretariat in Japan to Hubei province in China.

cartons sent from Jinan, Shandong Province, to Wako Prefecture in Siatama Province, Japan, a sailing ship connotes a smooth journey, while moonlight and river water emblematize a pure mind and the indivisible unity of all people linked in harmonious relationships.

A banner hanging from a truck delivering masks donated by the Chinese Embassy in South Korea to the inhabitants of Daegu (North Gyeongsang Province, South Korea)

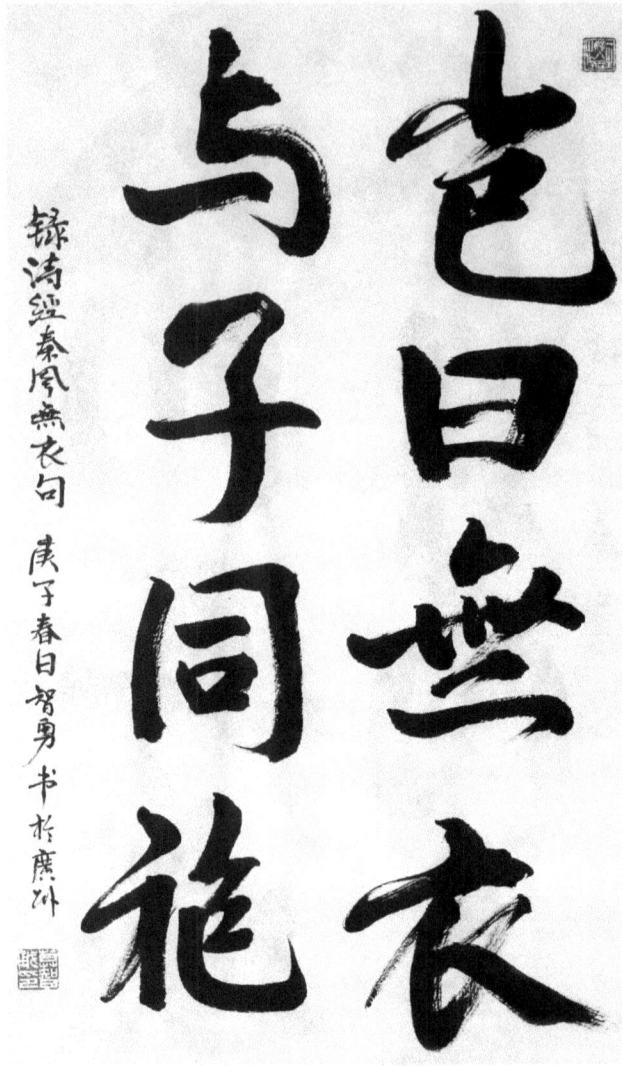

Figure 2: 豈曰無衣, 與子同裳 (How can you say you lack clothes? Don't worry, I will share mine with you). This excerpt lauds the camaraderie of soldiers by depicting a soldier sharing his armor with his comrade during a battle. It comes from the *Book of Songs*, the first collection of ancient Chinese poetry. From NOP Renxin Association, in Japan to Central China's Hubei Province.

reads: 'Dao is not something distinct from human life and nationality no longer matters' (Figure 5). These lines were written by Choe Chi-won (857–915), a well-known Korean scholar who, for several years, studied in China during the Tang Dynasty. The Xinhua News Agency translated the lines as 'Great distance cannot separate us; we all live in

天臺立本情無隔
一樹花開兩地芳

庚子年全球抗疫
彰顯天下情懷
智勇 書

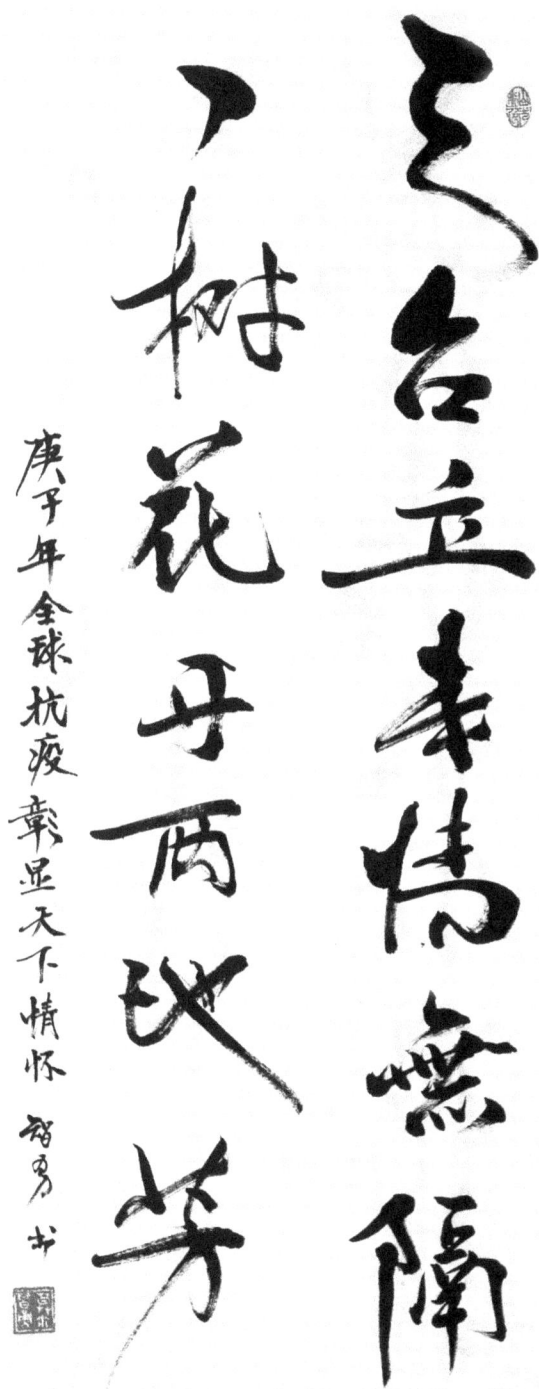

Figure 3: 天臺立本情無隔,一樹花開兩地芳 (Tiantai was built, witnessing the mutual affection; A tree blossoms, fragrant scents pervading everywhere). By Juzan 巨贊 (1908–1984), a Buddhist scholar, sent to Yushin Hosoi, the chief executive of the Libon Temple of Nichiren-shu in Japan. On supplies Zhejiang Province donated to Shizuoka Prefecture Government of Japan.

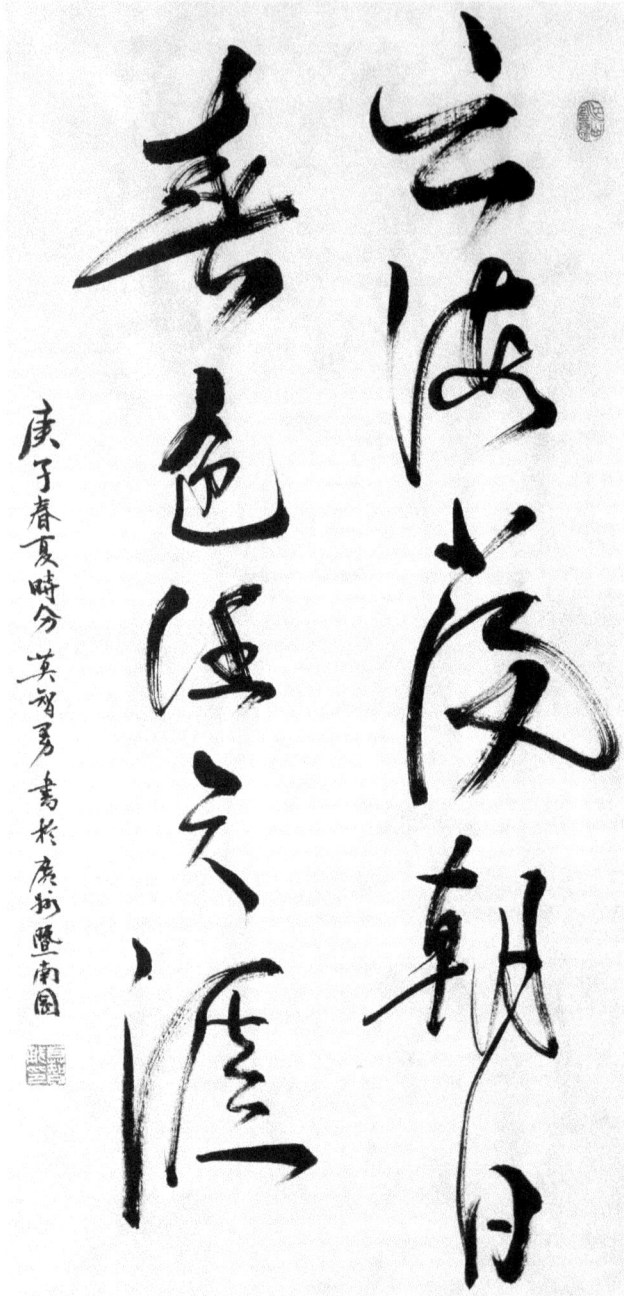

Figure 4:　雲海蕩朝日, 春色任天涯 (The sun rises in the sea of cloud; the spring is endless). By Li Rihua 李日華 (1565–1635), Chinese art critic from Jiaxing, during the late Ming Dynasty, to Matteo Ricci (1552–1610), the Italian Jesuit missionary. Supplies sent by China to Italy.

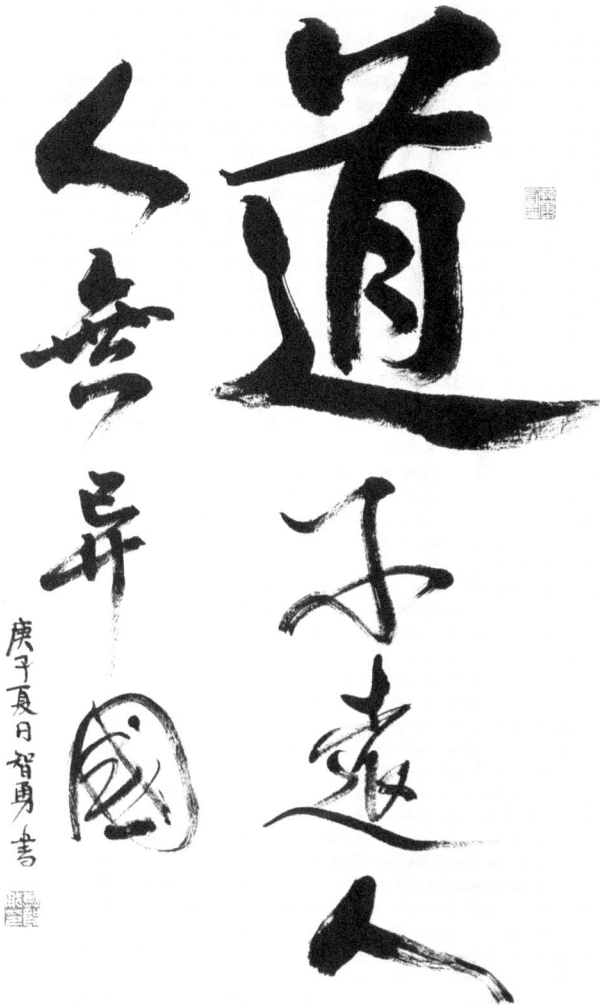

Figure 5:　道不遠人, 人無異國 (Great distance cannot separate us; we all live in a united world). By Choe Chi-won (857–915 CE), a Korean scholar who, for years, pursued study in China during the Tang Dynasty. Sent by the Chinese Embassy in South Korea to the city of Daegu.

a united world,' emphasizing the shared destiny of mankind. In another instance, Choe Chi-won's lines, 'outside the window, evening rain; lamp, and concern with the people miles away' (Figure 8) are used to convey China's solicitude for the Korean people during this bleak time. Another couplet, partly adapted from a letter by Qian Liu (852–932), was printed on the donations to Seoul from Fosun Foundation, Shangai: 'Flowers by the road are blooming; the sea is tranquil, and it is nearing dawn' (Figure 10). Qian Liu was the founder of the Kingdom of Wu-Yue and wrote the first line to his wife, urging her to come home. The second line is adapted from a poem by the Ming poet,

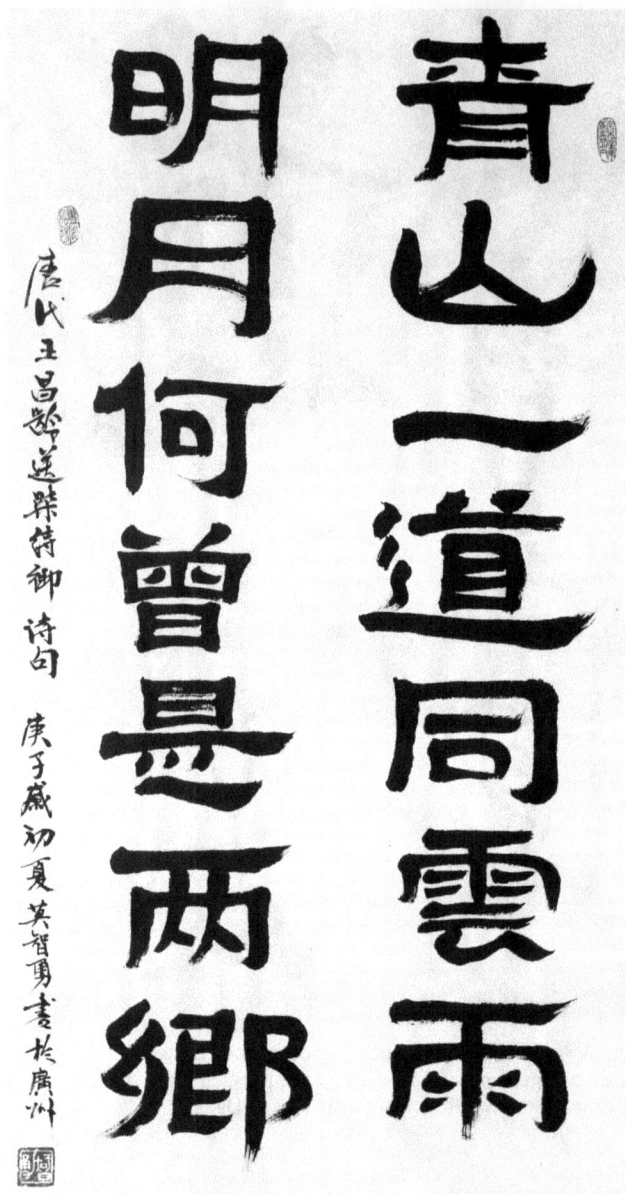

Figure 6: 青山一道同雲雨, 明月何曾是兩鄉 (You and I are of different lands, but the same clouds and rain fill our sky. Look up, the Moon is the same also). By Wang Changling 王昌齡 (698–756), a major Tang dynasty poet. Supplies sent from Maizuru, in Japan's Kyoto prefecture to China.

Chen Ruyan, which was dedicated to a friend's mission to Goryeo. The two lines combine to express the wish that all the medical workers will return home safely when the epidemic is over.

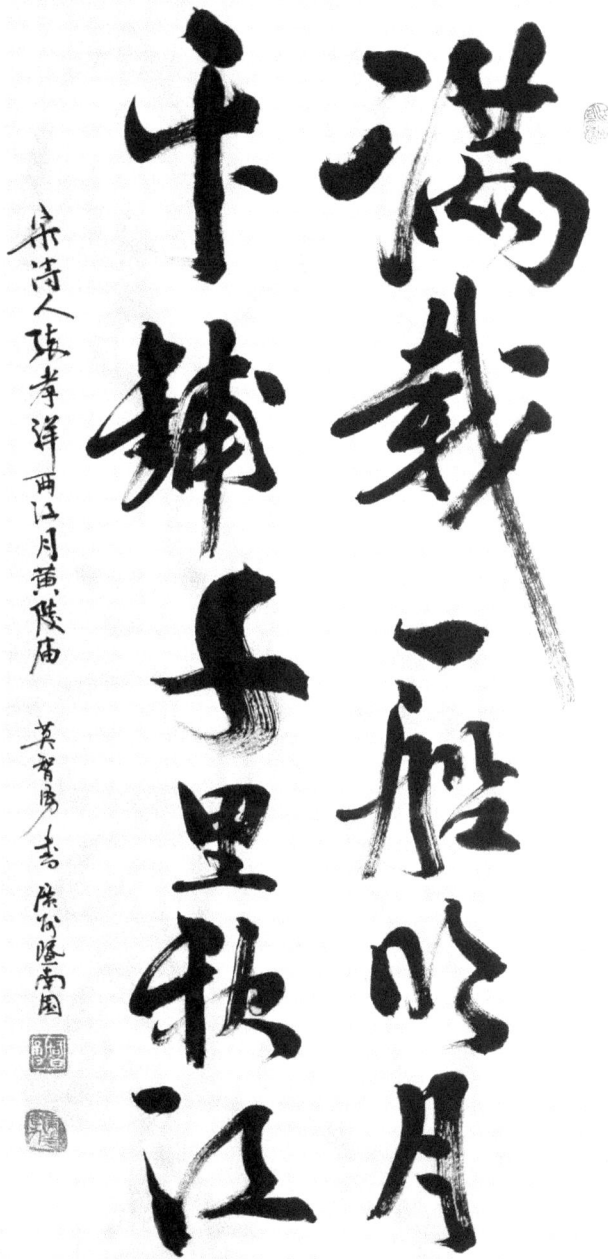

Figure 7:　滿載一船明月, 平鋪千里秋江 (A boat carries the moonlight; smoothly spread miles of autumn river). By Zhang Xiaoxiang 張孝祥 (1132–1170), a poet in the Southern Song Dynasty. On supplies sent from Jinan, Shandong Province to Wako Prefecture.

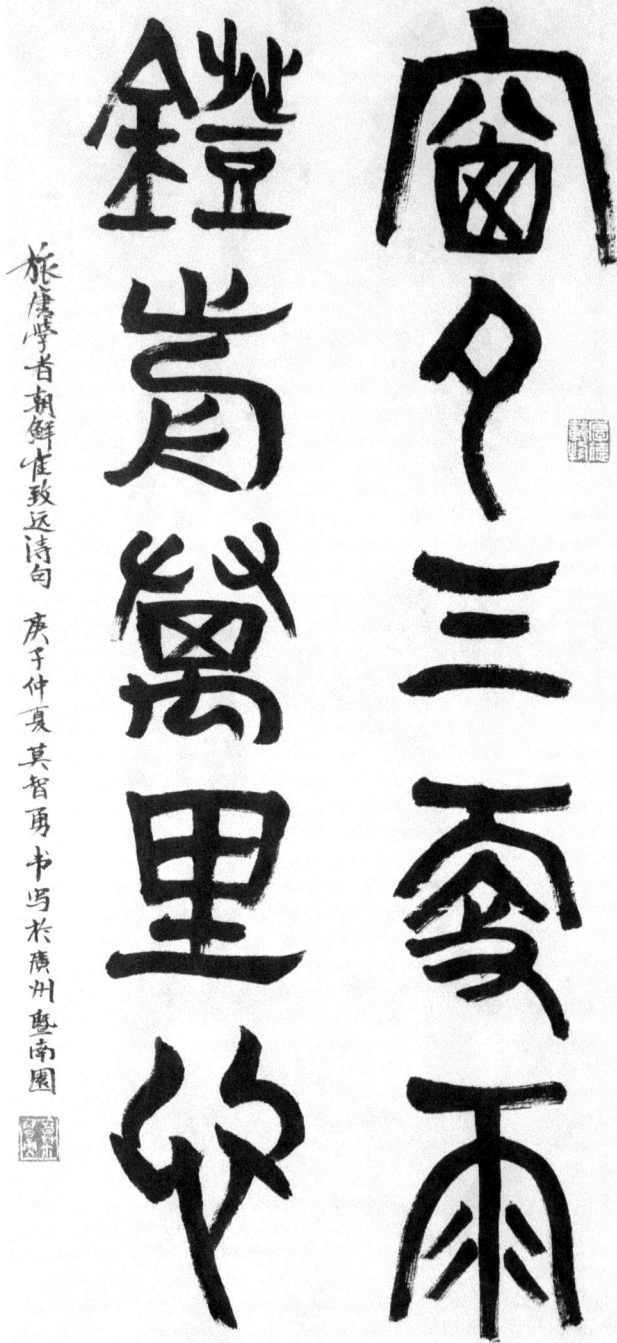

Figure 8: 窗外三更雨, 燈前萬里心 (Outside the window, evening rain; lamp, and concern with the people miles away). By Choe Chiwon (857-915 CE), a celebrated poet and scholar of the Unified Silla kingdom, who pursued study in China during the Tang Dynasty. Supplies sent from Yangzhou, China to Gyeongju, South Korea.

尼蓮正東流，西樹幾千秋

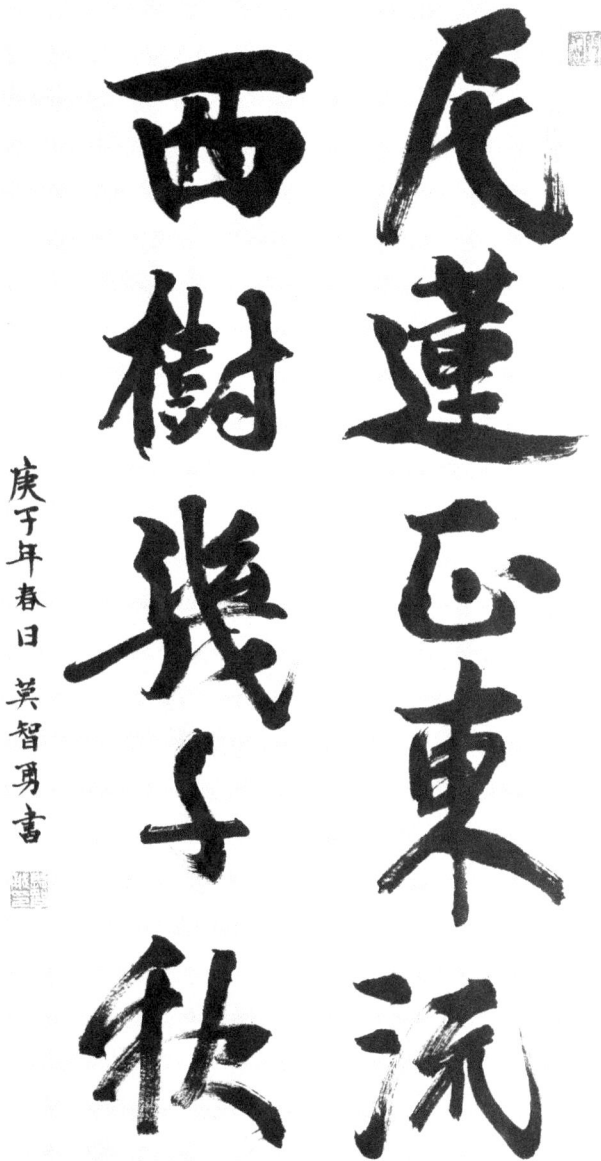

Figure 9:   尼蓮正東流, 西樹幾千秋 (By the Holy Lotus River in which pure gold flows east. Looks back to the western shore at Buddha's sacred grove for many thousands of autumns). By Buddhist monk Xuanzang 玄奘 (602–664). On supplies sent from China to India.

A Chinese foundation donated PPE and medical supplies to India, in which the pandemic was proving widespread and devastating. The words on the packaging were adapted from a poem by Xuanzang (602–664), a Tang Dynasty Buddhist monk and translator of the Sanskrit

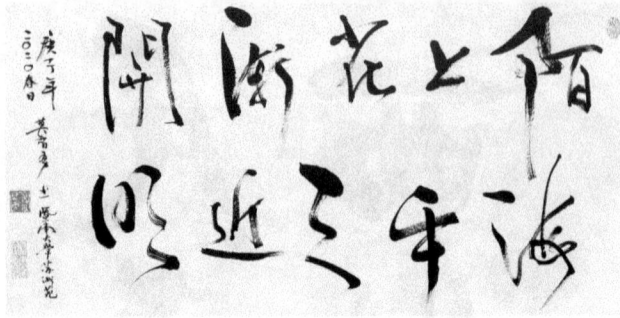

Figure 10: 陌上花漸開, 海平天近明 (Flowers by the road are blooming; the sea is tranquil, and it is nearing dawn). The first line is adapted from a letter by Qian Liu 錢鏐 (852–932), the founder of the Kingdom of Wu-Yue, to his wife. The second is adapted from a Ming poet, Chen Ruyan 陳汝言, dedicated to a friend's mission to Goryeo. Supplies sent from Fosun Foundation to Seoul.

scriptures into Chinese. These lines allude to the fact that after it was introduced into China, Buddhism became one of the most widespread faiths — 'By the Holy Lotus River, in which pure gold flows east. Looks back to the western shore at Buddha's sacred grove for many thousands of autumns' (Figure 9). Acknowledging China's indebtedness to India, these lines point towards the long history of the two nations' collaboration and mutual support.

The use of ancient Chinese poetry on COVID-19 supplies was not limited to donations across East Asia. Chinese donations to Italy carried lines which evoke the resplendent sunrise and the exuberant spring: 'The sun rises in the sea of cloud; the spring is endless' (Figure 4). These lines were written by a Ming scholar, Li Rihua (1565–1635) to Matteo Ricci (1552–1610), an Italian Jesuit Missionary, who is an icon of the friendship between China and Italy.

Generally stated, then, poignant and fitting lines from classical Chinese poetry were chosen to evoke a sense of civility, empathy with fellow humans and our collective yearning for a beautiful life. Gifting poetry along with tangible aid fostered a sense of care and concern by evoking long national histories of interaction and mutual support. The printed lines were both inspirational and aspirational: they reached into people's hearts and spirits, while also suggesting ideas and principles necessary to build a global future based in cooperation and shared values. It is centrally important that these lines were calligraphic. Chinese Calligraphy is a paramount visual art form and tradition in China. Creating a series of calligraphic artworks not only invokes transnational histories and traditions, it also records, commemorates and celebrates the strengthening of international solidarity. This has been central in campaigns against COVID-19. Chinese calligraphy is a lifeline connecting history to the present while pointing the way towards possible, enlightened futures.

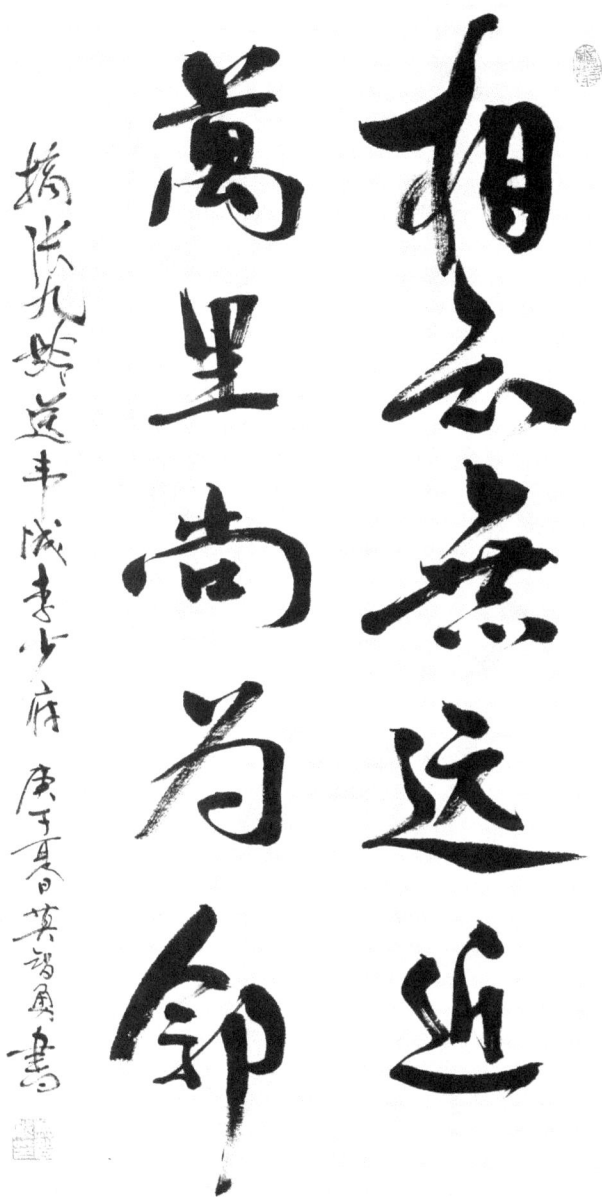

Figure 11: 萬里尚為鄰,相扶無遠近 (Friends no distance, thousands of miles apart). By Tang poet, Zhang Jiuling 張九齡(673-740). Supplies sent by Ma Yun Public Welfare Foundation to Iran.

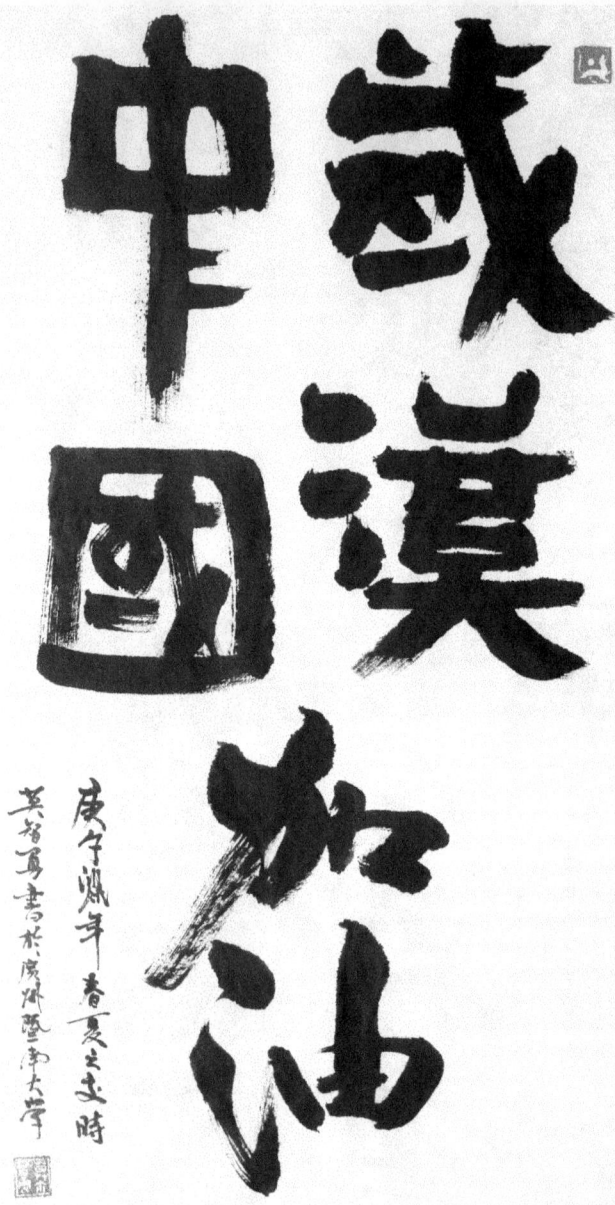

Figure 12:　中國武漢加油 (Wuhan, China, Stay strong)

Funding

This essay is supported by the *14th Five-Year Plan* project for the development of philosophy and social sciences in Guangzhou under the grant number 2021GZGJ254.

Note

1   This essay is indebted to the relevant reports in *China Daily*, *Global Times, CGTN*, *The Asahi Shimbun*, *The Straits Times*, *the World of Chinese*. In these sources, Yang Meng emphasizes the invigorating function of poetry while Zhao Wuji and Zhang Xiujuan use the case of gifting poems to explore the connection between cultural identity and image building. Liu Xin and Hu Yuwei first suggested that these poems figured the cultural ties between China and Japan. Chen Xi, on the other hand, examines East Asian ways of managing intercultural relationships and also observes that these classical Chinese poems are 'strategically' selected and often encode the message that 'common ground is shared by different countries' (570–71).

Works Cited

Chen, Xi. 'Fighting COVID-19 in East Asia: The Role of Classical Chinese Poetry'. *Multilingua* 39(5), 2020:565–576.

Liu, Xin and Hu Yuwei. 'Chinese poems on Japanese donations show cultural ties'. *Global Times*. 12 February 2020. https://www.globaltimes.cn. Accessed on 12 July 2021.

Yang, Meng. 'Poetry Conveys Hope During Coronavirus Pandemic'. *CGTN*. 21 March 2020. https://news.cgtn.com. Accessed on 12 July 2021.

Zhao, Wuji, Zhang Xiujuan. 'Cultural Identity and Image Construction in the Epidemic Discourse from the Perspective of Communication Rituals'. *Communication and Copyright* (7), 2020:133–35.

Will the COVID-19 Crisis Lead to a Fourth Wave of Neo-nationalism?

Eirikur Bergmann ⓘD

Abstract

In this paper, I analyze whether the COVID-19 crisis might lead to a new wave of neo-nationalism. History teaches that socio-economic crises tend to pave the way for populist nationalists to seize the moment and place themselves as saviours of the people/nation against both an external threat and the domestic elite. In previous research, I detected three waves of nativist populism, emerging into what I call neo-nationalism in the post-war era, each rising in the wake of crisis. The characteristics of the current crisis are in many ways reminiscent of those that have previously led to the rise of nativist populism, which defines much of contemporary politics in the West, and indeed around the world. It is therefore timely to contemplate whether the crisis resulting from governmental responses to COVID-19 might ignite the fourth wave of neo-nationalism.

Introduction

Over the past half-century, neo-nationalism – populist nativism, which is distinct from earlier versions for nationalism – has emerged as a prominent force in world politics. In previous research, I have detected three waves of neo-nationalism in the post-war era, each rising in the wake of crisis (Bergmann, *Neo-nationalism*). By the time of the COVID-19 crisis in 2020, this prolonged neo-nationalist surge had, for example, brought populists to power in all of the four largest democracies in the world, in the United States, Brazil, India and Indonesia. However, prior to the current crisis, we had started to witness the slow emergence of a new counter-wave, a kind of anti-populist pushback against the nativists and their populism. With the progression of the new crisis, spurred by the virus, many indicators show that nationalist sentiments are mounting once again – as I explore in this paper.

The COVID-19 crisis might not be the most vexing predicament the world has faced since the Second World War, but it may thus far have been the most ubiquitous. The virus reaches all corners of the world and so does the economic and political calamity that follows. This is a multi-phased and multi-layered quandary, and it disrupts many of the most vital structures of modern societies. COVID-19 is a global outbreak that prompted a highly nationalistic response in many places.

These are precisely the sorts of circumstances in which neo-nationalists can find success. Socio-economic crises tend to pave the way for populist nationalists to seize the moment and position themselves as saviours of the people/nation against both an external threat and the domestic elite. As I explore in this paper, the characteristics of the current crisis are in many ways reminiscent of those that led to the rise of nativist populism, which defines much of contemporary politics in the West, and, indeed, around the world. It is therefore timely to contemplate whether the COVID-19 crisis might lead to a fourth wave of Neo-Nationalism rising.

Varying Responses

Governments around the world responded in various ways to the disease. Some imposed draconian lockdown measures, even suspending traditional human rights. Restrictive measures taken by many governments – mainstream and populist alike – have also raised significant concerns regarding democracy and human rights around the globe. Many of them in effect violated the core principles of liberal democracy. Other governments limited their actions to issuing only general guidelines to the public and urging caution. In several cases, such as in the United States and Brazil, chaos reigned.

The vastly differing and sometimes contradictory responses to the same core problem illustrate a highly fragmented global system, a weakness that unscrupulous populists might attempt to exploit. In Hungary, for example, Viktor Orbán and his Fidesz government went for a quick power grab, almost completing the transformation to authoritarianism. As I will discuss later in the paper, the government was able to rush through emergency legislation that allowed it to bypass parliament and rule by decree.

When the virus was ripping through the United States, it left Donald Trump's reputation as a successful steward (according to a significant swathe of the US population) in tatters. Erratic decisions led to turmoil and reactions to the pandemic turned into fierce infighting between many governmental actors across the country. The president started out diminishing the threat, then offering at best questionable remedies to it, while at the same time dismissing the knowledge of specialists – that is, before he, in effect, surrendered to its spread and left it up to each state to deal with the pandemic's effects. Throughout the crisis, the US president turned to conspiracy theories to excuse the ominous situation at home.

In this paper, I examine several examples indicating that populist politics might be on the rise once again. First, briefly, it is necessary to map the evolution of neo-nationalism over the past half-century before looking into examples of an increased spread of conspiracy theories, disinformation, varying response to restrictions and vaccine nationalism.

Three Waves

After two devastating world wars, the West embraced a new system of liberal democracy. In addition to increased systemic state co-operation and pooling of sovereignty, the post-war, liberal democratic system rested on shared values, including the rule of law, firm division of power, free trade across borders, respect for human rights, wide-reaching civil rights, unbiased and professional administration and a free and independent media. This was the liberal aspect of the post-war democratic order installed to protect individuals and minorities from oppression by the majority. These basic rules of liberal democracies were respected across the political spectrum, and the system indeed celebrated human diversity. It actively and persistently countered collectivity.

Three distinct waves can be identified in the last half-century when nativist populist political parties have contested this post-war liberal democratic order. At the height of these waves, these parties travelled from the fringes to the mainstream in European and American politics. All of these waves were ignited by crises.

The first rose in Western Europe in the wake of the oil crisis in the early 1970s. The second began after the fall of the Berlin Wall, first mainly in opposition to migrants from Eastern Europe seeking work in the West. Far-right populism travelled east in the 2000s, when the promise of prosperity accompanying new-found liberal democracy was failing to materialize in many places. The third wave was triggered by the financial crisis of 2008. On the back of the refugee crisis of 2015, in the wake of the Syrian War, anti-immigrant and far-right populism found foothold even in Germany, where such sentiments were assumed to have been suppressed after the fall of Nazism (Bergmann, *Neo-nationalism*).

In previous research, I identified a threefold claim that nativist populists put forth in their support of the people: first, they discursively tend to create an external threat to the nation; second, they accuse the domestic elite of betraying the people, often even of siding with the external aggressors; third, they position themselves as the true defenders of the 'pure people' they vow to protect, against both the elite and these malignant outsiders, that is, against those that they themselves have created.

When contemplating whether the current COVID-19 crisis might lead to a fourth wave of neo-nationalism, several underlying currents must be kept in mind. One of the most prominent has been the avalanche of disinformation, which has been spread with greater force than ever before.

The Politics of Disinformation

Public discourse around COVID-19 and the crisis that it brought has festered with all sorts of fabrications and false information, which has often proved to be fertile breeding ground for populism in politics. Before examining examples of fake news tactics in the current crisis-ridden political environment, it is first necessary to lay the ground for understanding the politics of misinformation (Bergmann, *Populism*).

The proliferation of fake news and conspiracy theories coincided with the emergence of digital media, which has grown to dominate the distribution of information in the new century. Distribution of bogus tales is not, in itself, a novel act. Rumours, urban legends, folklore and other kinds of oral transmissions have always existed in human societies. Fabricated news was also spread by mainstream media outlets in the twentieth century. Spreading lies and fabricated news stories to demonize political opponents is nothing new. However, the emergence of 24-hour rolling news broadcasts proved to be especially fertile for conspiratorial populists in transmitting distorted information. The take-off for these tales was accelerated by the rapid growth of online outlets and social media platforms that followed. Since 2016, conspiracy theories, disguised as news, were blazing like a wildfire across the political scene on both sides of the Atlantic.

This is a fundamental shift in the way we learn about the world and how we come to foster opinions. The revolutionary change in the media mechanism, which the world developed in less than two decades, has served to enable conspiratorial populists to bypass the previously powerful gatekeepers of the mainstream media, and instead bring their combative and polarizing political messages directly to the public.

This overflow of unscrutinized information can render the public incapable of properly interpreting the large amounts of data to which they are being subjected. This has opened up a space for misinformation to thrive, leaving the democratic space highly vulnerable to manipulation. Indeed, this has led to the emergence of a new political culture, which has been branded post-truth politics. Distorted information has impacted political discussion to the extent that public debates have increasingly come to revolve around false stories.

Alongside these debates, the manipulation of information has been weaponized in political campaigning. The world has, thus, entered an era of information warfare. This is the politics of disinformation, based on the more general flow of misinformation. In the face of the diminished gatekeeping capabilities of the mainstream media, it becomes ever more difficult for people to distinguish between factual stories and fictitious news, as both can be presented in the same guise.

It can be argued that debates around the COVID-19 crisis have been inundated with misinformation and fake news, where the glut of fabricated information has now infiltrated into more traditional media, which often reports fabricated news as facts, citing the bogus tales as a credible source. Here, the mainstream media is turned on its head to become a far more powerful vehicle for fake news than social media outlets were ever able to do on their own. Only when picked up by the mainstream media does the distorted data find full credibility.

The pandemic invoked fear, and as fear is the main ingredient of both conspiracy theories and populism, it was perhaps not unexpected that the crisis brought many conspiracy theories. The world not only faced an unprecedented health scare, and a deep economic recession, but we all also had to navigate a sea of distorted information. In many instances, the new crisis has simply been used to reaffirm and re-produce conspiracy theories that were already afloat (Bergmann, *Conspiracy*). Often, conspiracy theorists argued that the outbreak was simply the result of their own favourite tales coming true. Let's take a look at a few examples.

Against Outsiders

At the start of the outbreak, several governments resorted to blaming the spread on outsiders. In Eastern Europe, many pointed fingers at the Gypsy population, particularly in Bulgaria, Slovakia and Hungary. In Hungary, Viktor Orbán also blamed Muslim migrants: he referred to the first known COVID-19 patient in the country, a student from Iraq, as proof that the spread of infection stemmed from outsider populations (Katsambekis and Stavrakakis). The response was to target infected infiltrators.

Both Matteo Salvini of Lega, the Italian populist political party, and the Flemish Block in Belgium blamed immigrants crossing the Mediterranean for spreading the disease (Wang). In France, the National Front blamed a combination of globalism and migration for the spread of COVID-19. Even in Denmark, the prime minister of the mainstream Social Democratic

Party said that it was unacceptable how many people who were 'not of a Western decent,' as she phrased it, were roaming around the streets while infected.

Several anti-Semitic conspiracy theories were also fabricated to explain the pandemic. One such theory cast the American businessman of Hungarian origin, George Soros, as its main villain – a role often imposed on him by far-right conspiracy theorists in the West. In the US, several theories argued that the pandemic was part of a Zionist plot to dominate the world (Buarque). Across the Middle East, many suspected Jews of covertly controlling the spread of the virus (Frantzman 2020).

Since blaming outsiders is one of the key features of neo-nationalism, it may be concluded that the pandemic has supported its rise in that regard. Let's now look at conspiracy theories from specific areas.

Out of Russia

In recent years, conspiracy theories have become increasingly prominent in Russia (Yablokov, 2018). Many have revolved around suspicions of a Western plot to emasculate the Russian state. Such conspiracy theories were heavily reinforced during the pandemic. Early in the pandemic, a tale spreading in Russia insisted that the UK government had already developed a vaccine against the virus, and that they would roll it out only at the height of the pandemic, for their own maximum gain. Another story went that COVID-19 had been developed as a weapon by the US Central Intelligence Agency (CIA).

Studying stories like these can be amusing for the researcher, but we also need to understand their effect in society. Spreading these sorts of conspiracy theories has an impact. In March 2021, an opinion poll published by Reuters showed that 64% of Russians believed that the virus had been made in a lab. Many suspicions were also raised against vaccines, leading to a clear majority of Russian responders being hesitant to receive one (Reuters 2021).

Against China

Many conspiracy theories accused China of wrongdoing. This was perhaps not entirely unexpected as the virus had first been detected in a notorious wet market in the Chinese city of Wuhan. As it happens, Wuhan is also home to a virus lab that had been known for studying coronaviruses. This, of course, raised many eyebrows.

Many people sounded legitimate concerns about the incredible coincidence, asking whether the virus might accidentally have escaped from the lab. However, in addition to these reasonable doubts, several actors delved into a full-blown conspiracy theory, insisting that the Chinese government had developed the virus as a biological weapon in their fight against the West (Pattillo 2020).

Several stories also revolved around suspicions of China's involvement in projects to build infrastructure for 5G communication networks in Western countries. Many feared that authorities in China were using the network for distributing the virus.

To begin with, these rather far-fetched conspiracy theories were distributed exclusively from the periphery, by marginalized people. Increasingly, these kinds of stories would also be voiced by people in power. In the US for example, Republican Party senator Tom Cotton maintained that the virus had indeed been made in the Chinese lab in Wuhan precisely to hurt Donald Trump in America. The US President himself flirted with this theory. The *New York Times* ran a story maintaining that the President ordered his secret service agencies to find proof that backed this theory (Mazzetti et al. 2020). Often, however, he made do with blaming China more generally for the pandemic, calling it the 'China virus', or, in an attempt at a pun, the 'Kung Flu'.

Anti-Chinese stories were also blazing in Europe, especially propagated by the populist far-right. Amongst those voicing concerns about Beijing's possible involvement in deliberately developing the virus as a biological weapon was, for example, Marine Le Pen of the Rassemblement national in France (previously named *Front National*). More than a quarter of the entire French population was found to believe the story, and 40% of those were supporters of Le Pen's party (Camus).

From China

China has not only been the target of conspiracy theories in this pandemic. Beijing has also been active in distributing their own versions of events regarding the pandemic in world media. Academics analyzing Chinese propaganda found that Beijing has been engaged in supporting favourable media outlets around the world, and even operating their own, facilitating the spread of their own bogus tales (Lim and Bergin 2020).

The American think tank, Freedom House, concluded in their 2021 annual report on freedom and the state of democracy in the world that China has indeed used the pandemic to increase its global influence, and was, in its actions, often operating against democracy and liberal rights. Chinese authorities have, for example, been found to be behind distribution of similar stories to those in Russia discussed above. In one of these, the story of the Wuhan lab is turned on its head, with Beijing actors claiming that the virus was indeed created in a foreign lab, pointing instead to facilities controlled by the CIA producing the virus as a weapon against China (Sardarizadeh and Robinson 2020).

Gates-gate

Some of the most prevalent conspiracy theories in the pandemic have revolved around suspicions of Bill Gates, billionaire founder of Microsoft. Many conspiracy theorists suspected Gates of manufacturing the virus so that he could covertly inject the world population with microchips when people were being vaccinated (Wakabayashi, Alba and Tracy 2020). In the wake of the vaccine campaign, as the story goes, Gates and his clandestine collaborators could monitor the entire world population and manipulate their behaviour for their own gain.

Gates was initially suspected of wrongdoing in the pandemic as he had already in 2015 warned of an imminent risk of a worldwide pandemic caused by the spread of viruses or bacteria. During the COVID-19 spread, his prior warnings were misconstrued and taken as proof of Gates leading a global cabal of evil-doers, plotting world domination. These and other stories were, for example, prominent on QAnon, discussed in the next segment.

Despite how far-fetched the microchip theory must sound to most people, versions of it have been upheld by people in power. For example, it was suggested to be true by the US President Donald Trump's prominent campaign adviser, Roger Stone (Goodman and Carmichael 2020).

QAnon

The once obscure QAnon conspiracy theory platform grew increasingly influential during the COVID-19 pandemic. Like so many others, followers of QAnon suspected Bill Gates of malignant intentions. From there, a story circulated that Gates, in conjunction with the UK-based Pirbright Institute, situated southwest of London, spread COVID-19 for the purpose of reducing the world population (Broderick 2020). This is especially interesting as the aim of the Pirbright Institute is actually the prevention and control of viral diseases. Once again, actors are suspected of upholding goals that are the precise opposite of their official objectives.

During the pandemic, QAnon turned into a cacophony of conspiracy theories. Many on the platform followed Trump's lead in dismissing the threat stemming from the virus, insisting that the whole thing was a hoax. Others suspected the 'deep state' of having developed the virus in its ongoing warfare against Donald Trump.[1] Some insisted that Democrats in the US were plotting the same in conjunction with Beijing for the purpose of undermining the strong domestic economy and, thus, preventing Trump's re-election.

Prior to COVID-19 hitting, QAnon had been a fringe phenomenon in the US. However, over the course of the crisis, several prominent Republican Party members, including congressmen, started to spread its conspiracy theories. Even the President himself flirted with some of their unsubstantiated tales (Rosenberg 2020).

Manifestation

Above, I selected several examples of conspiracy theories floating around in the COVID-19 crisis. As discussed, prolonged undermining of professionals and specialized knowledge by populists in the last decades has enabled misinformation to proliferate in public discourse. This can also be viewed as a systemic and powerful distribution of disinformation, often spread from powerful actors. This was demonstrated by Donald Trump in America, who was prone to distorting facts, to the extent that the President's spokesman branded his unsubstantiated falsehoods as 'alternative facts'.

This trend in public discourse had by the time of the pandemic, perhaps, weakened people's resilience in critically processing distorted information. The relentless dissemination of misinformation, including several conspiracy theories spreading around the globe alongside the pandemic, had serious effects. Opinion polls conducted in many countries around the world indicate that large swathes of the world population believe in one or more of such conspiracy theories. For instance, in the US, more than a third of the population has proved susceptible to conspiracy theories. In South Africa, more than half of the population voices doubts about vaccines (Henly and McIntyre 2020).

The anti-Asian discourse that rose during the pandemic had its own effect. Around twenty million people of Asian origin live in the US. Inquiries into the effect of the COVID-19 crisis on Asian Americans indicate a massive spike in harassments and violence against the group across the US (Bieber 2020). This was perhaps similar to what Arab Americans experienced in wake of the 9/11 terrorist attacks, when hate crimes against people considered Muslim spiked in the US.

Social unrest grew in the US alongside the spread of the novel coronavirus. The summer of 2020, for example, saw renewed racial tension after an African American man, George Floyd, was suffocated to death by a policeman. White civil militia gangs were seen roaming freely around the streets in many US states and repeated acts of violence were becoming increasingly frequent.

After it became clear that Donald Trump had lost the presidential election in November 2020, many of his supporters took up arms and attempted to reverse the outcome of the election. Tension turned to violence in early January 2021 when armed and angry mobs, incited by the outbound President, stormed the US Capitol in Washington, DC in a chaotic attempt to prevent Joe Biden from being confirmed as the next US President. In an extremely ill-planned coup, lacking in coordination and resources, this insurrection was an attack against American democracy.

What is perhaps most interesting, and what needs monitoring in the coming years, is how fast norms and conventions were being eroded by means of disinformation and populist actions in US politics.

Power Grab

Several countries used the pandemic for a power grab at home, another indication of a renewed rise of neo-nationalism. Hungary is amongst the countries moving further in that direction. Viktor Orbán and his Fidezs government was able to rush through emergency legislation that allowed authorities to bypass parliament and rule by decree. One new decree stipulated that anyone who opposed authorities in the pandemic, with what the government deemed falsehoods, ran a risk of incarceration. Later, the government replaced the legislation with what was called a 'state of medical crisis'. Although the new stipulation no longer allowed the government to change laws on its own, or restrict fundamental rights, it still allowed the government to issue a host of decrees. Furthermore, the state of medical crisis could not be lifted by the parliament (Bayer 2020).

With actions like these taken in Hungary and elsewhere in mind, it was, thus, perhaps not entirely unexpected that recent analyses have indicated a clear deterioration of democracy around the world during the course of the pandemic. Freedom House, the US think tank mentioned earlier, found that democracy and freedom was served a massive blow in 2020, shifting the balance in the world in favour of tyranny. In their examination, Freedom House found not only that countries experiencing democratic deterioration 2020 outnumbered those showing improvement, but that those countries which deteriorated did so by the largest margin since 2006, when the current negative trend began. The year 2020 marked the fifteenth consecutive year of decline in global freedom. The institution also concluded that the impact of the prolonged democratic decline was extending its global reach. Democracy had improved in only 28 countries out of the 195 in their study; deterioration of freedom and democracy was detected in 73 countries. According to their measure, three quarters of the world's population were living in areas facing deterioration of democratic practices, while only a fifth of the global population was now living in what they counted as legitimate democracies (2021).

The Civil Liberties Union for Europe reached similar findings in its 2020 report, saying that democracy and the rule of law had suffered across many European countries in the pandemic. The report found that civil liberties, including the right to protest, had been curtailed in a bid to stop the spread of the virus. Freedom of media and civil society was found to have been undermined in many counties. In addition, law-making was increasingly pushed through by fast-track procedures, with limited possibility for civil society to get involved in the political process. The report also found the executive putting increased pressure on the judiciary in several countries in the eastern part of the continent, mainly in Bulgaria, Hungary and Poland (CLUE 2021).

Moving away from freedom and civil rights towards a new wave of neo-nationalist rising has not occurred only in countries that recently turned to democratic practices, such as in the former-communist states in Eastern Europe, but such trends have also been detected in countries that were deemed established liberal democracies. In Denmark, for example, the Social

Democratic government introduced new epidemiology legislation that allowed the government to bypass traditional civil rights when facing current and future pandemics. Amongst its many stipulations, the legislation made it mandatory for people to provide authorities with delicate personal information, and to disclose their travels and with whom they had associated. The Copenhagen-based mainstream daily, *Politiken*, described the legislation as entailing 'forced research, forced hospitalization, forced isolation, forced treatments, forced cleansing, forced quarantine, forced detentions' (Kjeldtoft 2021).

International Tension

In addition to eroding liberal democratic norms, and political discourse falling victim to disinformation tactics, the pandemic has also brought increased tension among countries. States, for example, competed for medical equipment and fought fiercely over vaccines, in campaigns that have been branded vaccine nationalism. The international institutional order clearly gave way to national governments who acted primarily for the benefit of their own populations, irrespective of whether that led to prolonged global difficulties. At the time of writing, even old alliances were experiencing increased tensions, such as in a serious vaccine row between the United Kingdom and the European Union. Even closely knit areas like the Nordic five, who usually enjoy unison and strong ties, experienced increased suspicion across their borders. One indicator of that was found in an opinion poll showing a starkly negative attitude towards Sweden during the pandemic amongst their Nordic neighbours (Sveriges Radio 2020). Whether those tensions will escalate into any sort of conflict or whether they will subside with the progression of vaccine campaigns remains to be seen.

Internal tensions were high in other countries, too. Voices opposing severe restrictions, for example, were gradually growing louder. Initially, those criticizing government-imposed restrictions in the pandemic had very limited reach. Protests against restrictions were indeed firmly kept on the periphery in most societies. Yet, with the progression of the pandemic, which prolonged restrictions, more people grew concerned. Frustration brewed in many societies. This led to increased public protest and other means of demonstrations in Berlin, Paris, Vienna, London and elsewhere.

Two Caveats

I have argued that the COVID-19 crisis could produce a fertile breeding ground upon which nativists and populists may rise, and that it might even lead to a fourth wave of neo-nationalism taking off. However, in the current crisis, populists around the world are faced with two caveats. First, populists are in power in many countries. They are thus no longer solely placed as outsiders challenging the ruling elite, and, in many countries, have become the ruling elite. Reverting to the traditional populist tactics of attacking the ruling elite from the periphery is, thus, more difficult in several places.

Populists in power have indeed faced difficulties in navigating the crisis, and their responses have been somewhat erratic. Both Donald Trump in America and Jair Bolsonaro in Brazil attempted to place themselves as outsiders, seen in their attempts to defy lockdown measures of local and regional governments. They flirted with several conspiracy theories of both external evil and internal traitors, and they blamed everyone but themselves. Numerous examples like these existed in which populists in power undermined proper and professional administration when dealing with the crisis. It can be argued that erratic decisions and a lack of coherent and coordinated policymaking served to deepen the crisis.

The second caveat is found in the nature of this crisis. Around the globe, populists tend to offer simple solutions to complex problems. They are also prone to dismissing the wisdom of specialists and discrediting established knowledge. Both Trump and Bolsonaro scorned scientific warnings regarding the disease and dismissed most concerns raised by experts. The crisis fast undermined the image of Donald Trump as a robust leader who gets things done, and eventually contributed to his political demise in the November 2020 Presidential elections in the US. That many populists dismissed scientific findings and displayed careless leadership might prove problematic to overcome in this particular crisis, as COVID-19 is a complex global quandary to which there are no simple solutions. It became clear early on that only a unified cross-border effort by world-leading scientists could remedy this truly global crisis.

A High Tide

Although these conditions around this current crisis might disrupt the populist message, and thus hinder an otherwise unrestricted rise of neo-nationalism, nativist populists might still be able to bypass these difficulties and find a way to blame the situation on their usual culprits: external evil and the traitorous domestic elite.

As I document in the book *Neo-nationalism: The Rise of Nativist Populism*, history teaches us that a crisis of this magnitude can lead to the rise of a tide that becomes arduous for the mainstream to control. Bearing in mind the forces that have triggered the rise of populism in the wake of previous crises, it is not unimaginable that the current calamity might be of a magnitude that could allow populist politicians to overcome the caveats discussed above and lead us towards another surge of neo-nationalism.

Note

1   The deep state conspiracy theory insists that a covert band of officials in government and military are controlling states behind the scenes, effectively rendering those democratically elected as powerless.

ORCID

Eirikur Bergmann ⓘ http://orcid.org/0000-0002-0274-6354

Works Cited

Bayer, Lili. 'Hungary Replaces Rule by Decree with "State of Medical Crisis"'. *Politico.* 18 June 2020.   https://www.politico.eu/article/hungary-replaces-rule-by-decree-controversial-state-of-medical-crisis/. Accessed on 18 June 2020.

Bergmann, Eirikur. *Conspiracy & Populisms: The Politics of Misinformation.* New York: Palgrave Macmillan, 2018.

Bergmann, Eirikur. *Neo-nationalism: The Rise of Nativist Populism.* New York: Palgrave Macmillan, 2020.

Bergmann, Eirikur. 'Populism and the Politics of Misinformation'. *Safundi: The Journal of South African and American Studies* 21(3), 2020: 251–65

Bieber, Florian. 'Global Nationalism in Times of the COVID-19 Pandemic'. *Nationalities Papers*. 27 April 2020. https://doi.org/10.1017/nps.2020.35. Accessed on 24 July 2021.

Broderick, Ryan. 'QAnon Supporters and Anti-vaxxers are Spreading a Hoax that Bill Gates Created the Coronavirus.' *BuzzFeedNews*. 23 Jan. 2020. https://www.buzzfeednews.com/article/ryanhatesthis/qanon-supporters-and-anti-vaxxers-are-spreading-a-hoax-that. Accessed on 24 July 2021.

Buarque, Beatriz. 'How the Pandemic is Used to Legitimise Anti-semitism Through Conspiracy Theories'. *e-Extreme* 21(2), 2020: 12–14.

Camus, Jean-Yves. *Right-wing Populism and the COVID-19 Crisis in Europe: Frace.* n.p.: Friedrich Ebert Stiftung, 2020. The Profiteers of Fear.

CLUE. *EU 2020: Demanding on Democracy: Coutnry & Trend Reports on Democratic Records by Civil Liberties Organisations Across the European Union.* n.p.: Civil Liberties Union for Europe, 2020.

Frantzman, Seth J. 'Iran's Regime Pushes Antisemitic Conspiracies about Coronavirus'. *The Jerusalem Post*. 8 Mar. 2020. https://www.jpost.com/middle-east/iran-news/irans-regime-pushes-antisemitic-conspiracies-about-coronavirus-620212. Accessed on 24 July 2021.

Freedom House. *Freedom in the World 2021*. Freedom House, 2021.

Goodman, Jack and Flora Carmichael. 'Coronavirus: Bill Gates "Microchip" Conspiracy Theory and Other Vaccine Claims Fact-checked'. *BBC News*. 30 May 2020. https://www.bbc.com/news/52847648. Accessed on 24 July 2021.

Henly, Jon and Niamh McIntyre. 'Survey Uncovers Widespread Belief in "Dangerous" Covid Conspiracy Theories'. *The Guardian*. 26 Oct. 2020. https://www.theguardian.com/world/2020/oct/26/survey-uncovers-widespread-belief-dangerous-covid-conspiracy-theories. Accessed on 24 July 2021.

Katsambekis, Giorgos and Yannis Stavrakakis (Eds.). *Populism and the Pandemic: A Collaborative Report*. Spec. issue of Populismus Interventions (7), 2020: 3–56.

Lim, Louisa and Bergin, Julia. 'China is Reshaping the Global News Landscape and Weakening the Fourth State'. *The Guardian*. 25 June 2020. https://www.theguardian.com/world/commentisfree/2020/jun/25/china-is-reshaping-the-global-news-landscape-and-weakening-the-fourth-estate. Accessed on 25 June 2020.

Kjeldtoft, Sebastian Stryhn. 'Eksperter: Ny epidemilov er styret af krisetænkning og hastværk.' *Politiken*. 18 Feb. 2021. https://politiken.dk/indland/politik/art8102989/Eksperter-Ny-epidemilov-er-styret-af-kriset%C3%A6nkning-og-hastv%C3%A6rk. Accessed on 24 July 2021.

Mazzetti, Mark, et al. 'Trump Officials Are Said to Press Spies to Link Virus and Wuhan Lab.' *The New York Times*. 30 Apr. 2020. https://www.nytimes.com/2020/04/30/us/politics/trump-administration-intelligence-coronavirus-china.html. Accessed on 24 July 2021.

Pattillo, Ali. 'Coronavirus, November 2020: What it Could Look Like in America'. *Inverse*. 28 Feb. 2020. https://www.inverse.com/mind-body/coronavirus-usa-2020. Accessed on 24 July 2021.

Reuters. 'Over 60% of Russians Don't Want Sputnik V Vaccine, See Coronavirus as Biological Weapon: Reuters Poll'. *Reuters*. 1 Mar. 2021. https://www.reuters.com/article/us-health-coronavirus-russia-poll-idUSKBN2AT2XK. Accessed on 24 July 2021.

Rosenberg, Matthew. 'Republican Voters Take a Radical Conspiracy Theory Mainstream'. *New York Times*. 10 Nov. 2020. https://www.nytimes.com/2020/10/19/us/politics/qanon-trump-republicans.html. Accessed on 24 July 2021.

Sardarizadeh, Shayan and Olga Robinson. 'Coronavirus: US and China Trade Conspiracy Theories'. *BBC News*. 26 Apr. 2020. https://www.bbc.com/news/world-52224331. Accessed on 24 July 2021.

Sveriges Radio. ,Undersökning: Sverige tappar i anseende i Norden'. *Sverigesradio.se*. 23 Mar. 2020. Accessed on 24 July 2021.

Wakabayashi, Daisuke, Davey Alba and Marc Tracy. 'Bill Gates, at Odds With Trump on Virus, Becomes a Right-Wing Target'. *New York Times*. 17 Apr. 2020. https://www.nytimes.com/2020/04/17/technology/bill-gates-virus-conspiracy-theories.html. Accessed on 24 July 2021.

Wang, Zhongyuan. 'From Crisis to Nationalism?: The Conditioned Effects of the COVID-19 Crisis on Neo-nationalism in Europe'. *Chinese Political Science Review* 6(1), 2021: 20–39.

Yablokov, Ilya. *Fortress Russia: Conspiracy Theories in Post-Soviet Russia*. Cambridge: Polity, 2018.

THE ROOM

Kobus Moolman ⓘ

It is all happening in a room. This small room to be precise.

Day after day. For months now. It has been happening. Maybe even years. I have lost complete track of time. When was yesterday? Day after day sitting at the same old pine desk beneath the window. The bare desk with nothing inside its drawers. Sitting on the same high-backed chair with the broken seat. A narrow pine bed in the corner of the room with a bare mattress and a dirty pillow. Are now and here, here and now? Staring out of the same rectangular window. Day after day. Through the same dusty blinds. At the same dismal scene. Will the future ever break down these doors to get through to me?

It is a small square room with a high ceiling and a worn carpet and with two old-fashioned doors. The one door, directly behind me, opens onto the main ground floor reception of this derelict institute where years ago I ended up somehow, after being on the streets. The other door, on the right, leads onto the front veranda with its concrete benches and tables, its tattered umbrellas and faded bunting I once used to sit beneath and sleep in the sun.

But I haven't dare open either of these doors for quite some time now. I don't know how I have survived for so long. Have I in fact survived? Or am I just an echo?

After the announcement by the World Health Organisation that the crown of the virus had mutated – that it was now not only more virulent but also more resistant to the vaccine – after this announcement there was no way I could risk going outside. Into the garden, along the old pathways, the way I used to. Collecting all my little things. My little stones and my seeds, my bottle-tops and my cigarette butts. And then putting them all back again. I couldn't risk it. Not with my hypertension. My shortness of breath, which made wearing a mask almost impossible, and my allergic reaction to things. All kinds of things. My hands, for example, would turn raw from the alcohol sanitisers we were forced to use whenever we went out. Anywhere. Even just into a neighbour's room.

But I doubt that my neighbours (or anyone else for that matter) are still alive in this building. It's as silent as the grave out there, and as forlorn.

I am more than likely the last.

And yet there were times. Oh yes! There were times when I did hear singing. And clapping. And ululating. Once upon a time. Outside my door. When they used to bring me my daily meal, since I could not leave my room to eat in the dining hall. The attendants in their stiff white dresses and white tennis shoes. And their little paper caps on their round heads.

But now … nothing. Behind and ahead. This side and that. Only nothing. The same. Over and over.

So that in the end the only thing left still to happen, and the only thing still happening, is the small room. And the story of the room that is the story that I have to tell. That only I can tell. While I still have some strength left in my arm.

But wait. Listen! There. The wind is picking up. The sky is closing over. Dark rain and heavy wind again. I just pray the old rusted roof sheets hold out a bit longer. Just until … And that these cracked trees stay standing. One old oak came down on the back of D-Wing some time ago. Yesterday. Long ago. Whenever. When I could still push myself around on my wheels. Up and down the corridors and the wards. Collecting all my little things. And then putting them all back again.

But I am getting distracted. I must return. I must return to the subject of the room.

For it is the room, this room, out of all the other rooms in all the other wards in this abandoned institute, that my story is about. And to be more precise, the resemblance between this room, this configuration of tired and constrained details, and the configuration of another room, almost the same, but from my childhood at 82 Greyling Street. My own room at that address. Which first had been the room of my Oupa, my father's father, until he passed away in hospital from old age or lack of oxygen or any of the other diseases known to a ten-year old.

And then I moved into the room.

The room that had a rectangular window with long green blinds and an old pine desk beneath the window and a narrow pine bed in the corner with a colourful duvet, and a wooden floor with a small hole in one plank and a high ceiling. The same high ceiling and wooden floor as in this room. The same pine desk and narrow bed that sit here now. The same high-backed chair with the broken seat. Even the same black bakelite pull-cord light switch on the ceiling without its long string.

Stop.

I'm sure I have said all these words somewhere else before. Words like room. And window. Like bed. And floor. Like father's father. Like hospital. These words sound so familiar. Everything in me now is coming out the same. Am I condemned to forever repeat myself? The same palimpsest of bored selves sliding along the floor on their arse. Day after day. Always and ever only talking about doors and windows and desks and floors and ceilings and beds and doors and windows.

About what I see now. And about what I saw. Two simultaneously existing worlds. Inseparable as the sides of a sheet of paper. Through the big rectangular window with the green blinds that opens suddenly onto the street of my childhood.

Buses travelling in the dark street with their lights on inside. The milk-delivery man in his white outfit dragging the sound of bottles up the street. Tall plane trees on either side of the road. The ground choked in sharp seed balls. Mother with a scarf over her head, knotted below her chin with a big bow. A slightly sloping driveway that my brother and I used to race up and down on our little tricycles. Father arriving home from work in his brown Ford Cortina. Wearing a short safari suit. Streetlights coming on at five o'clock in winter. The heavy smell of chocolate from the factory two blocks away. The sound of trains shunting in the distance. Dogs barking at strangers from behind fences and walls and gates.

And now.

This room. The small room where it is all of everything left taking place. The final story. With no food anymore. And water low. Power intermittent. Entire cities sealed off with electric fences and high walls and all-night curfews. Sealed off and left completely to their own devices. Soldiers in masks patrolling the perimeter to make sure the inhabitants stay on the inside.

Only a single bare oak tree outside. Against the dirty brown sky. The gravel driveway and the parking lot covered in rubbish and leaves. A smashed wardrobe and some rusted filing cabinets and office chairs. Cars stripped and abandoned. Pale thin fever trees trembling. And not a single bird. The empty swimming pool choked in leaves and rubbish. Bands of ravenous dogs roaming up and down the streets, looking for a way to get into the sealed buildings.

And inside?

Me on the floor all over again. For the last time this time. And with me on the wooden floor the four empty drawers from my old pine desk. The same four empty drawers that keep turning themselves over searching for the old love letters and dog-eared photographs, the mementoes and little keepsakes, blunt pencils and out of date coins, broken pens and aeroplane seating tickets, that proved that once upon a time, yes, I was indeed alive. That my life happened. That it mattered. And that for some time also, once upon a time, long or short, I was not the only one for whom it mattered.

But now there is just me and myself on the floor all over again. The same. Over and over. And the pressed ceiling looking down, white, with inlaid floral designs. A smell that should be the smell of piss on the old mat, the smell of sweat and dirt, but isn't the smell of anything because I cannot smell anything anymore. I gave up tasting long before. And the white pressed ceiling pressing down on my chest. Pressing down with its knee. With its inlaid floral designs. Pressing down with its knee on my chest.

I can't breathe, someone shouts.

Who shouted that? Someone shouted, I can't breathe.

A sweat has broken out on my forehead. A cold sweat. And a tightness in my chest. Something. Something. Something stuck. Making it difficult. To breathe. And me too thin, too weak to move, as if strapped down to the ground. As if wrapped tightly in plastic. Like the corpses in the mortuaries. Like those in the hospitals and institutions just like this one strapped down to their beds to prevent them running out into the streets in their final hours and spitting their contamination everywhere. Strapped down in their slow decomposition while the staff and everyone died around them.

I can't breathe, someone whispers.

What? I can't hear you. Say that again. I lost signal then. There is a ringing in my ears. Your sound is off. I saw your lips move but I could not hear what you were saying. There are too many voices in the air. And the sound of rushing water. My legs feel like two lead balloons. Only heavier. And dressed from hip to foot in solid white. Year after year. Into which dirt I scratched with my long nail. Into which I still scratch. And with the whiteness came masks and voluntary unconsciousness. The masks of men and women who bent over me. In white masks and plastic gloves and paper caps. Pushing their gloves into my skin. Their needles into the secrets of my flesh. And me in my single pine bed by the window with the colourful duvet. Sitting with my back against the wall and my leg lifted up on pillows, and peering sideways through the green blind at the bare trees and the ground choked in brown seed balls and the military band that came down the avenue blowing their horns and the fires on the hillside and the helicopters and the loudspeakers with their feedback and the sirens.

And through the window I finally see myself on a stretcher and people running alongside me. Looking down at me. Looking up at where we're going. And down again to see me going. A mask over my mouth and my nose. A pipe that makes the sound of breathing for me. Before the knee on my throat. When I suddenly see it all so clearly. But so far away. My body wrapped tightly in plastic on a steel table. Next to so many others. Waiting for the lorries to take us to the giant incinerators.

And through the same window at the same time I also see all the windows closing up and down my street. All over the city. Large square windows. Long rectangular windows. Small portholes. Windows with arches. Bay windows. Louvered windows. And windows with long green blinds. Windows with no people anymore. Abandoned desks. Fallen chairs and empty beds. No stretchers running. Nor masks breathing for anyone. Just ravenous dogs getting in everywhere. Feasting all the way to their red back teeth.

ORCID

Kobus Moolman 🆔 http://orcid.org/0000-0002-3778-4246

Fever Dreams: Surveying the Representation of Plagues and Pandemics in South African Speculative Fiction

Crystal Warren

Abstract

This paper provides an overview of the representation of outbreaks of infectious disease in South African speculative fiction. The focus is on novels by South African authors (even if some are set in the US) which envision a future plague or pandemic, from AIDS to flu-like viruses to a zombie outbreak. This is not an in-depth analysis of individual texts but a survey of the ways in which future plagues are envisioned, including in young adult fiction and popular fiction.

As COVID-19 spread across the world in 2020 with successive countries instituting lockdowns, a frequent remark made was how it felt as if we were in a science fiction film or novel. Empty cities, people in hazmat suits, disturbing scenes of mass graves, overcrowded hospitals, the constant climate of fear – these did indeed evoke images from dozens of films, or scenes from novels. Plagues and epidemics are a regular feature in science fiction, and have been explored from the beginning, with one of the earliest science fiction novels, Mary Shelley's *The Last Man,* being published in 1826 and imagining a 21st century world ravaged by a pandemic.

South African literature is not immune to this tendency, with many novels depicting a dark future world devastated by disease. As a rule, South African speculative fiction tends towards dystopia or apocalypse. Critics such as Michael Titlestad and Ralph Pordzik have traced early developments in South African dystopian literature. Titlestad posits three periods of dystopian literature: the years before and after 1948 and the rise of Afrikaner nationalism, the 1970s to 1990s against a background of armed anti-apartheid struggles and the increasingly repressive government, and the post 1994 period where fears of a post-apartheid state are revealed. While two of the novels discussed here do fit into this framework – Peter Wilhelm's 1994 novel, *The Mask of Freedom*, and Eben Venter's *Trencherman*, first published in Afrikaans in 2001, and can be read as pessimism about a post-apartheid state and fear of the future of white South Africans – these concerns are not revealed in the other texts. I would suggest a fourth period of speculative fiction, from 2000 onwards as South African exceptionalism diminishes and writers are freed to simply tell stories without the weight of political messages. This period allows for a wider range of possibilities and concerns to be presented.

The past two decades have seen an ever-expanding corpus of South African speculative fiction, whether it be fiction with a strong South African feel, such as novels by Marcus Low and Jayne Bauling, or fiction whose only South African link is the nationality of the author, such as that by Joanne Macgregor and Rob Boffard. This period has also seen a rise in the publication of popular fiction, and while many of the novels under discussion provide social commentary or would be classified as 'literary fiction,' many combine speculative fiction with the thriller genre. Of the plague narratives under discussion, none of the later novels depicts a concern about race or anxieties about post-apartheid South Africa. While some depict the collapse of government and breakdown of society (for instance, *South* and *Fever*), these are in the minority, and this collapse is attributed to contagion rather than corruption or revolution. In some futures, the government is depicted as repressive, for example in *Moxyland*, *Recoil* and *New Keepers,* while in others such as *Zero G*, *Afterland* and *Asylum,* the government might be flawed, but is doing its best.

Prior to the rollout of antiretroviral medication in 2004, a diagnosis of HIV/AIDS was in effect a death sentence; so it is not surprising that in novels of the time dystopian visions of the future are filled with images of decay and disease. The slow deterioration and increasing weakness of AIDS patients was perhaps an apt metaphoric vehicle for fear and pessimistic thoughts about the future of a post-apartheid nation. As AIDS moved from death sentence to manageable illness, writers turned to other options if they wanted to narrate the death of large numbers of people. Recent and recurring outbreaks of diseases such as Ebola, Sars, Bird flu and rumours of biological weapons in distant countries fed the fevered imagination of apocalyptically-minded authors.

Peter Wilhelm's novel *The Mask of Freedom* was published in 1994, yet it displays none of the 'rainbow nation' optimism. Set in a future post-revolutionary South Africa beset by poverty, an oppressive and increasingly bankrupt government, secret police, revolutions and counter revolutions, against a backdrop of an out-of-control AIDS epidemic, illness is not the focus of the story, but a backdrop to the world inhabited by the characters. Bodies are left in the street where they fall, giant crematoria work constantly to burn the dead, there is a Ministry of Health with the power to arrest those who are ill, prostitutes are required to have certificates of health and so on. When the protagonist helps a woman who has escaped from the police, they find themselves leaving Cape Town and joining the revolutionary army of Captain Freedom. In the countryside, Jason is aware of the frailty and surrealness of the army filled with the ill and dying marching past mass burials and wraith like figures waiting to die.

Similar figures throng the landscape of Eben Venter's *Trencherman*, first published in Afrikaans in 2001 as *Horrelpoort*. In Venter's reworking of Conrad's *Heart of Darkness*, Martin Louw, known as Marlouw, returns reluctantly to South Africa to find his nephew, Koert, who has become a semi-feudal lord on the family farm. He finds a country ravaged by corruption, mismanagement, violence, poverty, disease and despair. AIDS is the prime focus of the fear, but there are references to other diseases as well, for example the first outbreak of mouse disease. Marlouw is warned that four out of five people are infected. An explosion at the Koeberg nuclear power station had triggered the disastrous situation, leading to the collapse of central government, with the country now divided into factions and without finances to treat the rampant illness, and the interior ruled by crime syndicates. Some critics have read this as indicative of white anxiety about black rule. However, the young white man Koert is a parasitic figure, infecting the farm with his illness and corruption. Against the backdrop of the emaciated victims of disease, Koert is shown to be obscenely obese and suffering from gangrene.

Garth Kitching's young adult novel *Bracelet 12-005-35700,* published in 2001, is set in the near future (2012) where the HI virus is constantly mutating and growing stronger, and diagnosis is a death sentence. South Africa has enacted draconian measures for dealing with the disease by segregating and stigmatizing the infected. There are strong messages warning against sex, and compulsory monthly tests at schools for HIV. Those with HIV are provided with free treatment but subjected to monthly blood tests, and, once AIDS is detected, are required to wear a metal bracelet proclaiming their status. Frikkie notes "'I was a "red person" now. I didn't even have a name anymore, only a small set of red numbers.'" Frikkie is shown progressing through the stages of grief, displaying anger, denial, fear and so on until by the end he is able to accept, and live what is left of his life fully. The novel is somewhat didactic and fits with much of the youth literature of the time on HIV/AIDS, which was dominated by warnings of the dangers of sexually transmitted diseases.

Moxyland, Lauren Beukes' debut novel published in 2008 and set in 2018 shows the lingering effect of the HIV/AIDS epidemic, with one of the central characters an AIDS orphan who had been raised in a corporate orphanage/trade school. Yet AIDS is not the most pressing problem in this near-future society of genetic manipulation and biotechnology, repressive government control, ruthless corporations, inequality and hyper connectedness. There are references to quarantine riots and an outbreak of something that everyone thought was going to be the 'big one'. A character returning from Namibia is pulled over by police on her return as someone on the plane had reported her coughing and she is required to prove her health. Most ominous is the use made of diseases by the police force, who enforce obedience through the ability to use people's cell phones to shock them into submission or to disconnect their phones, leaving them unable to access money, enter their homes and so on. When these tactics do not work at a protest turned violent, the police spray a lethal but noncontagious virus onto protesters and innocent commuters at the station, with those infected forced to present themselves at a government quarantine station for the cure. In this all too familiar future world, disease is both a threat and a weapon.

If Beukes' debut seemed prescient in predicting the near future, especially our reliance on our phones for many aspects of life, her most recent novel, published in early 2020 upped the ante. There was something particularly chilling about reading a novel about a worldwide pandemic during the early stages of our current crisis. In *Afterland,* a flu outbreak spreads around the world, but with mild enough symptoms that few register it. Until a few months later when men and boys start to die. The virus has triggered prostate cancer and will eventually kill 99% of the male population. The novel follows a South African woman who had been in the US when the outbreak occurred and her pre-teen son, who is one of the few male survivors. With the young boy disguised as a girl, they flee across a devastated US, trying to find a way to return to South Africa, while pursued by the government and criminal elements all wanting to use the boy for their purposes. While certainly postapocalyptic, the world Beukes presents is not dystopian. The government is doing its best to cope with the crisis, even if at some cost to personal liberty — for example, male survivors and their female relations have been interred, partly for their own protection and partly to enable scientists to try to use their immunity to find a cure. Reproduction has been made illegal until a cure is found. Beukes also avoids the cliché of a world without men as a feminist utopia. Crime and violence persist, with the gangs continuing, now led by women, and the protagonists are pursued by those wishing to kidnap the boy, now a valuable resource. Yet most of the women are simply doing their best to survive in this strange new world, building new lives as they mourn the men and children they have lost. The novel is a fast-paced thriller that touches on reproductive control, human trafficking, and other issues. It is also one of the few novels to give a more international perspective, showing different countries coping with the plague. There are references to an absence of coffee, a result of Colombia's backlash against America's elimination of the drug trade. The potential buyer of the boy is a Saudi Arabian woman looking for a son, and pseudo-documentary evidence breaks the story, including reports of how the remaining men are being treated in other countries. It is implied that the US is being particularly draconian; Cole's desperate attempts to return suggests that they will be freer in South Africa.

The government in Marcus Low's *Asylum* also adopts heavy-handed measures to contain a crisis by quarantining sufferers of the disease. The central character is in an isolation hospital in the Karoo, being well cared for, but knowing that there is no cure. As the novel progresses, we learn that there are legal challenges against the forced quarantines as well as failing financial resources and, by the end, the hospital has closed, with patients being removed to home-based care. Some of our current challenges getting people to self-isolate are shown when a group of highly contagious inmates plan an escape. Barry joins in rather apathetically, for something to do, seeming not to care if he infects others. *Asylum* is the most literary of the recent plague narratives. Written in lyrical prose, it employs a split narrative; the story told through the journals of a patient, with occasional interjections of a later scholar who is doing research on the journals which are now preserved at the Museum of the Plague. *Asylum* is one of the few novels to show the outbreak as it occurs, but this framing narrative gives some distance, and, even in this case, Barry has been at the hospital for a few years and is shown to be an extremely unreliable narrator.

Under Ground, a thriller by Sarah Lotz and Louis Greenberg writing as S.L. Grey, is another novel that shows the outbreak in real time, although in many ways the pandemic is merely the inciting incident without being a central part of the story. When a vicious flu-like virus spreads across the world, several American families flee to a luxury underground bunker. We see the initial chaos as it reaches the US, with borders closing, and the outbreak forms a running background on TV screens within the bunker. When the property developer and manager is found dead, having sealed the bunker doors, the inhabitants of the bunker discover that they are locked in. And as the body-count rises, they realize that they are trapped with a murderer. While more trapped-room thriller than social commentary, there are elements that feel remarkably familiar, from the crowded airports, visuals of mass graves, to the beliefs that it is all a government plot or was started deliberately by China; a view that sparks anti-Asian racism shown towards the American Korean characters. Like Beukes, Grey sets the novel in the US but includes a South African character, the young au pair to one of the families, who is forced to join them when her flight home is cancelled. There is an irony in the name of the virus, AOBA, with *ayoba* being South African slang for something good or cool. An unrealistic aspect of this novel, as well as *Zero G* by Rob Boffard, that might not have attracted attention before we all became armchair epidemiologists, is the speed with which a cure is developed.

Boffard sets his thriller *Zero G,* the sequel to *Tracer,* far in the future, on a space station where the last remnants of humanity live after a nuclear war and the loss of all communication with earth. The space station, Outer Earth, is rundown and crowded; it was never intended to house so many people for so long. An outbreak of disease in such an environment would be disastrous, and this is so when a virulent disease, Resin, spreads rapidly, killing most of the population within two days (although the space station is blessed with extremely efficient scientists who come up with a cure within hours of discovering the source of the plague). Some of the conspiracy theories of COVID-19 are anticipated here, when it turns out that the disease was accidentally created by scientists using genetic manipulation of plants to enhance food production. The main character is dealing with multiple threats: the deadly outbreak, a blackmailer threating her life and her loved ones, and a plot by dissidents to escape to earth, an attempt that will cripple the space station.

Jayne Bauling's award-winning youth novel, *New Keepers,* is also set in the distant future, several generations after a series of disasters have destroyed life as we know it. The litany of disasters is repeated several times, 'the flooding then the salting then the contagion'. Once the teenage protagonists leave the city, they learn that there was an additional aspect, 'the purging'. After an unspecified disaster involving rising sea levels, lost continents and a great wave sweeping across the land, drowning vast numbers and leaving the land salted and unusable, with the survivors clustered in a small area of Gauteng, there was a great contagion. It turns out that the plague was engineered to reduce the population. But it was not random. Those selected to survive for their perceived value were given an antidote. One of the Elders resisted, giving the antidote to as many as he could. When caught, all those who survived against the plan were marked with a 'stain' on their face, to be passed down to all their descendants, another form of contagion or plague. At the time of the novel, the stained are forced to live on the outskirts of the city, Gauzi, and are stigmatized. Everyone knows that the stain is punishment for something their ancestors did, but nobody remembers what it was. Jabz, a young, stained man, follows his ancestors' lead in rebelling against the current oppressive regime.

Governments using or releasing plagues is a plot device that occurs in several novels. Joanne Macgregor's trilogy of youth novels, *Recoil, Refuse* and *Rebel,* is set in a near-future US in the aftermath of a biological terror attack. The first wave featured biological suicide bombers who infected themselves with a deadly and highly contagious disease, and then ventured into dense populations. The second wave entailed the release of plague-infested rats, which continue to spread the disease. Four years later, millions have died, the borders are closed, and the virus has mutated. People are confined to their homes as much as possible, with decontamination stations at the entrance of each building, school is online, everyone wears masks, and teenagers spend most of their time playing an online interactive game. The central character, Jinxy, is recruited, through the game, to join an elite group of teenagers trained as snipers to kill infected rats. As they are trained to shoot and kill, the parameters stretch to killing infected people, to put them out of their misery. Jinxy soon discovers that the government is using the plague to control the population, and the teenage snipers to eliminate protesters. As in Bauling's novel, as the teenage protagonists rebel, they discover the full extent of the government's betrayal, but must also confront the ways in which the rebellion is willing to use them as much as the government.

In Frank Owen's novels *South* and *North,* the government involvement in the plague does not need to be discovered; it is a basic fact of life and death. The novels are set in an alternate world where the American states did not unite after the Civil War, and talks of unification in contemporary times have triggered a second civil war. During the bloody war, the Northern states, under a strongman, Renard, built a wall dividing North from South, and then when the South seemed to be winning, they embarked on biological warfare. The South is now devasted by disease, with new viruses appearing on the wind all the time. Scattered survivors struggle in small settlements, taking shelter whenever the wind blows. One of the main strands of *South* is the quest for a cure, against a backdrop of the North having inoculated their own soldiers against the viruses let loose on the South. In *North* the quest is to destroy the source of the viruses. The main characters find themselves in the North, which is not the paradise they had anticipated. Renard entrenches his hold on power by constantly discharging new viruses into the air, keeping the people safe through antivirals in the water, and telling them that the diseases come from the South. The Southerners join the Resistance in an attempt to destroy the virus factory. As with Grey and Beukes, the novel is set in the US but one of the central characters is South African. And like Grey, Owen is a pseudonym for a writing team, in this case Diane Awerbuck and Alex Latimer. While the novels are set several decades after the initial outbreaks, new viruses keep circulating and are an ever-present threat. In each novel one character tells of events at the time of the war, showing the devastation the first biological attacks caused. The books are gripping yet bleak.

Deon Meyer moved away from his established genre of crime fiction into speculative fiction with *Fever*. A devastating plague has wiped out the majority of the world's population. The new world is seen through the eyes of a young boy whose idealistic father assembles a community of survivors. Although set in a devastated world, it is not a dystopian novel. It offers a rare glimpse of people working together and trying to rebuild a working society while confronting political infighting within the community. Despite threats from marauding gangs and mysterious soldiers, most of the survivors are trying to work together. Part coming-of-age story and part mystery, it is revealed early in the book that the father has been killed, leading to tension as the story progresses and the reader waits to learn when and how. The ending is at once abrupt and rather unsatisfying as it emerges that the plague has been manufactured and released onto the world, in a highly successful attempt to reduce the population.

If governments are often blamed, and frequently rightly so, for causing or at least using plagues, Lily Herne's fictional world places a whole new spin on that concept. Herne, the penname of Sarah Lotz and her teenage daughter Savannah Lotz, wrote a series of teenage novels, the *Mall Rats* series. The first book, *Deadlands,* published in 2011, is the first South African zombie novel and was followed by *The Death of a Saint* and *The Army of the Lost.* The books are set in 2020, ten years after the zombie apocalypse has struck. Strange beings known as Guardians stepped in to save the remnants of humanity who now live in a fortified settlement, surrounded by the deadlands, where the zombies live. The Guardians control the zombies as well as providing food, shelter, electricity and so on to the humans and allowing them to self-govern in return for a sacrifice of teenagers each year. It is revealed that the teenagers are turned into Guardians, through the spreading of a silvery substance found inside the Guardians and the zombies – the ultimate contagion. Only teenage bodies can survive infection. The first novel is set in Cape Town. When the central character discovers that she can move undetected through the deadlands, she joins a group who get black-market goods from the surviving mall (Canal Walk, identified by the rollercoaster nearby). In the second novel, the characters leave Cape Town, and we see how the rest of the country has fared. In the third novel, they arrive in Johannesburg, where those with their abilities are enslaved and used in power struggles. A recurring theme is that while the threat of contagion is ever present, in many ways the main characters have more to fear from fellow humans than from the zombies.

South African authors have drawn on the themes of disease and plagues in a range of fiction, from literary texts to thrillers to young adult fiction to speculative fiction. As we live through a worldwide pandemic it is interesting to note how many of our experiences are explored in fiction, for example conspiracy theories about the cause of the illness, distrust of government (in some cases with obvious justification), hoarding, and so on. Reality has proved stranger than fiction as none of the books depict the COVID-19 denialism, anti-mask and anti-vaccine sentiments hampering the real-world battle against the pandemic. It will be interesting to see if they will show up in future fictions (along with the previously unexplored trope of hoarding toilet paper). There is some reassurance that a year into the COVID-19, we have not seen a full-scale descent into dystopia, which many of the novels suggest our future to hold.

Works Cited

Bauling, Jayne. *New Keepers*. Cape Town: Tafelberg, 2017.

Beukes, Lauren. *Afterland*. Cape Town: Umuzi, 2020.

Beukes, Lauren. *Moxyland*. Johannesburg: Jacana, 2008.

Boffard, Rob. *Zero G* London: Orbit, 2016.

Grey, S. L. *Under Ground*. London: Macmillan, 2015.

Herne, Lily. *The Army of the Lost* London: Much-in-Little, 2013.

Herne, Lily. *Deadlands*. Johannesburg: Penguin, 2011.

Herne, Lily. *Death of a Saint*. Johannesburg: Penguin, 2012.

Kitching, Gareth. *Bracelet 12-005-35700*. Malvern: UmSinsi, 2001.

Low, Marcus. *Asylum*. Johannesburg: Picador Africa, 2017.

Macgregor, Joanne. *Rebel*. Johannesburg: KDP, 2016.

Macgregor, Joanne. *Recoil*. Johannesburg: KDP, 2016.

Macgregor, Joanne. *Refuse*. Johannesburg: KDP, 2016.

Meyer, Deon. *Fever*. Translated by K.L. Seegers. London: Hodder & Stoughton, 2017.

Owen, Frank. *North*. London: Corvus, 2018.

Owen, Frank. *South*. London: Corvus, 2016.

Pordzik, Ralph. 'Nationalism, Cross-Culturalism, and Utopian Vision in South African Utopian and Dystopian Writing 1972-92.' *Research in African Literature* 32(3), 2001: 177-197.

Titlestad, Michael. 'Future Tense: The Problem of South African Apocalyptic Fiction'. *English Studies in Africa* 58(1), 2015: 30-41.

Venter, Eben. *Trencherman*. Translated by Luke Stubbs. Cape Town: Tafelberg, 2006.

Wilhelm, Peter. *The Mask of Freedom*. Johannesburg: Ad Donker, 1994.

An End in Itself: Genre, Apocalypse and the Archive in Deon Meyer's *Fever*

Devin William Daniels

Abstract

What are the affordances of reading apocalyptic fiction under apocalyptic conditions, when a realism without apocalypse hardly seems realistic at all? What does it mean that our attempts to imagine a future beyond capitalism seem tethered to such an apocalyptic event, and what might these attempts tell us about the present – and the past – from which they emerge? While apocalyptic fiction contends to imagine a world beyond capitalism, I argue that it is more effective at exposing the apocalyptic nature of our present. I tether my analysis to a novel as prototypical of the genre as it is exceptional: *Fever* by the South African crime novelist Deon Meyer. I explore this protean text through a variety of generic frames – as fictional memoir, as Bildungsroman, and as multi-genre hybrid – to consider what the post-apocalyptic genre is and can be. Ultimately, I propose that, by rerouting our readings of post-apocalyptic and other speculative fictions towards what they reveal of our present cultural logics, this literature and our readings of it hold the capacity to escape the confines of anticipatory mourning towards the politically urgent task of recognizing and reckoning with the world of late capitalism and the affective trap of capitalist realism.

Our contemporary moment is typified by the pairing of a radically insecure future and a profoundly stagnant present. While climate disaster and global pandemics were once the domain of computer models and science-fiction, the COVID-19 pandemic and the increasingly palpable and material effects of climate change make dystopian conditions an almost everyday experience, well within the domain of literary realism. In our mainstream imaginary, however, the radical political, social and economic change that this sense of quotidian disaster would seem to demand is dismissed as 'unrealistic'. Mark Fisher describes this as 'the widespread sense that not only is capitalism the only viable political and economic system, but also that it is now impossible even to *imagine* a coherent alternative to it' (2). What somehow persists is the sensation that, in Fisher's paraphrase of Fredric Jameson, 'it is easier to imagine the end of the world than it is to imagine the end of capitalism,' even as capitalism threatens to actualize that very end of the world, whether through climate change, nuclear disaster or other unforeseen means (2). It is hard to deny we are still living under capitalist realism, but what happens when the end of the world ceases being a matter of the imagination? What does it mean to read apocalyptic fiction under such conditions, when a realism without apocalypse hardly seems realistic at all? I hope, in this essay, to query exactly what we are imagining when we imagine the end of the world, rather than merely pining for what we are not imagining. In short, exactly what is the post-apocalyptic genre? What defines it, generically and ideologically, besides the diegetic presence of some disaster that precedes the moment of narration? What does it mean that our attempts to imagine a future beyond capitalism seem tethered to such an apocalyptic event, and what might these attempts tell us about the present – and the past – from which they emerge?

Paul Saint-Amour describes how the 'nuclear condition,' which dominates the post-apocalyptic genre after 1945, 'afflicts humanity with a case of anticipatory mourning, a mourning in advance of loss because the loss to come would nullify the very possibility of the trace' (25). The sense is not just that the world might be destroyed but that the archive of that world might be effaced; without any archival trace, that future is – or will be – unable to tell its own story. The future must be grieved before the fact because it may not be possible to grieve it after. This sense of anticipatory mourning also typifies climate fiction, which is forced to imagine and thus elegize a world undone by a 'potential' disaster that seems less an idle possibility and more a statistical inevitability. Peter C. van Wyck has noted how this need to consider radically distant futures bends the conventional temporalities of grief:

> the future itself is no longer secure … . The decisive accident may *already* have taken
> place. And paradoxically, because of this, the future itself comes under the domination
> of the present as the projective field of its ethical responsibility … . (61)

This ethical responsibility to a future that is always-already disclosed by the current system, paired with the lack of alternatives to that system that characterizes capitalist realism, leaves anticipatory mourning as the only theoretically available action.

The post-apocalyptic text would seemingly offer an avenue for this grief: through the discreet event of disaster that separates its world from our static present, it is able to depict and thus archive a world that might otherwise outlive cultural and institutional memory, offering it up for pre-posthumous meditation. However, this future-oriented theorization belies the retrospective mood that typifies actual post-apocalyptic narratives, exemplified by a novel such as Cormac McCarthy's *The Road*. While McCarthy's novel does take up the ethical responsibility of archiving and mourning for the future, the text, once occupying that future diegetically, finds itself gazing backward, with a tone of elegiac nostalgia, as the world-that-was slowly fades away. This narrative structure of gradual decline is one way of 'plotting' the post-apocalypse. In lieu of a sudden upheaval or an event of rupture, we witness the remnants of society, represented by the fractured and partial familial unit of a father and son, as they persist, romantically, in spite of their inevitable doom. This nostalgic tone is captured in a scene where the father insists his son drink a salvaged can of Coca-Cola, to which the son responds, 'It's because I wont ever get to drink another one isn't it?' (20). Michael Titlestad describes this scene as an elegy not just for humanity but capitalism: 'Not only has the father's childhood, sun-filled world of trout fishing ceased to exist, this is also the end of the line for the world of commodities that flowed in such abundance from the great corporations of the past' (95). As a typical example of its genre, *The Road* seems to confirm Jameson's aphorism that it is easier to imagine the end of the world than the end of capitalism – or, rather, that it is only possible to imagine the end of capitalism *through* the end of the world. The problem with both of these 'ends' is that they are never quite reached, only asymptotically approached. We do not see the 'after' of capitalism or the world but their last gasps. Even when imagining the apocalypse, *The Road* and texts of its ilk do not imagine a way 'out' of this conundrum; they merely look back on the present from a future anterior that is itself only hypothetically posited. If this future has any positive spatial content, it is in the blank margins of the novel's final page that the text itself can only gesture toward.

While we might thus conclude that we have reached the dead end of narrative possibility, I hope to query how the post-apocalyptic novel might encounter and (re)negotiate these supposed limits through the consideration of a novel that is as prototypical of the form as it is exceptional: *Fever*, an out-of-character foray into the genre by the South African thriller novelist Deon Meyer. *Fever* is the story of a father and a son in post-apocalyptic South Africa after a mysterious disease known as the Fever has decimated the world population. *Fever* seems at first to be following *The Road*'s path step for step, as Nico Storm and his father Willem navigate a desolate landscape, scavenging for canned goods and avoiding violent gangs. However, it quickly exceeds the boundaries of McCarthy's plot, as Willem establishes a colony called Amanzi in an attempt to reconstitute civilization. Across 500-some pages of meticulously catalogued salvaging, infrastructural work, military training and political intrigue, Meyer unfolds an almost impossibly complex plot that climaxes with the murders of Willem and Domingo, a mysterious ex-criminal who acts as Amanzi's head of security and as Nico's secondary father figure. In the wake of these murders, Nico reunites with his mother, thought deceased, who is revealed to be the architect behind the Fever. The Fever itself is revealed to be a genetically engineered disease intended to thin the world's population in the face of climate change. Previously immunized, upper-class individuals live in isolated cities, keeping away survivors through false stories of nuclear meltdown and lethal radiation. Nico briefly considers joining his mother in one of these cities before having second thoughts, jumping out of a helicopter, reuniting with the love of his life and taking over his father's colony, essentially choosing his father's philosophy of democratic progress over his mother's Malthusian vision. Meyer's text resists even an elliptical summary, however, filled as it is with stunted, half-explored plots and generic false starts. Throughout, Meyer utilizes the conventions of a number of genres to 'plot' the post-apocalypse in a way that avoids a narrative of gradual decay. To gain a handle on such a protean text, I aim to meditate upon it through a variety of generic paradigms – as memoir, as Bildungsroman and as multi-genre hybrid – to consider what the post-apocalyptic genre is and can be. I hope these meditations contain lessons on what implications the practice of 'apocalyptic reading' will have for real-world practice.

One of the most striking ways *Fever* differentiates itself from more prototypical post-apocalyptic texts is through relating its plot in the form of a memoir and through imagining its own status as a material text within the universe of its narrative. The physical book's initial page identifies it as 'Fever: The memoirs of Nicolaas Storm, concerning the investigation of his father's murder' – though on the title page proper it is called 'Fever: A Novel'. By imagining itself as not only a memoir but a material memoir, *Fever* evokes a long tradition in apocalyptic narrative. In describing 'nuclear fantasia,' the dominant post-apocalyptic genre of the Cold War period, Saint-Amour identifies two main sub-genres:

> The first envisions human beings surviving a nuclear war but undergoing a profound loss of 'civilization' emblematized by the end of literacy and numeracy .... The second type of nuclear parable ... imagines a catastrophe *without* a survivable aftermath ... an archive that should not have survived is read by the absolute other, an alien inhabitant of a future inaccessible to the extinguished species. The nuclear condition, with its warped temporality, has required such contortions in the scene and chronology of reading its remains. (135)

At issue in this archival anxiety is thus not only the preservation of the archive itself – as physical, material remnant – but the preservation of legibility. *Fever* participates in this concern but does not narrate it: the novel is never read within its own plot. Rather, *Fever* is itself this archival trace, and the reader, despite their present temporality, is placed without diegetic explanation in the position of the 'absolute other' of Saint-Amour's second form of fantasia. While McCarthy, in *The Road*, merely narrates information that no living narrator could possibly relate, *Fever* gives a first-person account that foregrounds its physical form. Nico self-consciously struggles with the memoir as a genre, hoping to tell the 'truth' but not being sure how to separate it from the flawed subjectivities of memory. He writes,

> I am forty-seven years old today. The age my father was when he died, in the Year of the Lion. Perhaps that offers enough distance from the events of the time, though I don't know if I will ever develop the necessary wisdom and insight, but I worry that I will begin to forget many of the crucial events, experiences, people. I can't postpone this any longer. (1)

The inability to postpone reflects Nico's sense of urgency to record and archive his story in a world of such radical precarity. Yet his capacities are challenged in this post-apocalyptic world so overdetermined by an eventful disaster, a singular traumatic event. He recalls his father telling him, "'We remember the moments of great trauma the best. Fear, loss, humiliation ... You will see, one day'" (23). Nico confirms this:

> *Now* I see. Now, as I try to write this memoir, now that I want to recall *everything*, not just the trauma. Also the events in between. It's not that easy ... when it comes to the memory river's more troubled waters, you are reliant on your own, sometimes unreliable and prejudiced memories, and the stories of others. You are exposed to the urges (and fears) of the ego, which wishes to include only select events. And exclude others. (23)

Nico wishes for his text, *Fever*, to be a perfect archive, to collect everything, yet the moment of apocalypse obscures it. While Nico wants to tell, in his words, 'the story of what happened *after* the Fever,' the text can only be read in light of that event (23).

In its frustrations and preoccupations with the archive, Nico's memoir might be diagnosed with a different brand of fever, the *mal d'archive* – or archive fever – that Jacques Derrida finds at the core of not only the archival process but also memory itself. Derrida writes that '*every* archive ... is at once *institutive* and *conservative*. Revolutionary and traditional ... it keeps, it puts in reserve, it saves, but in an unnatural fashion' (7). The unnaturalness of archiving means that that which is archived is not only preserved but somehow changed; the archive, in removing that which it archives from its original context, destroys that context, instituting a new arrangement, position, or interpretation. Derrida relates this archival drive to Sigmund Freud's death drive, writing, 'There would indeed be no archive desire without the radical fini-tude, without the possibility of a forgetfulness that does not limit itself to repression' (19). Destruction thus serves as both the motivating force and the method of archivization; one cannot archive everything, so some things will be destroyed so others can be preserved. While this line of approach might risk reducing Nico's frustrations with memory to a metaphor for archivization, Derrida locates, in Freud's writing on the 'mystic writing pad,' the capacity to think of these two systems as operating under a shared logic: 'the hypothesis of an *internal* sub-strate, surface, or space ... it prepares the ideas of a psychic archive distinct from spontaneous memory' (19). The mystic writing pad, as a model of consciousness, considers memory as an internal prosthesis that does not fully correspond with consciousness but supplements it. This internal 'rupture which is ... originary with nature' allows us to consider psychoanalysis itself as 'a theory of the archive and not only a theory of memory' (19). The archive would be, for Derrida, an additional layer of prosthesis to the internal process that is memory itself. In recog-nizing its archival logics, we might consider how memory resists stable assignation and preser-vation. Rather than merely depositing memories into the material archive of the memoir, Nico finds that the very act of remembering is itself a process of archivization, continuously producing – and reproducing – the very meanings it would inertly preserve. Here Nico confronts that destructive, feverish drive that he describes in aptly Freudian terms above: 'the urges (and fears) of the ego, which wishes to include only select events. And exclude others'. The memoir may be considered an archival genre in itself, but *Fever* literalizes this connection by producing – not only in our world but in the world of its plot – the very physical tome in which Nico's memory is materialized, linking the archival instabilities of internal memory to the material precarity of the physical archive – the potential destruction of which we are forced to consider as imminently possible.

Oddly, in its attempts at mitigating these problems, the text ends up looking not much like a fictionalized memoir at all – if we understand a memoir as a first-person account of an individ-ual's life. Nico's narrative is consistently interrupted by italicized passages from a variety of per-spectives – though never his father or mother's – that are noted as being part of the 'Amanzi History Project,' a series of oral histories, recorded first by Willem and later continued by Nico, which are then transcribed by Nico into the narrative proper.[1] Nico's text seems to crave these additional voices as archival supplements to assist his search for 'truth,' and Meyer must thus explain the material conditions of their inscription so as to maintain *Fever*'s status as a – fictionalized – material text. The text's simultaneous stability and instability are further reflected in its incredible number of chapters, one hundred and twenty in all, which strike the reader as a series of archival documents that have been placed in a certain order. Each chapter is extremely contained, and Meyer's narration is likewise meticulous. We are treated to intricate, excessive detail in a hyperrealist style; we do not deal with 'guns' but 'R4 DMs,' not cars but 'Toyota Prados'. In most cases, we know the specific dates and locations of events, and the events themselves, particularly the military expeditions, are related in almost step-by-step fashion. While the Fever has rendered this world new and much emptier, it has not rendered it in any way illegible; Meyer is instead faced with a surplus of details, objects, and processes. The book's overlong, overstuffed nature reflects, on Meyer as well as Nico's parts, a tendency towards collecting and scavenging that is typical of the post-apocalyptic narrative. Much as the characters rely on a remnant archive of canned goods and military stashes that they collect and refashion, Meyer/Nico present a seemingly endless stream of technically specific memories in the hope of producing a 'truthful' memoir, yet this is a goal that necessarily eludes the text. The novel's hijacking of the memoir genre seems to limit it to a somewhat pathetic process of archival accumulation. Even the end of the world provides inexhaustible detail to be catalogued, and its final gasp is thus deferred through the asymptotic progress of meticulous record keeping.

While succumbing to the temptation of archival description, *Fever* does manage to proceed in a way a text like *The Road* cannot: first, through its adoption of the Bildungsroman as a form; and, second, through its restoration, in a post-apocalyptic context, of the correspondence the Bildungsroman draws between the development of the individual and the development of the nation-state. In his work on the Bildungsroman, Jed Esty notes that 'the tension between the open-ended temporality of capitalism and the bounded, countertemporality of the nation,' which is, 'a formative condition of both the classic (national-era) and the modernist (global-era) bildungsroman,' can no longer be cleanly negotiated under the uneven development of modernity (5). Esty maintains,

> a national-cultural system in the emergent phase of European industrialization could mediate between unevenly developed regions (e.g., city and country) in ways that, during a later phase, neither a multinational imperial state nor a capitalist world-system could. (26)

The 'nation' as a category is able to stabilize these problems through 'appeal to a common culture, language, and destiny,' and the Bildungsroman is able to conceive of this national development following in step with the maturation of its protagonist, who enters the stability of adulthood not only as a mature individual but as a national subject (26). As Esty demonstrates, however, across a thorough investigation of modernist narratives of arrested development, 'such claims cannot really be sustained by the inorganic entities of the modern state, the baggy empire, or the acultural world-system,' for which the Bildungsroman-as-national-allegory proves an unstable and incoherent genre (26). Meyer, however, pursues this outmoded 'classic Bildungsroman' with a great deal of fidelity, as Nico's growth from an unskilled adolescent to a sharpshooting political leader (and author/archivist) directly follows the establishment and development of the Amanzi colony. As it grows in population, technological sophistication, and military power, so grows Nico. Indeed, it is only through the founding of Amanzi that *Fever* escapes the stasis of its opening chapters, which read as a rewrite of *The Road* set in South Africa. We might dismiss Meyer's usage of the Bildungsroman as anachronistic and stubborn, merely out of step with the larger cultural trends Esty traces, but Meyer's adaptation of this otherwise outmoded form into a post-apocalyptic novel, as a strategy for lending an otherwise entropic narrative a sort of forward propulsion, reveals the logic and limits of the post-apocalyptic genre's understanding of disaster.

Fever's sudden plague, like the floods, storms and atomic blasts of other disaster narratives, is treated as punctual and interruptive. Willem explicitly laments the Fever for interrupting what had been, in his eyes, the gradual and teleological progress of modernity:

> 'The Fever, it's horrible, the billions who died … but I wonder if the greater harm wasn't the interruption of what we were on the road to accomplishing. We had such huge

problems before the Fever. Political and social and ecological, but we were finding solutions, as we have always done.' (224)

Willem views history as a single temporal line of development that is interfered with, from the
outside, by a discreet moment of disaster. He harkens back to a time before the Fever when the
eventual, if gradual, culmination of modern society was just a matter of time. Meyer contrasts
Willem's gradualist model of history with the apocalyptic logic of the Gaia One organization
that is eventually revealed to have designed the virus to quell climate change through a
sudden, artificial decrease in the world population. While Meyer's resistance to this Malthusian
idea, connected to what Titlestad calls 'the apocalyptic logic of strands of "progressive" politics,' is admirable, he nonetheless adheres to a problematically progressive conception of
history (101). Aníbal Quijano describes how this view of history – which he calls Eurocentric
– allows Western powers to conceive themselves as the culminations of 'a linear sequence of
universally valid events,' such that their dominant position is inevitable and incontestable
(198). Such a perspective, rather than recognizing underdevelopment as an actively generated
aspect of modernity, temporally displaces colonized subjects to a 'premodern' past: 'the Europeans generated a new temporal perspective of history and relocated colonized populations,
along with their respective histories and cultures, in the past of a historical trajectory whose culmination was Europe' (201). Willem views the Fever as an isolated interruption of this linear
progression. He is thus unable to account for the unevenly distributed violences of the pre-apocalyptic past, which become mere steps on the path of universal progress.

The virus, however, actively enables Willem's conception of history by creating a situation
in which everyone appears to be equally under threat (though this is an appearance that Nico's
discovery of the Gaia One conspiracy will ultimately undermine). The apocalyptic event at the
heart of *Fever* does not actually interrupt a narrative of universal development – which, as Esty
demonstrates, has already been thoroughly interrupted by the late capitalist world-system.
Rather, the apocalyptic event revitalizes the Bildungsroman's formal capacity to serve as a
national myth. Only through the supposedly clean slate of the apocalypse is the unity
between individual and national destinies restored. Given the dissolution of any previous state
apparatus, the founding of Amanzi can be imagined as a linear, developmental narrative, escaping even the historical entanglements of a postcolonial Bildungsroman like Salman Rushdie's
Midnight's Children. Thus, while *Fever* rejects the Malthusian politics of Gaia One, it is
through this apocalyptic logic that Willem's pining for a model of progressive history gains
coherence as an alternative position. We might read the book's optimistic final line, 'I was
glowing with knowledge, and anticipation for what lay ahead, the adventures to come,' as a nostalgic pining for a world in which this progressive model has not been dismantled (530). This
nostalgia is oddly unbothered by its indebtedness to a mass extinction event, reflecting the indifference of the pre-apocalypse to the underdevelopment it precipitates in peripheral zones. The
apocalypse does not undo capitalist modernity. Rather, it gives it another shot.

Despite Willem and Nico's shared moments of optimism, the text does somewhat undercut
its investment in an apocalyptic new beginning by gesturing towards lingering agencies of the
pre-apocalyptic world that have not been effaced. Due to the Fever, Cape Town's nuclear reactors have been abandoned and are no longer maintained, resulting in a supposed 'meltdown' that
renders the entire area irradiated and uninhabitable. This meltdown is ultimately revealed to be a
ruse by the Gaia One organization to keep outsiders away from their Cape Town base, which
remains powered by these very reactors. Nonetheless, Meyer calls attention to the fact that

the sudden disappearance of humans cannot in fact return the planet to a so-called state of 'nature'. Humanity, even posthumously, will continue to assert agency in the world through its infrastructural remnants. Nuclear development has rendered the planet into a built environment that requires constant maintenance to avoid deterioration, and this need for maintenance complicates the desire for a 'clean start' in which the apocalyptic imagination indulges. Simply stated, when it comes to the Anthropocene, there is no going back, only different ways of going forward.

Does this mean, then, that the post-apocalyptic text is doomed to incoherence and deconstruction? Can it do anything besides somewhat pathetically accumulate records of the world's dissolution, as in McCarthy's elegies of capitalist commodities and Meyer's prevarications over traumatic memory? I would contend that, while these considerations of *Fever* help us to address the somewhat incoherent logics of the text's political and psychological aims, there is more to *Fever* than its instability – or, rather, *Fever*'s instability has something more to it. In *The Archaeology of Knowledge,* Michel Foucault defines his own understanding of the archive as 'the first law of what can be said, the system that governs the appearance of statements as unique events' (129). The post-apocalyptic genre, in positing a radical rupture point between the world as it is and the world as it will be, seems motivated at escaping these archival logics, yet, as discussed above in relation to the Bildungsroman, they remain a condition of its enunciability – and narratability. Thus, despite its 'post-' designation, the genre is ultimately less successful at imagining new, radically changed worlds than it is at exploring the structural logics of our present world with a certain imagined distance. Foucault notes that 'the archive is also that which determines that all these things said do not accumulate endlessly … they are grouped together in distinct figures' (129). The archive is not a matter of raw accumulation but also organization, and it is those specific, historically contingent manners of organization that one must seek to describe, though Foucault cautions that 'the archive cannot be described in its totality; and in its presence it is unavoidable. It emerges in fragments, regions, and levels, more fully, no doubt, and with greater sharpness, the greater the time that separates us from it' (130). By imagining a radical, historical rupture point, the post-apocalyptic text attempts to speculate about what of the archive will remain and how it will be refashioned, allowing us as readers, perhaps, to glean, in this new context, the cultural logics we fail to see in our present moment. In other words, while anxiety over the precarity of the cultural archive might preoccupy the post-apocalyptic text, in imagining the destruction of that very archive, the genre seeks to view that archive in greater clarity.

Of course, these clarifications are ultimately the products of writerly imagination, and so for our purposes it is perhaps most interesting to ask what we learn about the ideologies of our moment from the way we imagine their fracturing. For a text like McCarthy's, this serves towards creating, in Titlestad's terms, a 'clarifying limit-experience,' through which 'the veil has been lifted on the complexities of the quotidian revealing the essence of the human condition, figured in a chosen few' (97). That essence, for McCarthy, is one of a bare bones world in which good and evil are clearly distinguished, with the social and political institutions stripped away. *Fever*, however, provides less a 'clarifying limit-experience' and more a tangle of generic hybridity. The lingering cultural logics of the Foucauldian archive are reflected in the great number of genres that emerge in stunted, half-familiar forms throughout the text. Whereas the Bildungsroman and the memoir are the genres that most seamlessly map onto the whole of the novel, it is at times a murder mystery, a war epic, a love story and a political thriller, suggesting a variety of potential narrative paths that are not fully explored. On one such path, the novel seems, for a great while, to be heading towards a dramatic clash between Amanzi and a mysterious army of looters known as KTM. Through a series of skirmishes, KTM are revealed to not be a simple army but rather a decentralized conglomeration of criminal enterprises called the Sales Club. The villains behind KTM, then, are not the wandering rapists and murderers of *The Road* – and the opening scenes of *Fever* – but capitalist middle managers. Meyer makes this association rather explicit through the organization's corporatist lingo:

> The man and woman's radio call signs were 'Number One' and the 'Chair'. They used many hiding places and Sales Conference venues. They were very clever, because everyone wanted to eliminate them. They were the middlemen, they had all the contacts, they controlled everything. (284)

Here, a would-be war epic turns out to be a story of the lingering logics of late capitalism. These middlemen, however, are never found, and the dramatic clash of civilizations never occurs. The murders of Willem and Domingo precipitate a subsequent foray into a detective plot that is likewise never 'solved,' as Nico's detective work is subsumed by other concerns: the Gaia One organization is revealed and his long-dead mother reappears. Though Willem's murderer is incidentally revealed in the novel's denouement, the conventions of the detective story have long been abandoned; the circumstances of the murder are not deduced by Nico but merely revealed to him by his mother. The Sales Club, meanwhile, fades into the background, though Nico gestures towards this and other loose threads on the novel's final page, just before the novel's vaguely open final line: 'there were secrets to unravel, about spies, and the Sales Club ... but there wasn't time for that' (530). These various genres have given the novel a way of narrating itself through to Nico's adulthood, but they are not in themselves avenues to be fully realized.

In exploring these genres, Meyer approaches the question of how one narrates the post-apocalypse when it is defined by endings, not progress. The surplus of genres might suggest confused indecision in the face of this question, but I view this generic uncertainty as an aspect of the novel's developmental logic itself. Just as Amanzi is fashioned out of vaguely remembered science and collected refuse, *Fever*'s narrative is fashioned out of generic detritus. While no one genre is able to dominate the novel, neither can the novel escape these generic logics; imagining a truly new genre is outside its capacities; or, rather, to the extent its genre is new or unique it is through this archival combination of generic and material elements. We are unable to narrate the post-apocalypse in a truly new way because it lies beyond the limits of our episteme.

Fever is unable to escape the generic/archival logics of its moment, yet its multi-genre narrative of reconstruction does enable Meyer to explore the structures of our current apocalyptic imaginary. The text's overstuffed nature prevents it from offering a coherent ideological statement. This makes it a uniquely rich text for considering the Foucauldian archival method, in which varying statements are considered alongside each other towards identifying the shared discursive rules that govern their enunciative possibility. Meyer's popular text collects, somewhat indiscriminately, from contemporary discourse to fashion its post-apocalyptic world, and thus makes apparent the larger discursive relationship that allows for such a collection of statements to be made. In this way, we might reconsider the text's clash of the liberal progressivist Amanzi and the apocalyptic Gaia One in a different light. Both these positions seek to avoid disaster in different ways, but they both accept a notion of disaster as something in the future to be avoided, rather than something that is present, active and continuous. The wish to mitigate the risk of the potential disaster of climate change is strong enough, for Gaia One, to justify the elimination of billions of people. This is a shocking position, but it shares a future-oriented understanding of 'disaster' with the opposition. This opposition, represented by Willem, believes the (future) threat will be averted by the gradualist measures of liberal governance. Neither side recognizes climate change as an event that is already here. This future-orientation is enabled by the fact that *Fever* imagines its universalized narrative from a privileged position of two white South Africans, for whom the disastrous effects of modernity had previously not been felt. While the tragedy of the Fever is supposedly its mass scale, the consequences of this scale, for the narrative, are that it brings effects of climate change to the doors of the formerly untouched protagonists. Proving it exists in the same discursive formation as the apocalyptic logic it would critique, this liberal vision can only think of disaster on a generalized, global scale, without accounting for the differentiated, uneven ways that disaster, particularly ecological disaster, is already distributed across the globe in the present.

We might thus ask if Mark Fisher is not asking the wrong question about whether we can imagine an end of capitalism. I would instead question if we can even imagine capitalism itself, in its present instantiation. Do we possess the imaginative capacity to truly recognize, comprehend and narrate the slow, distributed disasters of contemporary globalized capitalism, in all their specificity, or do we still conceive of disaster – ecological or otherwise – as something *to come* that must be mitigated and deferred, rather than presently dealt with? Ultimately, I propose that, by rerouting our readings of post-apocalyptic and other speculative fictions towards what they reveal of our present cultural logics, this literature and our readings of it hold the capacity to escape the confines of anticipatory mourning towards the politically urgent task of recognizing and reckoning with the world of late capitalism and the trap of capitalist realism. We cannot get 'outside' – or past – capitalism without understanding its incongruence with the simple temporality of pre- and post-apocalypse. The apocalyptic effects of capitalism – and the climatological change it has helped to bring about – are not only anticipated and emergent but in many ways already here, albeit in uneven distributions. The apocalyptic picture painted by a writer like Deon Meyer thus proves to be the reflection of our world in a carnival mirror: reversed, swollen and extended, but not quite transformed.

Note

1   While *Fever* is, for its bulk, quite meticulous in making clear the material status of its additional narrative perspectives, as the text goes on the 'Amanzi History Project' tags sometimes do not appear before these passages, though they are still italicized. I am unable to fully explain the ontological status of these passages within the novel's universe, a puzzling conundrum that *Fever* forces us to consider (yet which we of course encounter, without anxiety, in the 'immaterial' narrations of free indirect discourse in countless other novels). The inconsistency of Meyer's practice perhaps unwittingly betrays the unwieldiness of the attempt to stave off the archival anxiety of post-apocalyptic fiction under the supposedly stable and contained genre of 'memoir'.

Works Cited

Derrida, Jacques. *Archive Fever: A Freudian Impression*. Translated by Eric Prenowitz. Chicago: The University of Chicago Press, 1998.

Esty, Jed. *Unseasonable Youth: Modernism, Colonialism, and the Fiction of Development*. New York: Oxford University Press, 2012.

Fisher, Mark. *Capitalist Realism: Is There No Alternative?*. Washington, USA: Zero Books, 2009.

Foucault, Michel. *The Archaeology of Knowledge and the Discourse on Language*. Translated by A.M. Sheridan Smith. New York: Vintage, 2010.

McCarthy, Cormac. *The Road*. New York: Vintage, 2006.

Meyer, Deon. *Fever*. Translated by K.L. Seegers. New York: Atlantic Monthly Press, 2016.

Quijano, Aníbal. 'Coloniality of Power, Eurocentrism, and Latin America'. *Coloniality at Large: Latin America and the Postcolonial Debate*. Edited by Mabel Moraña, Enrique Dussel and Carlos A. Jáuregui. Durham, NC: Duke University Press, 2008. 181–224.

Saint-Amour, Paul K. *Tense Future: Modernism, Total War, Encyclopedic Form*. New York: Oxford University Press, 2015.

Titlestad, Michael. 'The Logic of the Apocalypse: A Clerical Rejoinder'. *Safundi: The Journal of South African and American Studies* 14(1), 2013: 93–112.

Van Wyck, Peter C. 'An Archive of Threat'. *Future Anterior: Journal of Historic Preservation, History, Theory, and Criticism* 9(2), 2012: 53–80.

Plagues in Palimpsest: Historical Time and Narrative Time in Diane Awerbuck's *Home Remedies*, Marcus Low's *Asylum* and Russel Brownlee's *Garden of the Plagues*

Beth Wyrill

This article takes as premise that the onset of the COVID-19 pandemic in 2020 has left South Africans, along with the rest of the world, feeling acutely aware of their own historicity. The idea of historical self-awareness coalescing around major social and historical shifts has been expertly theorized already, but I hope to offer a reading of this phenomenon through three post-2000 South African novels that deal with the theme of plague. A reading of Ricoeur's work on time and narrative, combined with Bakhtin's theorization of polyvocality in the novel leads me to suggest, following Gérard Genette, Ken Barris and Ronit Frenkel, that the idea of the palimpsest in South African writings has particular potency for thinking about historical change. I propose that these ideas are skilfully fictionalized and rendered imaginatively accessible in Diane Awerbuck's *Home Remedies* (2012), Marcus Low's *Asylum* (2017) and Russel Brownlee's *Garden of the Plagues* (2005).

In an opinion piece for the *Guardian* in January 2021, nearly a year after the onset of the COVID-19 pandemic, Jonathan Freedland muses, '[O]ne day, not soon perhaps, we will speak of the pandemic in the past tense. When that time comes, how will we remember the plague that visited death upon us?' (2021). There is a curious movement of tense across this sentence, casting forward into a future in which we might look back upon the present moment; a transformation of the present lived moment into an imagined history of the future. Freedland suggests that it is difficult to remember pandemics clearly because '[t]hey sprawl the entire globe. And the facts can take decades to emerge' (2021). Historians of the Spanish flu suggest that because that virus took victims 'across social, sexual and ethnic lines' (Honigsbaum in Freedland 2021), it 'lack[ed] the essential ingredients of a story: clear heroes and villains with intent and motive' (2021). Similarly, because those self-same elements are absent in the COVID-19 story, there is a risk that 'the current pandemic could eventually be enveloped in the same cultural amnesia that surrounded the one that struck a century earlier' (2021).

There has been a fair amount of media speculation about how this historical moment will be memorialized. Stephen Moss, also writing for the *Guardian*, tells of recent additions to museum collections that curators hope will someday denote the lived moment of the pandemic as remembered history. This penchant for live collecting reflects a similar temporal movement – casting forward to the time when we will be able to look back, so that the artefacts become 'manifestations of our strange current reality that we can see and touch, although not for the moment. They are our message to the future' (2021). Freedland speculates that this anxiety around remembering, this shoring up of objects and stories against loss, speaks to the presently deferred moment of collective mourning of the COVID dead. Such a suggestion gestures, again, to the temporal no-man's-land of the present moment.

It is my contention that the novel as a storytelling form offers writers the space for an array of useful creative techniques that might better express our apprehension of tectonic historical shifts. From the midst of this temporal vortex, novels might offer imaginative inroads into historical time in the absence of easily digestible, linear narratives. I investigate the intersection of storied time and history in three South African novels that play self-consciously with ideas of plague, creative fiction and the historical artefact: Diane Awerbuck's *Home Remedies* (2012), Marcus Low's *Asylum* (2017) and Russel Brownlee's *Garden of the Plagues* (2005).

Time, Narrative and the Idea of the Palimpsest

The novels under consideration all play with temporal layering in distinct ways, but an idea that has potency across all three is the concept of the palimpsest, which offers a way to consider historic time spatially rather than in linear terms. It will be useful to consider briefly the concepts of time, narrative and the idea of the palimpsest before embarking on analyses of the novels in question.

Ricoeur illustrates the connection between lived time and narrative as follows: 'narrativity is the mode of discourse through which the mode of being which we call temporality, or temporal being, is brought to language' (*Reader* 99). He shows, further, that the temporal being to which he refers is ill-served if it is expressed in purely chronological terms. This is because chronology 'takes into account neither the centrality of the present as an *actual* now nor the primacy of the future as the main orientation of human desire, nor the fundamental capacity of recollecting the past in the present' (100). So, if we think about time as a linear, chronological progression, we fail to consider that our experiencing, present-tense selves often orient our perspective backwards through memory or forward through desires for our future selves. Heidegger calls this a 'dialectic of intentionalities,' which describes a 'threefold present: a present about the future, a present about the past, and a present about the present' (qtd in Ricoeur 100). All three intentionalities are at play both in the way that Freedland is thinking about the current pandemic, and in the creative engagements with historical ideas around plague offered by Awerbuck, Low and Brownlee.

As Ricoeur understands it, 'history and fiction each concretize their respective intentionalities only by borrowing from the intentionality of the other' (*Time and Narrative* 181). It is from this mutual support of fictive and historical genres – each occasionally borrowing the compositional techniques of the other – that Ricoeur's idea of time and the idea of the palimpsest might be usefully conjoined. Ricoeur contends that story-telling, particularly of the metatextual kind exemplified in the work of Awerbuck, Low and Brownlee, allows us to distinguish between the '*abstract representation* of time as linear [and] the *existential interpretation* of temporality. Story-telling achieves that in a fundamental way by revealing the existential traits of within-timeness over and against the abstraction of linear time' (*Reader* 108–9). Interestingly, in trying to move away from a linear temporal epistemology, Ricoeur draws on spatial diction – prepositions such as 'over,' 'inter,' 'paralleled' and 'within' proliferate – so that the idea of the historical narrative begins to take on dimensional rather than temporally progressive properties (108–9).

Writing about Awerbuck's short story 'Phosphorescence,' which takes as a narrative focal point the historic location of Graaff's Pool in Cape Town, Ken Barris describes

> a notion of time that fails to keep to its appointed linear order, but allows past moments and events to loop back into the present, rendered visible by the markers of age and wear, or made audible by the accumulation of narratives around a particular site. … The markers of past time become influential within the dynamic of perception, as in a palimpsest, and thereby change the meaning and aesthetic of the scene for an observer, detached or otherwise, as its visible surface becomes more layered. Depth then becomes co-legible with surface, so that whatever cognitive or perceptual values one reads into it might form a plurality. The implication … is that past and present coexist as partner terms of an ambiguity, rather than as opposed ends of any given string of time. (60–61)

In the novels under consideration, there are moments where time and history coalesce in the fashion described by Barris, 'as in a palimpsest' (61), around certain historical artefacts and places. This is true of the remains of the 'Fish Hoek Man' in *Home Remedies* – '[h]e [is] at once twelve thousand years old and thirty, the same age as [Joanna] would be soon' (28). It is also true of the description of the Company Gardens in *Garden of the Plagues*, where the garden is shown as distinct from its surroundings: 'All around the settlement now the earth is dry and the mountain has black scars from the fires that begin for no reason. But in the garden the trees have reached such a height that they give shade, and there is the sound of water from the modest stream in its cobbled furrow' (13). The present-day Company Gardens present a similar break from their surroundings in the heavily urbanized city bowl. Readers might read real life narratives around these sites into the fictionally rendered versions, so that the present of the reader and the historical past invoked by the novel converge.

If Ricoeur's ideas about time are brought into conversation with Bakhtin's notion of heterology and polyvocality, then it is conceivable that Barris's idea of the palimpsest might take on a discursive layer. All three of the novels chosen for consideration are unquestionably polyvocal. In Bakhtin's theoretical sense, all novels, even single-voiced writings, by which he means novels which maintain one consistent narrative focalizer, are by design polyvocal. This is because he views other literary forms *as* an 'uttering act whereas the novel *represents* one' (qtd. in Todorov 65). The act of uttering in the novel is doubled: 'In the novel, language does not merely represent: it is itself an object of representation' (qtd in Todorov 66). However, these novels are perhaps especially and self-consciously polyvocal because their narratives are delivered by multiple focalizers, representing a diversity of discursive positions. In the case of Awerbuck's novel, the narrator Joanna Renfield is persistently interrupted by her snarky, quick-witted male alter ego, Dr Renfield. In Low's *Asylum*, the main narrative of James Barry is deftly framed by imagined academic commentary on the found artefacts of Barry's notebooks, which form the bulk of the narrative. In *Garden of the Plagues*, we hear from a motley crew of characters found at the colonial outpost of the Cape of Good Hope, from gardeners to governors.

Bakhtin also rejects the idea that any information can be unidirectionally exchanged in the novel form, situating each utterance in 'a complex choir of other voices already in place' (Todorov x). In this way, one might envision layers of discursive dialogism coalescing around things and places in the same way that layers of historical time accumulate for Barris, such that the 'cognitive [and] perceptual values' of both characters and readers 'might form a plurality' (Barris 61).

Defined literally, a palimpsest is a visual impression left by the action of partial erasure and overwriting on a piece of parchment or vellum. It is easy to see how the term has come to have useful applications in literary studies, as well as in architecture and archaeology, as a metaphor for reworking or adding new content or meaning to a historical assemblage, while still leaving the older work partially visible. Baldick defines the figurative application of 'palimpsest' as pertaining to literary works that have 'more than one "layer" or level of meaning' (158). The idea of the literary text revealing 'layers' of meaning to the perceptive reader is not new. Roland Barthes reminds the reader that 'to read (to listen to) a narrative is not merely to move from one word to the next, it is also to move from one level to the next. .... It is proposed to distinguish three levels of description in the narrative work: the level of "functions" ... the level of "actions" ... and the level of "narration"' (259–60). The palimpsest trope develops this understanding from the intra- to the inter-textual level.

Gérard Genette's *Palimpsests: Literature in the Second Degree* (1992, French original 1982) is the first scholarly text to explore rigorously the many ways in which texts might work with intertexts and historical context as in a palimpsest, although Genette prefers the term 'hypertextuality' (5). He differentiates between intertextuality, metatextuality and hypertextuality based on degrees of abstraction, considering all terms to fall under the umbrella of the 'architext' (1) – the textual environment in which a narrative is crafted and to which it must respond. Given that all texts, consciously or not, must exist in conversation with the architext in which they are created, it follows that '[a]ny text is a hypertext, grafting itself onto a hypotext, an earlier text that it imitates or transforms; and writing is rewriting; and literature is always in the second degree' (Prince ix). Genette thus limits his work to those texts which are, 'more visibly, massively, and explicitly' (9) hypertextual. As such he spends much time in *Palimpsests* exploring genres such as parody and pastiche.

Chantal Zabus's more recent work on the palimpsest in *The African Palimpsest: Indigenization in the West African Europhone Novel* (2007) uses the concept to think about post-colonial europhone language use in African literatures. Zabus contends that '[w]hen "the empire writes back to the centre," it does this not so much with a vengeance as "with an accent," by using a language that topples discourse conventions of the so-called "centre"' (xv). Reviewer Maïr Verthuy says that Zabus's work springs from the view that 'most African texts reveal, beneath the European writing, traces of various source languages, an assumption translated into the striking metaphor of the palimpsest' (207). It is interesting to note that Zabus cites Alain Ricard's work on African literary translation as the catalyst for *African Palimpsests*. Ricard has worked specifically on the publication and translation history of Thomas Mofolo's *Moeti oa Bochabela* (1907) and *Chaka* (1925), and although he does not invoke the trope of the palimpsest, the idea of layered and hypertextual literary construction has resonance for Southern African and post-colonial literary history. Thus, the idea of the palimpsest has provided rich figurative ground for describing literary production abroad, and increasingly, in specifically local ways.

In fact, the idea of palimpsest appears in Ronit Frenkel's theorization of the current period of South African literary production; a period that she and Craig MacKenzie termed 'post-transitional' literature in a much-cited 2010 article in *English Studies in Africa*, 'Conceptualizing "Post-Transitional" South African Literature in English'. The term, first suggested by Meg Samuelson in 2008, also in *English Studies in Africa*, is much contested, and even as it was brought into being by Frenkel and MacKenzie, it was critiqued in the same journal issue. Chris Thurman asks '[a]ren't we still in the process of transition from apartheid to something else? What is that something else?' (91), and Michael Titlestad posits that to use such a label is premature, and that in fact, '[w]e have been forever transitional and all indications are that we are condemned to that plateau of being and meaning' (121). Aghogho Akpome suggests that literature emerging in South Africa after 2000 be theorized as 'post-TRC' (39) instead. Perhaps in response to some of these criticisms, Frenkel invokes the palimpsest in a follow up article in 2013. In 'South African Literary Cartographies: A Post-Transitional Palimpsest,' Frenkel argues:

> The post-transitional can be read as a palimpsestic concept itself ... in that it enables a reading of the new in a way in which the layers of the past are still reflected through it. Rather than moving in a temporal linear fashion, post-transitional literature creates a palimpsest in which we can read the imaginaries circulating through and shaping South African cultural formations today. (25)

The development of thought about South Africa's contemporary literary production is thus acutely aware of the currents of historical time and the multiple ways in which past and future-present are interwoven in the wake of major historical shifts. There is evidence that the novel form in general and the South African novel in particular are sensitive to ways of 'reading the new' so that 'the layers of the past are still reflected through it' (25). What Barris's invocation of the palimpsest in the work of Awerbuck, specifically, does is move the concept from a strictly textual realm to a geographical, spatial plane. The works of Awerbuck, Low and Brownlee might offer insights into novel ways of conceiving the persistent historicization of the present that the COVID moment has highlighted.

Diane Awerbuck's *Home Remedies*

I have chosen to include Awerbuck's most recent novel because of its engagement with South African heritage, and its use of *muti* as a thematic referent, although there is not a direct treatment of the theme of plague. *Home Remedies* follows protagonist Joanna Renfield, who, at the opening of the novel, has just lost her job as a researcher at the Fish Hoek Valley Museum of Natural History. The unassuming provincial museum has won national attention for a brief moment with the return of Saartjie Baartman's[1] remains to South Africa. Baartman is, in the world of the novel, discovered to be a genetic relative of the museum's main exhibit, the preserved remains of the 'Fish Hoek Man' (28), a neolithic fossilized skull excavated from the nearby Peers Cave. In a moment of spite at the director of the museum, Joanna steals a small glass jar containing Baartman's preserved genitals. In fact, she steals it from a hiding place fashioned by the director, Viola, a woman of colour whose claim to the Baartman legacy irks

Joanna. The reader is led to believe that Viola had her own plans to take possession of the Baart-man remains. This much transpires in the first pages of the novel and what follows is a lengthy section depicting Joanna navigating her discontent in the domestic roles of mother and wife, a graphically rendered and brutal rape, and the loss of her child, James, in a road accident that is Viola's fault.

The series of disasters that befall Joanna are presumably meant to be read in some way as the revenge of Saartjie Baartman, as her body once again becomes the contested ground over which private and public battles are fought. Even more unsettling, Baartman's remains are foggily ren-dered, and it is unclear whether the stolen jar is meant to represent a kind of protective talisman, or a shameful and potent *muti*. Certainly, the reader is invited to draw parallels between the remains in Joanna's possession, brought into the house in the cardboard box into which she packed up her office, and another abandoned cardboard box that Joanna keeps spying at a bus stop in Fish Hoek: '"It's *muti*. It's definitely *muti*," she told Jan as they lay drinking tea one morning' (92). Later Joanna spells out her fears more explicitly: 'Did you know that the person has to be alive when they harvest the organs?' (93). Reviewers have been wary of tack-ling this narrative thread. Mary Corrigall, writing for the *Sunday Independent*, makes the most sustained attempt, and is worth quoting at length on the subject of Joanna and Viola's tussle over Baartman's body.

> [T]here is something very uncomfortable about [Joanna's] anger and resentment towards Viola. …
>
> It's uncertain whether Awerbuck aims to challenge political correctness or is interested in presenting a white female who refuses to acknowledge or understand the persistent victimization that others have endured. Is Joanna insensitive or does Awerbuck assume to excoriate an institutionalized form of victimization, which relies on exploiting abuses from the colonial era? This paradigm relies on establishing a heritage of victimi-zation that can never be transcended, which is a self-defeating gesture. It's slippery ter-ritory for sure, where both Joanna, and by proxy Awerbuck, risk appearing as if they are denying abuses of the past. (18)

I am inclined to give Awerbuck the benefit of the doubt. Joanna certainly regards herself as someone to whom the worst has already happened: 'she felt sorry for the people who still had to experience what she had endured the summer she was eight – the blistering year her mother had vanished' (46). As a result, she regards herself as living outside of time in some ways, such that at the beginning of the novel she believes that 'everything important in your life happened before you were eighteen' (46). The novel subsequently upends this assumption and plays quite self-consciously with ideas about comparative victimization. Further, as Bakhtin's theory of polyvo-cality reminds us, the character of Joanna need not stand in proxy for Awerbuck (as Corrigall suggests). Joanna turns out to be wrong about the box in Recreation Road – it has been placed not by a *sangoma* but by a pair of Fish Hoek Satanists, and contains a mutilated cat. Her investigation of its contents – opening Pandora's box – brings on her brutal rape. Neverthe-less, Corrigall's conclusion that Awerbuck fails to resolve 'a sticky political discourse that was half-heartedly raised' feels apt (18).

The level at which *Home Remedies* works best, however, is not as a politically cogent com-mentary on identity politics but rather as a variety show of historical ghost stories that are threaded through and newly recombined. Joanna tries to defend herself not against any literal plague, but against her own lingering fear of the loss of James, a fear which, when it is tragically realized late in the text, nevertheless comes as an unexpected body blow to the reader. The twinning of love and loss is pre-figured early in the novel with her anxieties over James' cough:

> It was the Armistice, they say, that brought the final wave of Spanish flu. In 1919 people were hugging in the streets and passing on the virus with each transporting kiss. Once she had heard that little ditty, Joanna had not been able to get rid of it, thinking of the children who had watched their healthy parents foam from the mouth, haemorrhage, turn blue and shit themselves. The kids in their Edwardian frills jumped rope and sang:
>
> *I had a little bird*
>
> *Its name was Enza*
>
> *I opened a window*
>
> *And In-flu-En-za.*
>
> …
>
> Nothing's changed, she thought. Now it's Bird Flu or Swine Flu or AIDS. Everybody's sick with something. (15)

It is useful to consider this moment in terms of the palimpsest. Although it is only a passing reference in the text, Awerbuck's invocation of historical plague as an intertext is worth exploring in some detail. The 'In-flu-En-za' (15) ditty functions as intertext in the narrow technical sense in which Genette uses it, namely, 'a relationship of copresence between two texts or among several texts: that is to say, eidetically and typically as the actual presence of one text within another' (2). Awerbuck inserts the quoted intertext 'In-flu-En-za' (15) into a broader consideration of historical epidemics. It is conceivable that these historical narratives could function as part of the 'architext' (Genette 1) to which Awerbuck is responding, that is, 'the entire set of general or transcendent categories – types of discourse, modes of enunciation, literary genres – from which emerges each singular text' (Genette 1). If that is the case, then this interchange of intertext with architext allows the quoted excerpt to skip lightly from the global to the local and from the historical to the contemporary (moving from the Spanish flu through to the AIDS epidemic).

The palimpsestic overlay happens, crucially, through the trope of plague. As Freedland, quoted earlier in this article, says; pandemics are terrifying precisely because their amorphous spread makes them difficult to narrativize. This excerpt offers a way of thinking about a moment that is at once undetermined (disease does not discriminate) and excruciatingly specific (Joanna translates the broad historic terror of plague on to her own baby boy). Joanna's solution implies its own impossibility: 'If you could just avoid contact! That was it, thought Joanna. Splendid isolation' (15). The point, of course, is that no person, or text, can exist in singularity. Layering the historical trauma of Baartman with Joanna and Viola's present-day struggles drives home this idea.

Joanna seems doubtful that a widely experienced history can affect the present-day individual so acutely. Viola suffers from 'Post-Colonial Syndrome' (17), says Joanna, her tone dripping

with cynicism. Awerbuck's wider narrative proves Joanna wrong; she becomes directly impli-
cated in these South African historical undercurrents, even though she dismisses Viola's personal claim to them. Musing on her work as a ghost-writer in producing a book about
Baartman, '*Saartjie's Ghost*' (18), Joanna thinks; '[m]aybe Saartjie had been at peace before,
and the attention, this insistence on addressing her directly, had called her up. Joanna was the
same as the rest of them, when you got right down to it, a grave robber' (20).

When Joanna steals the small jar containing Baartman's genitals away from Viola, she
becomes a literal as well as a figural grave robber. Besides the use of Baartman's remains to
link her bodily violation by French scientists to Joanna's white middle-class horror at the idea
of '*muti* murders,' Awerbuck also introduces the historic ghost of ritual sacrifice in the Satanist
narrative thread. Joanna's rape scene is prefigured by a 'toad moon' (172), where the flood of
toads migrating across Silvermine Road to the wetlands for mating season is part miracle,
part biblical plague.

Awerbuck's meditation on the primal fear of loss engendered by motherhood takes place at
distinctly palimpsestic sites. They occur in the present time of contemporary Cape Town but also
echo strands of historical experience. They are both real places and figures – the geography of
Fish Hoek, Baartman, the Fish Hoek Man – and fictional renderings of them. The ghost stories
are connected across time, place, culture in this way, and project future-facing anxieties as
much as historical sins.

Marcus Low's *Asylum*

While *Home Remedies* received a mixed reception upon its release, Low's debut novel *Asylum*
(2017) was roundly praised. Released at roughly the same time as the English translation of
Deon Meyer's extremely popular *Fever* (2017), another post-apocalyptic plague tale set in
South Africa, Low's more subdued literary offering seems to have been largely overlooked
despite its warm critical reception. Karina Szczurek calls it 'deft,' 'lyrical' and 'striking'
(2017), while Karin Schimke describes it as 'the most credible – and therefore the most disturbing – dystopian novel [she has] ever read' (2017). The novel tells the tale of Barry James, a
patient (or inmate) at the Pearson quarantine facility in the Karoo, a sanitorium set up to
house infected carriers of a lung disease, 'pulmonary nodulosis' (ix), which had struck the
globe sometime around or before 2020. After a suicide attempt, James is encouraged by the facility's visiting psychologist to keep a journal. The journal entries, delivered in the first person by
James, are framed by academic commentary on the narrative, cast from some time in the future
of James's narrative. These framing passages explain the motivation for the text's arrangement
and the provenance of James's notebooks, stored at the Beaufort West Museum of the Plague
since 2026. His narrative charts his uneventful existence and his delusional romantic attachment
to the psychologist (Ms Van Vuuren) until he is caught up in an escape attempt, mostly for lack
of anything else to do. James is shown up from the very first to be an unreliable narrator, thanks
largely to the commentary which precedes his tale. In this way, the novel plays with historical
and fictional narrative construction, and chronology, by using disease as a narrative focalizer and
central trope.

Both Gareth Langdon and Karina Szczurek pick up on the thematic concern with chronology, with Langdon noting that 'the lung disease serves … as a measure of time, counting down
the days to his death as it progresses, and as a parallel to his mental deterioration' (2017).
Szczurek suggests that '*Asylum* explores how one can deviate from a predestined plot by

dreaming, or telling stories' (2017). The novel certainly foregrounds the constructedness of narrative chronology from the very start, thereby making evident the imbrication of historical and fictive modes. The framing editorial voice informs the reader that 'compiling this volume has not been easy. Even though the notebooks are numbered, their lack of chronology is notable. Analysis of the sequence of events and of the writing style does, however, allow us to arrange the entries into at least a plausible chronology' (xii–xiii). That James is an unreliable narrator is also emphasized in the editorial 'preface':

> [A]s far as the novels contain a narrative arc, this arc hinges on misrepresentation. The literary power of Mr James' journals lies in the fact that he makes these misrepresentations seem an unavoidable outcome of his experience of the infection. ... If not an exact history then, the journals could be read as a meditation on the psychology of illness. (xi)

James' fictional notebooks are presented in the style of primary historical source in much the same way as can be seen in Brownlee's *Garden of the Plagues*, where Pepys-like diary entries are included from the back story of the character Adam Wijk, who prior to the timeframe of the novel has worked as a physician treating the plague in London. Although in both cases the 'artefact' sections are written by the authors of the respective novels, they are presented separately from the voice of the main narrative, so that the reader is asked to perceive them as intertexts. In both texts, the written artefact acts as the fictional history around which the narrative present is oriented. Conversely, the diary entries in both novels are written as though 'for posterity,' indicating the existence of future-facing 'intentionalities' (Heidegger qtd in Ricoeur 100) in the character's fictional past.

Of the three novels under consideration, Low's is the only one that might be considered speculative or post-apocalyptic. It has been important to include at least one speculative novel in a piece considering plague as a thematic referent, because most popular writing on the subject (I am thinking especially of Lauren Beukes and the aforementioned *Fever* by Deon Meyer) fall squarely into this genre. When interviewed about *Asylum*, Low suggests that the plot draws from contemporary realities, rather than projecting present anxieties into an imagined future. With a history working with the HIV/Aids Treatment Action Campaign in South Africa, and suffering from a degenerative loss of vision himself, Low's metaphoric use of disease feels immediate. In fact, for evidence of his direct inspiration, Low refers interviewer Karin Schimke to a *New York Times* article published in 2008, about 'the Jose Pearson TB Hospital in Port Elizabeth, where patients with multi-drug resistant strains of tuberculosis were kept behind high security fences which they often tried, and sometimes succeeded in, breaching' (2008). Low's work within the context of another global pandemic – HIV/AIDS – makes one wonder why he chose to invent a fictional plague framework within which to flesh out these contemporary problematics. Something about the blank slate offered by speculative fiction must be necessary for the imaginative undertaking, and so Michael Green's 1994 work on 'future histories' feels relevant here.

Writing about the dystopian fiction of Nadine Gordimer, Green links the 'future history' (14) to standard historical fiction as follows: '[m]oments of radical social transition throw the burden of historical interest on the future, reminding us that histories usually include, even if only implicitly, a prospective element that serves as an important structural feature for their retrospective interests' (14). This structure is directly mimicked by the *Guardian* pieces with which this article opens, and it is interesting that Green links the focus on prospective rather than retrospective history-making to moments of significant social change. Of course, the novels in question here are all responding to their own specific historical moments of production (such as the immediate pressures of disease in his own life, for Low), rather than to the COVID-19 pandemic, but in light of the onset of the pandemic, it is interesting and useful to read these historiographically reflexive stories through Green's frame.

In *Asylum*, the extent of James' unreliability as a narrator is exposed when it transpires that the ex-girlfriend, whose death he is mourning, is in fact alive, and that she has visited him at the Pearson facility. When James reflects on his conflicting versions of his own past as presented to Van Vuuren, he ties illness and delusion to historical veracity: "'But the past," she said, "I mean the past as it really was, surely some of that is worth holding on to?" "There is no past *as it really was* as you put it. That past is dead"' (197). If this seems a rather dire and hopeless conclusion, the exchange is followed by a beautiful rendering of one of James' recurring dreams:

> From the balcony, a Balkan waltz filled the ballroom with a sweeping melody, every now and again flirting at the edge of madness and dissonance. She and I danced, and it was intoxicating. And as we rose and fell, I saw that all those around us were also dancing, and that, like me, their clothes didn't fit them and their bodies seemed weak, that some had injuries, and that there was even a trickle of blood from Dugan's neck.
>
> None of the pain mattered. We danced, and it was as if all the world had fallen from us like dirt, as if the ballroom itself was about to take off and blur the snowy landscape outside the window into an indistinguishable mess. (201)

The implication is that there is space for glimpses of beauty and creativity even when travelling toward the most predestined of outcomes. If disease functions here as a fixer of absolute chronology (you get sick, and then you get sicker, and then you die), James' narrativized response offers retaliation against hard truth and the inexorable progression of time. Low's novel does not use place or historical event as a palimpsestic site, in the way that Awerbuck does, but one might argue that *Asylum* makes evident the discursive palimpsest that is enabled by the novel form. The polyvocal strands of dream world and real world, delusion and verified history, reliable and unreliable narration are all shown to speak through one another in the structure of the story.

Russel Brownlee's *Garden of the Plagues*

In Russel Brownlee's *Garden of the Plagues*, the author plays more with the idea of liminality as a descriptive technique than the layered effect of the palimpsest, but the notion of palimpsest is useful (as in Low's text) for thinking about the discursive focus of the novel. The tale overlays and pre-shadows an emergent positivist logic against and through herbalist, spiritualist sensibilities in a Dutch-occupied Cape of Good Hope, in the year 1685. Shaun De Waal says that 'Brownlee is able to examine how it was at the start of the period now ending – the Enlightenment' (1). *Garden of the Plagues* skilfully juxtaposes notions of modernity and pre-Enlightenment sensibilities and has ambivalence at its core. In struggling to lead their lives in a climatically challenging and geographically remote world, the characters must also contend with one another, and in this way an epistemological contact zone is established. Bakhtin's notion of polyvocality is constantly applicable among the contesting and disputing voices that make up the text.

This analysis will focus only on Adam Wijk's narrative thread, from the arrival of the *Tulp* at Table Bay – a ship thought to be carrying the plague – to Wijk's nursing a surviving passenger, the nameless 'Girl' back to health. Through this narrative the reader learns of Wijk's history as a physician treating the plague in London, before becoming disillusioned with the shaky science of medicine and resorting to botany. He ends his journey as we find him at the start of the novel, a gardener in charge of the Company Gardens under the administration of Commander Van der Stel, before he is forced to consider the nature of contagion once more in the case of the Girl. As with Awerbuck's novel, Brownlee counterpoises herbalist remedies and witchcraft with modern medical interventions. Like *Home Remedies, Garden of the Plagues* stages this clash over the body of a silent, dispossessed woman, who ultimately avenges herself upon her perse-cutors. Finally, both novels use the idea of disease as a locus around which to position charac-ters' sensibilities and anxieties.

From the first, the settlement at the Cape of Good Hope is figured as liminal and precarious, a place where new world rationalist sensibilities are not easily taken as given and are persistently haunted by something which escapes positivist logic. This is the metaphoric function of the dark whale in the bay with which the novel opens, and this is the sense of the topography of the bay itself. Flagman Abram Moolman describes the view from his position atop Lion's Head as follows: 'The heat makes the horizon shimmer. Dust blows from the dry northern coastline out over the sea, so there is a white haze that blurs the division between sky and water. The light is like salt' (41). In a landscape such as this, the briskly ordered world-view of the VOC, whose belief in civilization and progress is reflected in the neatly walled and pruned Company Gardens, is 'preceded and exceeded by a haunting' (Jamal 8). Ashraf Jamal explicates the idea of Southern African liminality, drawing on historical cartography and travel writing to position the Cape as 'Janus-faced,' since it figures only as a stopping off point 'between the riches of the East and West' (5). As such, the colonial inhabitants of this 'tavern of the sea' (4) are characterized by an 'abyssal in-betweenness' (6); they are 'neither here nor there; fac-tored in yet cancelled out, surviving under a morbid erasure' (5).

It is the threat of plague that comes to signify this unsettling counter to 'scientific and Pro-testant truth' (12) for the colonial inhabitants at the Tavern of the Green Door. The first retelling of the plague rumour by mutinous sailors from the *Tulp* is set up like a ghost story. The sailors 'lower their voices, cast eyes about the room for spies and traitors, then bring their audience on board with them, where on a night just like this, warm and breathless, Dirk the cabin boy is about to make a terrible, nay a gruesome, discovery' (Brownlee 28). The plague figures as frightening to the colonial authorities not entirely for its own sake, but because it signifies the incursion of a Machiavellian element in a land upon which the grip of order and stability is tenuous. Indeed, 'what bothers the Commander is that this *Tulp* has made a little hole in his dreams, it has fru-strated his plans' (26). In an interlude from an unnamed ship's captain, narrated in the second person, the impulse to instil 'order' at the Cape is explicitly linked to positivism:

> Whether it is keeping the dust out of the laundry or making a garden or building a farm, you will need to draw deeply on your single, shared belief – that your God is a lover of order and progress, that it somehow matters to this deity that people can write their history and count beyond ten. Without this you are lost. (66)

Without the colonial ordering of knowledge, the passage suggests, Southern Africa becomes 'an uncircumnavigable region said to exist outside knowledge and beyond any imagined retrieval'

(Jamal 2). In the world of the novel, plague exists as a question to which the new rationalist world order has no answer. As Wijk says, the 'Black Dog' (48) of the plague 'follows no rules that man can discern' (48) and he asks the inconvenient question: 'how can you trust your grand corpus of knowledge when there is something like me out there, striking left and right without pattern or reason?' (48–49).

The palimpsest of sensibilities, overlaying herbalism with the newly scientific approach to medicine beginning in the timeframe of the novel, makes evident that the progress from one knowledge system to another is not linear, or even necessarily progressive. Jamal argues that 'the two categories collide' (12). I would suggest that this is where the visualization of a palimpsest becomes useful, so that both categories may coexist without collapsing or resolving, overlaying and undergirding one another, or even surfacing and subsiding through one another. This idea is reinforced over and over in the character of Wijk. When asked to remedy minor ailments of the settlers, '[m]any times he has refused to answer the call, shouting through the door of his cottage … that they will have more luck bothering the witch Halsenbach for a charm or a spell than trusting themselves to a man tainted by knowledge of physic' (32–33). His collection of medical specimens in glass bottles hung from the rafters of his cottage are also described as belonging to the magical rather than scientific realm. It is worth noting the echo of Baartman's remains, preserved in a glass bottle and used to evoke the idea of *muti*, in Awerbuck's novel. Wijk's specimens are presented to the reader 'in ghostly outline against the darkness of the roof, their strange contents floating above the world in a supernatural suspension' (57).

Brownlee's novel, like Low's *Asylum*, uses a written artefact, Wijk's diary entries from his time as a doctor treating the plague in London, to draw attention to the novel's constructed chronology. The diary entries stand conspicuously separate from the rest of the narrative, marked out by a more archaic style. The section is introduced as '*Notes of an Ordinary Doctor in the Year of the Plague 1665 (For his own use, personal, and not for printing, even if this were to fall into unauthorised hands by theft, misplacement, etc)*' (144). The note seems to suggest cheekily that all written history, since retold using the tools of narrative construction, is arrived at by theft or misplacement. Further, the entries gesture to a version of the future that is still contingent, where Wijk's predictions may or may not come to pass. The diaries *have* been reprinted in the novel, in accordance with Wijk's fear that they might be, but Wijk's prediction that 'there is no reason for alarm as yet' (145) in the context of the Great Plague of London in 1665, turns out to be mistaken, both from the perspective of the narrative present in which the threat of plague at the Cape of Good Hope is profoundly alarming, and the reader's actual historical present which understands the Great Plague of London to have been devastating. The reader is asked to orient imaginatively their present positioning via the past into an alternative future, recalling Ricoeur's injunction that we distinguish between the '*abstract representation* of time as linear [and] the *existential interpretation* of temporality' (Ricoeur 108–9).

Conclusion

When Ronit Frenkel suggests that, in spite of all the criticism levelled against it, the term 'post-transitional' as applied to South African literature is still generically useful, she does so by invoking the idea of palimpsest. This is in deference to a recognition that history resists neat periodization, because even in the wake of a major historic and social shift, such as the dismantling of apartheid, or the onset of a global pandemic, reality is still read through what came before, and predictions of the future-to-follow will proliferate. Our cultural expressions of the present moment will always be layered through with historically generated anxiety and future-facing desire, and the South African cultural imaginary knows this acutely, understanding itself more than most to be in a state of suspended, perpetual transition.

Awerbuck, Low and Brownlee's novelistic engagements with questions of time and history are, helpfully, positioned from an imagined present (in *Home Remedies*), future (in *Asylum*) and past (in *Garden of the Plagues*). Their technical and discursive approaches to engaging history frequently overlap, and all three novels are well primed to help us imagine major historical shift more perceptively. All the novels use the idea of disease or plague as a metaphoric vector for imagining a loss of control, or an interruption of seemingly fixed ideologies. In Barris's writing on Awerbuck's work (which might be extrapolated as applicable to all three novels), he singles out a use of narrative time that is 'rendered visible by the markers of age and wear, or made audible by the accumulation of narratives around a particular site' (60). Perhaps he would contend that this sensory and perceptual overlap is engendered by the process of narrativizing time into story. The experience of living through a global pandemic demands that we contend with a persistent feeling of out-of-time-ness. It is perhaps comforting, in the face of such perceptual anxiety, to observe the process of embedding time and memory into history in the work of these skilful writers of fiction.

Note

1   I have used 'Saartjie' rather than Sara or Sarah, in accordance with its usage in the text.

Works Cited

Akpome, Aghogho. 'Towards a Reconceptualization of "(Post)Transitional" South African Cultural Expression'. *English in Africa*. 43(2), 2016: 39–62.

Awerbuck, Diane. *Home Remedies*. Cape Town: Umuzi, 2012.

Barris, Ken. ''Every Place is Three Places': Bursting Seams in Recent Fiction by Diane Awerbuck and Henrietta Rose-Innes'. *Current Writing* 26(1), 2014: 59–69.

Bakhtin, Mikhail M. *The Dialogic Imagination: Four Essays*. Translated by Caryl Emerson and Michael Holquist. Texas: University of Texas Press, 1981.

Baldick, Chris. *The Concise Oxford Dictionary of Literary Terms*. Oxford: Oxford UP, 1990.

Barthes, Roland. 'Introduction to the Structural Analysis of Narratives.' In *A Barthes Reader*. Edited by Susan Sontag. London: Vintage, 1982. 251–95.

Brownlee, Russel. *Garden of the Plagues*. Cape Town: Human & Rousseau, 2005.

Corrigall, Mary. 'Dour Tale of Domestic Drudgery'. *The Sunday Independent*. 17 February 2013: 18.

De Waal, Shaun. 'Garden of Tales'. *Mail and Guardian*. 12–18 August 2005: 1.

Dugger, Cecilia. 'TB Patients Chafe Under Lockdown in South Africa'. *New York Times*. https://www.nytimes.com. Accessed on 12 March 2021.

Freedland, Jonathan. 'History Suggests We May Forget the Pandemic Sooner than We Think'. *The Guardian*. https://www.theguardian.com. Accessed on 29 January 2021.

Frenkel, Ronit. 'South African Literary Cartographies: A Post-transitional Palimpsest'. *Ariel: A Review of International English Literature*. 44(1), 2013: 25–44.

Frenkel, Ronit and Craig MacKenzie. 'Conceptualising 'Post-Transitional' South African Literature in English'. *English Studies in Africa*. 53(1), 2010: 1–10.

Genette, Gérard. *Palimpsests: Literature in the Second Degree*. [1982] Trans. Channa Newman and Claude Doubinsky. Nebraska: University of Nebraska Press, 1997.

Green, Michael. 'Nadine Gordimer's 'Future Histories': Two Senses of an Ending'. *Wasafiri*. 19 (9), 1994: 14–18.

Jamal, Ashraf. ''Africa's Appendix': Distortion, Forgery and Superfluity in a Southern Littoral'. Unpublished paper presented at Rhodes English Department Seminar. 2009. Amazwi South African Museum of Literature. 1–19.

Langdon, Gareth. 'Review: *Asylum*'. *Aerodrome: Words That Matter*. https://thiswasaerodrome. wordpress.com. Accessed on 16 February 2021.

Low, Marcus. *Asylum*. Johannesburg: Picador Africa, 2017

Meyer, Deon. *Fever*. Translated by K.L. Seegers. London: Hodder & Stoughton, 2017.

Moss, Stephen. 'Vaccine Vials and a Virtual Hug: A History of Coronavirus in 15 Objects'. *The Guardian*. https://www.theguardian.com. Accessed on 21 February 2021.

Prince, Gerald. 'Foreword'. In *Palimpsests: Literature in the Second Degree*. [1982] Trans. Channa Newman and Claude Doubinsky. Nebraska: University of Nebraska Press, 1997. ix–xi.

Ricard, Alain. 'Towards Silence: Thomas Mofolo, Small Literatures and Poor Translation'. *Tydskrif vir Letterkunde*. 53(2), 2016: 48–62.

Ricoeur, Paul. 'The Human Experience of Time and Narrative'. In *A Ricoeur Reader*. Edited by Mario J. Valdés. Hertfordshire: Harvester Wheatsheaf, 1991. 99–116.

Ricoeur, Paul. *Time and Narrative: Volume 3*. Chicago: University of Chicago Press, 1988.

Samuelson, Meg. 'Walking through the Door and Inhabiting the House: South African Literary Culture and Criticism after the Transition'. *English Studies in Africa*. 51(1), 2008: 130–7.

Schimke, Karin. 'Custody and Consultation: Karin Schimke talks to Marcus Low about His Debut Novel *Asylum*'. *The Sunday Times*. http://bookslive.co.za. Accessed on 16 February 2021.

Szczurek, Karina. 'Review: *Asylum* by Marcus Low'. *Karina Magdalena*. https:// karinamagdalena.com. Accessed on 16 February 2021.

Thurman, Chris. 'Places Elsewhere, Then and Now: Allegory 'Before' and 'After' South Africa's Transition?' *English Studies in Africa*. 53(1), 2010: 91–103.

Titlestad, Michael. 'Tales of White Unrest: David Medalie's *The Mistress's Dog: Short Stories 1996–2010*'. *English Studies in Africa*. 53(1), 2010: 118–21.

Todorov, Tzvetan. *Mikhail Bakhtin: The Dialogical Principle*. Translated by Wlad Godzich. Minneapolis: University of Minnesota Press, 1984.

Verthuy, Maïr. Review '*The African Palimpsest: Indigenization of Language in the West African Europhone Novel*'. *Traduire La Théorie*. 4(2): 1991, 207–10.

Zabus, Chantal. *The African Palimpsest: Indigenization of Language in the West African Europhone Novel*. Amsterdam: Rodopi, 2007.

HERO

David Medalie

They have not lived together for almost forty years. Now, with the lockdown in place, they pool their isolation.

'Don't you think we should see this out together?' asks Eileen.

'I'm not leaving my flat,' says Vanessa. 'Everything is set up for me here.'

'Then perhaps I should come and stay with you?'

'Ok. I'll get the spare room ready.'

In the mornings and early afternoons Vanessa works online. She has the kind of computer which she speaks into, and which then turns her words into documents. 'It's called speech-to-text,' she explains.

Eileen does a little dusting and cleaning, but she's not permitted to do much.

'You're 83 years old,' Vanessa says to her.

'But there's nothing wrong with me,' replies Eileen.

'Nevertheless.'

Vanessa has a way of terminating conversations with a single word.

At first Eileen speaks on the phone to several friends every day, then the calls dwindle to only one or two. No one has any news and talking about the pandemic makes everyone gloomier. The platitudes grow ever more threadbare.

It makes one feel so helpless.

It's out of our hands.

When will it ever end?

Who would ever have imagined?

Eileen has the expected responses ready.

It does.

It is.

No one can say.

No one could.

'What's it like staying with Vanessa?' they ask.

'It's great. She's made me so welcome.'

'She's my hero,' enthuses one (who hasn't seen Vanessa since she was a child).

'She's extraordinary,' others say.

'She's a remarkable person. I'm so proud of her,' Eileen replies. 'Any mother would be.'

Vanessa is and has always been *extraordinary*.

But she's also extraordinarily stubborn. She can be abrasive. And now, in the time of plague, she isn't easy to live with.

she's my hero

Eileen thinks about it. Is Vanessa a hero? Heroes these days are as common as flies at a braai. The concept of heroism has been so diluted that it's hard to say what it means. It seems to be an offshoot of fame. And fame has become a very odd creature. People are famous now simply for being famous. You don't have to *do* anything. You announce yourself. You acquire followers. You become a household name. Before long you're a *legend*; you're a *hero*. Millions buy the clothes and cosmetics and perfume you endorse, mouth the same hand-me-down opinions. You become stinking rich. They try to *keep up with you.*

Eileen knows that Vanessa doesn't think of herself as a hero. She does what she has to do, moving at speed from room to room on her motorized scooter, lifting things, even heavy pots and pans, with her left hand, balancing them with the stump of the right arm. She cleans the flat efficiently, even wielding a small vacuum-cleaner from her scooter. She has lived in her home for years and has mastery over every inch of it. 'That doesn't go there,' she says to Eileen. 'I won't be able to reach it if you put it there.'

'Sorry,' says Eileen. 'I'm just trying to help.'

She should have known better. Vanessa has never asked for help from anyone. Her heroism – if that's what it is – has been cast in the forge of her daily life, where every task accomplished becomes an iron feat. It's a creature formed of necessity, thick-skulled and taciturn, filled with a determination nothing and no one can gainsay. But it's not pliable; it's not gentle. Eileen wishes that it were.

She's more than a little afraid of her daughter.

They watch TV together in the early evening, mostly the news. The President talks about social distancing, handwashing. He struggles to put his face mask on.

Vanessa has hot chocolate every night, which she drinks out of a chipped yellow mug adorned with faded kittens. Eileen cannot remember giving it to her and wonders where it comes from. It's a strangely childish object – and the drinking of the hot chocolate itself an unexpectedly child-like ritual – in one so unsentimental.

Sometimes they discuss the pandemic. Vanessa has done research and is well informed. She doesn't hesitate to correct her mother. 'Coronavirus is the virus,' she explains to Eileen. 'COVID-19 is the illness it causes. It's not the same thing.'

'Ah, I see.' Eileen wishes Vanessa would call her 'Mom,' but she never does. When she speaks to colleagues on the phone or on Zoom she says, 'Eileen is staying with me for the lockdown.'

'The evenings are getting cold.' Eileen shivers.

'I've got a throw in my room. You can drape it over you,' says Vanessa. She begins to lift herself out of the chair and onto the scooter.

'I'll go,' says Eileen. 'Just tell me where it is.'

Vanessa hesitates, then lowers herself into the chair again. 'It's in the bottom drawer of the chest of drawers. It's dark blue.'

Vanessa has a Degas print on the wall of her bedroom. It features a ballet dancer, stretching at the barre. She's wholly absorbed in the act of keeping her slender yet powerful leg in a precise position. Degas was so good at capturing movement, but this is a study in motionlessness. He has transformed the dancer into a still life: a flower forever unfurling.

There are no framed or displayed photographs, in this room or anywhere else in the flat, not even of Bob. Vanessa loved her father and he loved her – *my plucky girl* he called her – and she was distraught when he died, two weeks after her seventeenth birthday. At the funeral she wept bitterly, pushing people away when they tried to hug her. Eileen would have expected to see a photo of Bob on the bedside table. But there's nothing.

She finds the throw in the bottom drawer, where Vanessa said it would be. As she lifts it out a sheet of paper falls to the floor. She unfolds it. It's a photograph – more accurately, a photocopy of a photograph – of two people, a man and a woman. It's in black and white. The man she can see at once is John F. Kennedy. His smile is broad and toothy. But who is the woman? She stands next to the president, her arms lowered in front of her, clutching a handbag.

The photo must be important to Vanessa – why else would she have made the photocopy? Eileen has an idea that if she knew the answer it would tell her something about this closed-off daughter of hers, so fierce in maintaining the moat of her solitariness.

That night she struggles to sleep. She hears Vanessa moving around in her room, then there is silence. Living with her during this precarious time has renewed her admiration for her, but it has also made her feel a sorrow she has not allowed herself to indulge in before. She has never dared to pity Vanessa – and she doesn't pity her now. But the resourcefulness and independence she witnesses every day, the very qualities in her daughter that so many applaud, bring tears to her eyes. She grieves the fact that Vanessa is not grieving the loss of contact with people which the new regime of the pandemic has imposed. She's not longing for hugs; for the clasp of a hand. She and Eileen could touch each other – they are, after all, in lockdown together – but they never do. Vanessa, she realizes, is phlegmatic about isolation because isolation is habitual to her. It's an old and doughty companion. The imposed seclusion barely touches her because she has for years – for decades – led a sundered life. Oh, the pathos of it: to go into lockdown and to find that nothing changes.

Her thoughts return to the photocopy. Perhaps the woman in the photograph is receiving an award of some sort from the president? Yes, that might be it. But who is she? And why?

The next morning she trawls the internet, looking up information about President Kennedy: she begins by searching for people honoured by him and then, narrowing it down, women honoured by him. She doesn't find the photograph itself, but she finds other photos of the same awards ceremony. She knows now who it is.

Vanessa, it seems, may not be immune to heroism after all.

Dr Frances Oldham Kelsey, a physician and scientist whose name would forever be linked to the history of teratogens – drugs that cause birth defects – received the President's Award for Distinguished Federal Civilian Service from President Kennedy in August 1962. Decades later, in June 2015, shortly before her death at the age of 101, Canada, the country of her birth, conferred on her the Order of Canada. From the early 1960s onwards the word 'heroine' began to attach itself to her. Morton Mintz, writing in 1962 in the *Washington Post*, called her the 'heroine' of the Food and Drug Administration, who kept a 'bad drug' off the market, adding that Dr Kelsey 'prevented … the birth of hundreds or indeed thousands of armless and legless children.'

Despite considerable pressure from the manufacturer, Richardson-Merrell, Dr Kelsey refused to authorise the use of Kevadon, the trade name for Thalidomide. It was approved in Canada and more than twenty other countries, but never in the US. As a result, fewer than twenty Thalidomide children were born in the United States, while thousands were born elsewhere.

Eileen knows something of this story but not all the details. She reads several articles. What moves her more than anything is a comment made by a Canadian Thalidomide victim, who, when Dr Kelsey received the Order of Canada, said, 'To us, she was always our heroine, even if what she did was in another country.'

always our heroine, even if what she did was in another country

She did not save me, the woman was saying, yet I honour her.

Is the photo in the bottom drawer Vanessa's way of saying the same thing?

Eileen wants to talk about this to Vanessa, but how to broach the subject? They have so seldom spoken about Thalidomide, even though it has been central to both their lives. Eileen has lived for almost sixty years with guilt. It's something jagged that lies deep within her, splintering her heart anew every day of her life.

Vanessa has never blamed her. When Eileen once apologized to her, she waved the apology away.

'You're being silly,' she said. 'There's no point apologizing. You didn't know.'

'But it was my fault. I did it to you. Whether I knew or not. All because I wanted to get rid of the morning sickness. I am culpable.'

She tried to explain to Vanessa how bad the morning sickness was. It was the worst kind – *hyperemesis gravidarum*. She needed her to understand how desperate she was; how it wasn't just queasiness. She would vomit until there was nothing left to bring up; and then she'd vomit again, a dry retching which seemed to lacerate her throat. There were days when she couldn't get out of bed. She'd lie there groaning while Bob, reluctant to leave her but needing to go to the London Hospital, where he was doing his internship, hovered helplessly over her.

And with guilt there is regret. *If only* Bob hadn't gone to London to study further. *If only* they'd remained in South Africa, which recorded almost no Thalidomide cases. *If only* they hadn't been in the UK when Vanessa was conceived and born. *If only* she hadn't gone to that GP – the one who had rooms off Whitechapel Road, and who looked like a ferret. *If only* he had not told her of the new wonder drug for morning sickness, of how grateful his patients were to him for prescribing it …

'The culpability doesn't lie with you,' Vanessa had said. She mulled over it as if it were an abstract philosophical problem. 'It follows, therefore, that your guilt has no validity.'

This evening she feels the need to talk to Vanessa about it again. Perhaps it's because of the pandemic which is sweeping across the world. Plagues speak to plagues, they link cadaverous hands across decades and even centuries; comparisons are constantly being made between COVID-19 and the Black Death, the Spanish flu. The Thalidomide babies were not the result of a pandemic, a virus or an infection. But for those affected, it felt like a plague, biblical in its cruelty.

Vanessa was born in 1961 in the London Hospital. Eileen remembers Bob's stricken face. 'Oh, my God,' he said. 'Look at her, Eileen. Oh, God. What kind of life will she have? What place will there ever be for her?'

She wants to ask Vanessa about the photograph; about what Dr Kelsey means in her life. But how to raise the subject?

She thinks of an angle.

'I read something interesting,' she says. 'Did you know that Thalidomide is now given to cancer patients?'

'Yes. I know.' Vanessa takes a sip from the kitten mug.

'Strange to think that something so destructive is now being used to help people.'

'Yes.'

They fall silent. Eileen doesn't know how to move from this to talking about Dr Kelsey.

She looks at Vanessa, who sits beneath a curved wooden lamp. No other light is on; all four corners of the living-room are dipped in shadow. This gives the lamp a solicitous air as it arches over her. In stark light the lack of proportion in her body cannot be avoided – the full-sized head and torso contrasting with the tiny or absent limbs. But now the lamplight warms, softens, reconciles.

The scene is as still and quiet, in its own way, as the Degas print.

She wishes Bob were here to see this; to share this view of Vanessa, the shape of her mollified by the light. She longs for him to know what has become of their daughter, almost sixty years after her birth in London, fifty-eight years after they returned to South Africa. Vanessa owns her own flat. She has a degree. She has a job. She asks nothing from anyone. 'Your plucky girl *has* a life,' she would like to say to Bob. 'She *has* a place. It's not the life we might have wished for our child. At times it makes me weep. But it is worthy of respect.'

Vanessa breaks the silence. She herself brings Dr Kelsey into the conversation.

'When Dr Kelsey blocked Thalidomide, she could never have foreseen it would become a cancer drug one day. All she knew was that not enough testing had been done to ensure that it was safe. And so she dug her heels in.' She turns to look at Eileen. 'You know who Dr Kelsey was?'

'Yes, I do.'

'She saved thousands of babies. In America.'

'I know.'

Eileen hears again the voice of the Canadian victim. The words gather in the distance, draw closer, trail away.

always our heroine, even if what she did was in another country

'She was a hero,' says Eileen, eager to see how Vanessa will respond.

Vanessa takes a last sip of the hot chocolate and puts the mug down. 'I suppose it depends on what you consider a hero to be. These days every Tom, Dick and Harry is called a hero.'

'What does it mean to you?'

'Well, it must be someone who doesn't … who isn't swayed by anyone or anything.'

Eileen finds this very revealing. 'Interesting,' she says. 'Well, that does describe Dr Kelsey. She stood her ground.'

'And you?' asks Vanessa. 'What do you think a hero is?'

She pauses before she answers. 'I think a hero is someone who does something for the wider society. Brings people together. Provides wise leadership.'

'That's not how I would define it,' Vanessa says, adding, 'although to some extent that describes Dr Kelsey too.'

'Yes, it does.'

Eileen feels that something important has been discovered. It lies in the cleft of the two diverging conceptions: on the one hand, the hero as a lonely trailblazer, a soaring eagle spirit; on the other, the weaver of an intricate tapestry of consensus.

'Wise leadership,' says Vanessa. 'That's in short supply these days. There are lousy leaders aplenty but very few good ones. Just when we need them most. When the whole world is in crisis.'

'I couldn't agree more. It's one of the main reasons we're in such bad shape.'

Vanessa nods.

'And I hate to see some of the medical experts kowtowing to these awful leaders.'

'Oh, me too.' Vanessa is unusually animated. 'I can't bear it.'

'Dr Kelsey would have stood up to them.'

'I'm sure she would have.'

They're in full agreement. Eileen savours it. It doesn't happen often. She decides to push things a little further. 'Some people,' she says, 'describe *you* as a hero.'

'Do they? I hope you disabuse them of that notion.'

'I try. It isn't easy.'

'Just tell them that after being in lockdown with me, you know better.'

Eileen reaches for the remote to switch the TV on. It's almost time for the news. 'Yes,' she says. 'I know better.'

Dust Explodes for All to See: Narrating the Actual in a Time of Continuous Disaster

Kyle Allan

On 31 December 2019, scientists announced to the world the discovery of a new strain of coronavirus, COVID-19, in the city of Wuhan, China. COVID-19 soon spread globally, and by March had been declared a pandemic by the World Health Organization. In that same month, South Africa began a nationwide lockdown, which was divided into various stages, implemented according to the severity of the pandemic and its potential to cause extreme and rapid loss of life, particularly among South Africa's vulnerable populations. The impact of COVID-19 further exposed all the wounds and ruptures within contemporary society. Using the poetry of Mxolisi Nyezwa and Angifi Dladla as an analytical lens, this article critiques the distinction between a recognized state of disaster and the everyday state of violence in which the marginalized live and argues that the precarious are living in a state of continuous disaster. It recognizes the vitality and power of critique through literature that engages with the actuality of the present moment. Furthermore, it foregrounds the term 'the actual' as preferable to 'the real' or 'reality,' framed as those terms are by realist epistemologies and the heroic materialism of real capitalism.

On 31 December 2019, scientists announced to the world the discovery of a new strain of cor-onavirus, COVID-19, in the city of Wuhan, China. COVID-19 soon spread globally, and by March, had been declared a pandemic by the World Health Organization. In that same month, South African president, Cyril Ramaphosa, declared a National State of Disaster, anticipating a possible mass outbreak after local cases began to be reported. He followed this up with the announcement of a nationwide lockdown, which was divided into various alert levels that were accordingly implemented by government mandate depending upon the severity of the pandemic and its potential to cause extreme and rapid loss of life across South Africa's vulnerable populations. At the time of writing, March 2021, the death toll from COVID-19 in South Africa had passed the 50 000 mark. The fallout across different aspects of society included mass business closures, increased unemployment and massive strain on social infrastructure. What exacerbated this was the already fragile South African socio-economic context. However, it is worth noting that deaths from other major killers including HIV and TB continued during this period, and in the pre-COVID world, in 2016, according to the NICD and WHO estimates, 124 000 South Africans died from TB, of whom approximately 80% were HIV-positive. By contrast with the coverage most recently given to COVID-19, this catastrophic loss of approximately 330 people daily made very few headlines. In 2019, according to an Avert report, it was estimated that 72 000 South Africans suffered AIDS-related deaths.

Alongside the peaks of the global first wave of the COVID-19 outbreak, Black Lives Matter protests resumed with renewed strength in June 2020 as a response to the killing of George Floyd IV. The protests against yet another violent snuffing of a black life by the police soon spread, exceeding the reach and militancy of previous demonstrations and within days BLM had become a global movement. The image of George Floyd IV achieved iconic status. Echoing in many respects South Africa's Rhodes Must Fall movement, protesters across the United States, the United Kingdom and parts of Europe toppled or defaced statues of individuals who were associated with racism or colonialism. The protests briefly rendered the invisible or unseen intensely visible. The statues, once looked upon as unquestioned symbols or background features in social environments, had become visible as stark markers of oppression.

A resonant question emerges from this social upheaval: what does it take for us to recognize the state of disaster that we live in and oppose it effectively? How do we articulate the experience and reality of the everyday state of violence in which oppressed groups and individuals live; a submerged violence, seldom acknowledged, which affects deeply both individual lives and the polity? What, in this state of violence and precarity, can be defined as the real, or the actual? What form of truth, if any, exists across both the spectacular and the mundane? What is the role of a writer given these fluxes of uncertainty? Crucially, how do we guard against the limitations of critiques that are occasioned by the infrequent eruptions of large-scale protest and passionate challenge?

Mass and social media enable intense visibility of both modern protest movements and scenes of disaster; they also obfuscate their abiding causes and the scars they leave. Both mass and social media are more focused on the spectacular scenes of disaster and protest than they are committed to rigorous investigation and the rooted articulation of issues. And if the spectacular is recurrent, in depth, contextualized reporting recedes further into the background. After a while, news reporters and the public lose interest in additional victims, mounting casualties and waves of explosive protest – and so the hegemony they denounce remains unaddressed and unchanged. A critique that dwells only on the spectacular, or immediately immanent aspects of a scene or site of disaster, will not expose the graininess of 'what is'; it will fail to appreciate and represent the structural causes of oppression and inequality. Yet the reality for marginalized people is that oppression and suffering continue unabated, whether they are broadcast or not, whether they are given a catchy hashtag or not, whether they are photographed or remain unseen.

This essay highlights writing that foregrounds the slow death and slow violence that are irreducible but are non-events as far as the media is concerned. It recognizes literature that engages with the actuality of the present moment, which foregrounds the catastrophic effects of contemporary capitalism, yet defamiliarizes experience and its context by signifying an embodied response to oppression that topples the metaphoric statues of cliché and spectacle, revealing the otherwise invisible ideological structures of oppression. In this literature, slow and continuous disasters, which are frequently occluded and relegated to background noise, are revealed in all their violent immediacy.

Power in the 21st century is increasingly virtual, technocratic and intangible. Ideological – that is routine, ideational, disembodied – content only echoes hegemony. It cannot subvert oppressive systems and mechanisms, nor does it challenge the conspicuous consumption of the visual that is central in the formation of social consciousness. Yet an appeal to the visceral risks sensationalism: we quickly move from one image of violation to another, captivated, yet neglecting the structures of meaning of which violence is merely a symptom. A third mode of representation is what we might call 'dry realism': realism based upon direct reportage without promoting an awareness of underlying structures of meaning or causality. This is writing that seeks to duplicate surfaces and appearances.

Mxolisi Nyezwa and Angifi Dladla are poets who have distinct aesthetic approaches. Rather than dry realism or lapsing into sensationalism, their work develops a resonant sense of reality through using a range of poetic modes, even encompassing at times surrealism. Their poetics turns on defamiliarization, countering conventional representations, stock phrases and ideological cliché. Theirs is an intensely lyrical critique of socio-political realities that simultaneously exposes superficial readings of the contemporary. They reach beneath the conventional and ordinary to foreground the lived realities of subalternity.

Stark Ontologies

Angifi Dladla was born in 1950 and died in October 2020. He published two English-language books of poetry, *The Girl Who Then Feared to Sleep and Other Poems* (2001) and *Lament for Kofifi Macu* (2018). He also wrote plays and published *Uhambo*, a collection of isiZulu poems. He passionately believed poetry writing could be taught and he was director of the Femba Writing Project. Mxolisi Nyezwa was born in 1967 and has published three books of poetry: *Song Trials* (2000), *New Country* (2008) and *Malikhanye* (2012). He has also been the editor of *Kotaz* magazine since the 1990s. Dladla and Nyezwa belong to a group of poets who experimented with similar poetic commitments, most of whom were featured in *New Coin* poetry magazine during the 1990s, when it was under the editorship of Robert Berold. These poets have been described as

> ... the Poets of No Sure Place. This label represents the 'sense of imbalance and infinite disquiet in their poems' (Nyezwa, Message to Tom Penfold' n.p.) while simultaneously speaking of their innovation and different backgrounds. There is a united sense of apprehension and instability; a feeling that each poet is refusing to be publicly subservient while simultaneously working through their own personal dilemmas and grievances; a message of radical insecurity coupled with a call to rediscover the 'simple values' (Ramakuela 34) of life and in ourselves as individuals. (Penfold, 'No Sure Place' 505)

In various ways, these poets critiqued the inconsistencies, contradictions and entanglements of South African society, merging personal and political reflections, with *New Coin* as their primary forum. In fact, Robert Berold was inspired to co-found Deep South press in 1995 after realizing that most publishing houses were not prepared to take risks on the type of poetry that appeared in the journal, nor did these publishers have an understanding or appreciation of the new aesthetics at play. Both of Dladla's books and Nyezwa's *Malikhanye* were published by Deep South. Earlier versions of several of the poems in their volumes were previously featured in *New Coin*.

In these poets' work, form is dynamically shifted and tailored, and the content reflects the realities of South Africa. For Dladla,[1] poems such as 'the stubborn death' (15), 'so turned a taxi' (32), 'the dead' (68) and 'the building, the weapon and the way' (79), among others, capture moments of stasis (as opposed to the hegemonic notion of transition), continuous slow death and violence, as well as the ideological obfuscation of the real issues by the elite. For Nyezwa, poems such as 'things change' (*song trials*), 'it all begins' (also *song trials*) and 'the road ahead' (*Malikhanye*) evoke the uncertainty of, and ruptures within, existence, the slow death of the present moment, the stark ontology of oppressed life and the cruel optimism of tenuous futures. Yet there are also intimations of beauty and tremors of hope. Their poetry recognizes the 'ontological terror' (Warren 2018) of non-subjects who find themselves oppressed by socio-economic, racial and gender hegemony, which they subvert by elaborating an alternative aesthetics and engaging thematic concerns which subvert the structures of discrimination and bear witness to inequality and suffering.

> I like to think of my poetry as reflecting the dismal nature of politics and individual existence in the modern society, a reflection on greed and how capitalism and the financial system have devastated people's lives and cultures without shame. Poetry that identifies this kind of aggression, which is really driven by financial interests as the basis for corruption against human beings, must necessarily be bleak. The poetry must in turn invoke its unique form, impact the usual language extraordinarily, enmeshing flowers, human lives and global manifestations. In so many ways poets are writing to change the world. (Nyezwa 2012)

Both writers critique the economic status quo and highlight the emotional effects it has on those forced into the machine. Capitalism, as initially conceived by Marx and elaborated by Althusser and Adorno, entrances subjects through its glorification of production, consumption, entertainment and by inculcating a spirit of heroic materialism combined with love for the spectacular. This romanticism obscures the brutality of capitalism by overlooking 'slow death' (Berlant 2011), 'slow violence' (Nixon 2011) and promoting 'cruel optimism' (Berlant 2011). It encourages 'lifestyles' that can never be achieved and fosters desires that can never be fulfilled, or, if they can be, it is at too high a price. Furthermore, capitalism occludes its continual destruction of ecologies and the steady erosion of human freedoms in an increasingly technocratic world. Phrases such as the 'creative industry' and 'the production of knowledge' are cultural markers of this romantic capitalism. 'Outputs' are audited and evaluated in universities and by funding agencies, and utilitarianism and 'relevance' hang over the heads of intellectuals and artists like a sword of Damocles. All is about 'consumption' and 'incentives'. By contrast, Nyezwa and Dladla undermine the romanticization and ethos of capitalist life, stripping its various manifestations in lines of verse that cut across its logic and assumptions. This includes critiquing the complexes of production that dominate life spaces, turning them into death worlds:

> all i can make of my country
> is a sulphurous compound

a black room with two gigantic stars
as thoroughly silent as corpses (Nyezwa 10–13)

Spaces of consumption are predicated on class and racial power, as we see in Dladla's nightmarish depiction of the proliferation of malls, marked as they are by names designating geographical
cardinal points, and ending with the suffix of '-gate' (arguably connoting the gates of socio-economic power). They are described as bunkers whose escalators indicate not mobility but

phantasmagoria – whites
of all ages in all seasons
from sunrise to sunrise
with their apprentices
eat and eat and eat ... (Dladla, 'from sunrise' 9–13)[2]

And the arenas of entertainment, such as the literal physical places in the eponymous tavern in
'images from mamyang-chaza's tavern' (Dladla 50–54), are sites in which self-delusion and
psychological submission are apparent in a variety of forms. Bacchic behaviour only replicates
the damaged state of consciousness immanent in the political matrix of the continent, as the
tavern goers 'relax in prides / as if they are lions,' but end up being defeated in their dance
moves that put them,

on their knees, bellies
and backs - a classic
conquest and humiliation
as if they are africa (80–83)

Dladla even turns his eye towards the virtual plazas of amusement, evoking a haunting image of
fame transformed into delusory seduction by red carpets rendered as the audible 'sloshing on the
red / carpet of blood' (66–67) depicted in the poem 'in this world' (Dladla 75–77).

    Furthermore, both Nyezwa and Dladla expose the hypocrisies and contradictions of the
powerful, 'the real funders / of lies, germs and genocides' (Dladla, 'tomorrow' 21–22), depict
consumers as the living dead (Dladla, 'the dead' 68) and oppose the superficiality of intellec-
tualism (see Nyezwa, 'i want to be a university lecturer' 20). Their imagery punctures the
false consciousness of a supposedly liberated cognitariat (see Dladla, 'the building, the
weapon and the way' 79) and critiques romantic and liberal clichés used in representations of
the natural world. Whirlwinds, violent forces of nature and fire are used frequently in
Nyezwa's poetry, apocalyptic images that capture the travail and suffering of the precariat.

    Nyezwa and Dladla undermine a key aspect of romantic capitalism: the superficial materi-
alistic optimism that is manifest across society. They are aware of the cruel optimism of contemporary liberal democracy; the false hope constructed in the interests of capitalism, which in turn
shapes the prevailing constructs of race, gender and class – which serve the means of production
and mass consumption. These ontological underpinnings of romanticized capitalism, especially
as they prop up hegemony, are not simply critiqued; both poets present alternative ways of
feeling, thinking, acting and reacting. In addition to adopting a fatalistic tone in much of his
lyrical work, Nyezwa expresses his acceptance of the precarity of life and even depicts his
ecstatic embrace of vulnerability as he opens himself to the world:

but here there are only butterflies
only poles
which lack elasticity
skies
with bloodstains ('the sleepless world' 76–80)

Dladla observes bodies that are beset by fears, desires, multiple intentions, ambiguous identities, spiritual connections, childish souls and ancestors, and rejects the illusory abstract notions of self and secure individuality that are promoted by romantic capitalism. He foregrounds the dead in his verse, countering the understanding that they are no longer with us.

There is a particular focus on the casualties of history, with victims of apartheid and post-apartheid violence in poems such as 'morning after hiding' (24), where the intimate scene of a bedroom becomes an interior landscape of brutal assault, or, in 'impression' (22), in which, in the chaos of violence, a narrator sees someone who, once human, has become an

outsize
black wound
in the earth
where the tyre has nailed him,
human gravy in the sun ... (Dladla 4–8)

The phrase 'gravy in the sun' suggests that human subjects are consumable, trapped as they are within the dynamics of biopower and disposed of in the logic of 'necropolitics' (Mbembe 2019). Dladla notes the wide litany of casualties from contemporary forms of socio-economic violence, including, in 'so turned a taxi' (32), a chilling homage to the appalling death tolls from road accidents:

so turned a taxi
into a lightning bird
warming up,
but whirled in volumed flames
for failing to fly

we would later encounter
an unidentified object;
fused iron and bones. (1–8)

Aside from the shocking image of the traumatic dismemberment of people in a brutal accident, the poem also represents the most violent aspects of capitalism. Under prevailing neoliberal capitalism, the socio-economic sphere has become no more than the deadly trafficking of subjects – across which they 'fly' – in the interests of the elite. In the course of this coercive journeying, the system fails them; they are mutilated into 'unidentified objects[s],' distorted and compressed out of shape, becoming nothing more than 'fused iron and bones'. To use Cohen's trope (2012), they are reduced to the condition of the living-dead, the zombified, a drastically evacuated state of being. The 'social control complex' (Johnson 82) reduces these precarious, violated subjects to anthropological objects that are daily 'exhumed / for reburial' (Dladla, 'the dead' 3–4) and 'hunt, eat, drink and / ask extempore,' yet are carefully kept out of sight by the elite.

What stops Dladla's witnessing of violence from being simply a brutal litany of horror is the spiritual and emotional practice at the heart of his craft. With a keen interest in the application of *ku femba* healing to poetry, Dladla's poems can be conceived as analogous to that practice of channelling power to ward off 'evil spells in a society bedevilled by violence' (Bila and Abodunrin 1). His chant-like poems reflect more that the superficial witnessing of history; they represent a layered and integrated 'search for the essence of things' (Metelerkamp 76). Seeing beneath the surface of things is integral to the poetry of Nyezwa and Dladla; their gazes pierce the ordinary and familiar to represent the deep-seated pain of the marginalized. Their poetry's apparent simplicity drills through the superficial towards the heart of the matter.

> and inside each hemisphere
> in each visible landscape
> there is something immense
> solid to the eye –
> anguish, more anguish ('from a blue container in Motherwell' 25–30)

What is this clouded anguish, this reality only partially visible, partly intangible, that is simultaneously blatant and surreal? Further, how do these poems, written before the advent of the COVID-19 pandemic, relate to the present? Nyezwa in his epigraph to *Malikhanye* offers insight:

> sometimes there is just us, nobody else
> no bread, no language, no nothing.
> sometimes we lose ourselves over nothing
> haunted by the life we never had. (1–4)

These lines express ontological terror. They acknowledge the sense of non-being experienced by marginalized groups, capturing a haunted, crippled state of existence in which subalterns are prevented from 'becoming'. When originally published, 'sometimes there is just us, nobody else' spoke to a sense of psychic isolation, socio-political abandonment and the existential crisis of those experiencing marginalization and living precariously. Now it resonates with our reality of social distancing and self-isolation and the loneliness to which they have given rise. Similarly, 'no bread, no language, no nothing,' which concerns poverty, both literal and intellectual, and the failure of language (poetic or otherwise) to critique the structures underlying oppression, now aggregates new meanings: COVID-19 has impacted the vulnerable members of society disproportionately. They have suffered job losses (on top of obscene unemployment figures before the pandemic) and have been reduced to standing in food queues – 'no bread' – kilometres long, which have replaced the social connections that formerly achieved some measure of social cohesion. The present has also starved the marginalized of a language in which to express their suffering, not only because they have been forced apart by lockdown and distancing, but also because a new enervating disaster has simply been added to the perpetual disasters of poverty and alienation. The experience of subalternity that Nyezwa and Dladla set out to capture has been exacerbated in the present; new suffering simply added to the old. An, yet again, political promises have been hollow. Nyezwa's 'haunted by the life we never had' explores the cruel optimism of post-apartheid democratic life, suggesting that, for all the utopian rhetoric post-1994, reality did not improve for the precariat. The poem points towards their stunted or non-existent futures. The far-reaching socio-politico-economic and psychological repercussions of COVID-19 have further cauterized optimism since individual and social futures are now even more vexed and uncertain.

A Ghostly Black-and-White Tracing of the Invisible / What Do We Really See?

and during the many storms in my life
what happened?
what really happened?
during those nights
what did I really see? (Nyezwa, 14–18)

Branded as 'our "invisible enemy": a nightmarish, oneiric force that can't be seen, heard, or touched' (Frumkin 2020), COVID-19 is the ultimate example of what Slavoj Žižek describes as a 21st-century antagonist, whose essence is unseen (except microscopically) and yet with manifestations everywhere. This faceless enemy exerts force somewhere between the virtual and the actual, between the intangible and the tangible, its impact transforming slow disasters of the capitalocene into catastrophic crises, into blatantly visible disasters.

Information about the coronavirus and public mobilization have depended on visual representations of the invisible – the virus itself, vectors of infection, dangers of contagion, bodily affliction. CDC illustrations use colour schemes to capture attention and encourage preventative behaviours. Yet, apart from the mask, the icon of the pandemic is doubtlessly the image of a ball with crown-like (protein) spikes emanating from it. However, the use of x-ray crystallography generates another picture of the virus, one not so colourful but which yet has affective import. 'The process, in which the crystalline structure of the virion causes a beam of X-rays to diffract in many directions, allows researchers to construct an image of the molecule. The result is a ghostly black-and-white tracing of the invisible' (Frumkin 2020).

I have previously reflected that,

[m]uch as X-ray crystallography reveals a 'ghostly black-and-white tracing of the invisible,' so the contemporary writer strains to reveal even the invisible building blocks of reality; the seemingly intangible that hovers over a scene, changes everything, shifts names and identities, forges memories, changes fictions, loops and tangles narratives. (Allan, 'Editorial' 5)

The analogy suggests that writers who engage with – and are truly aware of – the spectrality of the past and the pervasiveness of contemporary oppression, recognize the priority of both 'the Event' and the longer history of ruptured time and slow death. Their texts construct a space in which written words are a 'black-and-white tracing of the invisible,' outlining the roots of power, the causes of conspicuous events, the energy and narrative undergirding appearances. They challenge the dominant myths of our time yet also tell alternative stories. They focus not only on what is trending and considered relevant, but also on what has been forgotten, buried or is even relegated to the categories of the 'disconcerting' and the 'uncanny'. They highlight the contradictions between appearance and reality, between cause and symptom. Through the use of foregrounding, defamiliarization and irony, these writers are able to reveal the disparity between the appearance of society in its various forms (the spectacular, the superficial and concealed ideological structures) and the essence of that society (degradation, oppression, divisiveness, discrimination). They strip the veil of familiarity from the world, leading us to discern the concealed, underlying real – which in the case of Nyezwa and Dladla is a materialist, historicized reality.

In 'granny's last lectures' (73), Dladla shares three life lessons taught by a grandmother to a younger person. The third of the lessons, subtitled 'on hell,' describes the implosion of heroes, in a way that evokes the collapse of a building:

> hear! echoing a storied-
> building, heroes, child
> of my child, implode.
> but dust, oh child
> of my child, explodes
> for the world to see ... (38–43)

Dladla skilfully moves away from criticizing individuals, which is the easier turn, and instead leads the reader towards broader contexts. Heroes are compared to a 'storied- / building,' which has a double meaning: a building with many floors, as well as a building that is heavily laden with stories and histories. Heroes fall, not only because of their own weaknesses or deficiencies, but under the pressure of the burden of (endlessly narrativized) history and systemic forces. But it is not simply the collapse of the building, but there is also 'the revelation of the previously unseen and the seemingly immaterial ... ; that within the body of the building, within the quotidian grains of dust there lies a deeper truth' (Allan, 'Witness' 118).

> Even the fall of the heroes does not reveal the vulnerability of individuals, but points to the frailty of all. In essence, the implosion is caused by a wilful denial of actuality which cannot be sustained. Dladla's 'sense of depth' (Penfold, 'Black Consciousness' 230) enables the reader to perceive the deeper truth(s). (Allan, 'Tribute' 104)

What are these deeper truths? Part of the truth is that the building was already unstable (like the edifice of South African society prior to COVID-19) weighed down as it was by socio-politico-economic fractures. Any additional pressure inevitably causes its collapse. The stress that fractures the structures is not only experienced passively; it is not only that to which the precariat is subjected. Political, socio-economic and spiritual ruptures in material and ideological infrastructure are leading increasingly to a struggle for decolonization and restitution. The building is coming down because of its own contradictions – but the vulnerable and exploited are also hastening its implosion by mobilizing around historical fractures.

Yet the dust of a collapsing building also obfuscates: if one visualizes the immediate after-effect of a building collapse, one imagines the dust cloud swirling in the wind, dense in places, more dispersed in others. Perhaps this is part of the truth: it swirls, flows, dissipates, gathers as particles are blown about on the winds of social change. The collapse of the building, a seemingly stable structure, lets loose the constitutive grains of dust. The implosion makes intensely visible both the tenuousness of society and the truths it has recuperated in its design and construction. Destruction and revelation are contiguous – as edifices collapse, the causes of the (inevitable and necessary) disaster are exposed.

And once the dust settles, what then?

> don't ask me about any of my poems
> for i will tell you that people are murdered in my country
> and their deaths arrive slowly as an illness
> as a desolate knock
> on a blank sky (Nyezwa, 'the road ahead' 1–5)

What does it say of a society that some have fought for the 'right' not to wear masks while vulnerable groups have suffered disproportionately from COVID-19 because they do not have access to PPE and vaccines and – given cramped living conditions – have been unable to self-isolate or socially distance? Ours is a society in which social geography was shaped by apartheid. Workers still live and work in different provinces, returning home in the holidays. As with TB and HIV, these movements have been vectors of COVID-19 infection. A population forced into migrancy and itinerancy inevitably spreads disease from one marginal population to another. Poverty – itself an affliction – becomes intrinsic to infection; disease, like wealth, is characterized by a steep gradient in South Africa, which is a patchwork of different societies that has always begged more questions than it provides answers.

> in every house where there lives a hurt child
> in every house where there is no future
> and men hang their misery on the wall
> in devastation
> at every turn they ask me
> *what do your poems speak to us?'* ('in every house' 1–6)

Nyenza dwells on this question in the 'Malikhanye' sequence of *Malikhanye*:

> i cannot understand
> why man exists
> and why things happen (1–3)

He immediately follows these lines with an image layered with presences:

> on the stairs i see
> someone is whispering
> the house is saying something
>
> on the stairs
> next to the wall
> something is written -
> someone is saying something (Nyezwa 4–10)

A close reading of these lines yields other layers of meaning. In the first of the two poems discussed above, the 'house' evokes and connotes pain, socio-economic precarity and the weight of history. In the second passage, not only does the line 'the house is saying something' refer to the present inhabitants, it also summons spectral voices from the past, perhaps ancestors or echoes from the organic world. The collapsing building was also a repository of individual and communal lives – a place of small lived experiences, families, communities, births, deaths, family gatherings, ordinary lives. While we incline to conceiving destruction as only loss – often apocalyptic disintegration – the collapse of structures also releases trapped voices and concealed experience. Even though these voices commonly express pain and suffering, stories of devastation and its causes can at least be heard; these wounds breathe life and truth into the present.

This relates to the question that is the title of the first poem, 'what do your poems speak to us?' The answer is possibly that they do not speak in comforting rhetoric or offer false solace, nor do they speak in the forms and flows of mass communication. Rather, they speak from a space that Unathi Slasha calls 'the Unlanguaged World,' 'a way of seeing, of reading, of creating, of criticizing the thing in the process of being created – of screaming, of faltering falling finding the voice of the dead' (2018). Nyezwa's 'the road ahead' might be read at face value as a poem about a poet's failure (there is another poem titled 'the poets failure' in *Song Trials*, which criticizes the failure of poets to articulate the contemporary moment). Interpretations should not be this categorical: 'failure' in this instance is staged to present the limits of signification, the 'unlanguaged' world that is concealed beneath or within the structures of familiar meaning. This is not a silent domain, though, but a space in which ancestral/spectral voices can be heard – whereby the hidden of history and being speak.

Actualizing/Reactualizing: Giving Substance to the Here and Now

Nyezwa and Dladla are both forthright about the evils of the world and their grievances. Yet they are not cynical voices, but writers who either offer hope or teach alternatives. As poets narrating actuality, they do not only make reality tangible but allow us to visualize the possibility of new and different things. This is key: analysis of, and opposition to, the structural causes of precarity exist alongside recognizing the potent energy of words. As Silvio Lorusso elaborates:

> The precarious condition is rooted in a series of virtualities that acquire more relevance than actuality. A plausible future and a romanticised past become more real than the lived present. The virtual dominates the real. If precarity is a ghost, a presage, an absence, or a void, maybe the way to break its spell is by reactualizing the present, by giving substance to the 'here and now'. (2017)

What is the 'here and now'? It is certainly not just the conspicuous world of 2021, a world of COVID-19 and the 'new normal'. It is also a world haunted and shaped by spectral legacies; a world shaped by the organic, a world of nature, floods, clouds, storms, earthquakes; a world of mass movements and hypnotic leaders; a world of trends and hashtags, Twitter and Facebook; it is a world shaped by dreams, visions, nightmares and hallucinations. To give substance to this here and now, to reactualize the present, is to employ a version of writing that embraces and evokes all of actuality, whether obvious or arcane, whether beautiful or painful. Instead of repressing the symptoms of reality, however horrifying they are, one must acknowledge them, traverse them. This entails acknowledging the past and its spectrality, without romanticizing or being overwhelmed by it. It means seeing alternative futures, rooted and centred in life's reality, rather than being lulled by optimism.

To give substance to the here and now is to foreground the marginalized aspects and occluded sights of our continuous state of disaster. The term 'foregrounding' originates from the Czech formalists, from the word *aktualisace*, which can be translated literally as (re)actua-lizing. By giving voice to the contemporary moment, to substance and scattered perceptions, sutures, wounds and pain, is how poetic language manifests the first intimations of possible change. This lyrical sensuousness is found in a poem such as 'to know you' (Nyezwa 32–37), which abounds in lucid imagery and stark juxtapositions while brushing up against precarious-ness and pessimism:

> i want to know you like a piece of joyous furniture
> like a desk
> or a swinging chair
> from one burnt out house
> to the next (25–30)
> …
> i want to find you in running water
> the way the poor drink cholera
> and tiny organisms
> from the earth
> which bring death
> and despair (36–41)

Giving substance to the here and now, these lines acknowledge that we are part of a spiritual-ecological world, made up of precarious and vulnerable lives. In contrast to the deluded opti-mism inculcated by capitalism, which leads to a steady brutalization of life and a destruction of meaning, this lucid and dynamic pessimism encourages open-mindedness, imagination, empathy and transcending binaries and capitalist ontology. This impulse is expressed most starkly and intimately in the 'Malikhanye' sequence in *Malikhanye*, where Nyezwa pays tribute to his son, Malikhanye Liyema Nyezwa, who died at the age of three months. In beautiful and simple yet layered lines, Nyezwa grieves in an outpouring of lyrical epiphanies that illumine life's precarity, and its entanglement within the contexts of socio-politico-economic hegemony. In the final poem of the sequence, Nyezwa concludes with impassioned questions:

> i want to know how the sea flows
> how the winds blow
> and how love is abandoned
> why things have to happen like this
> oh! so over and over again. (12–16)

Dladla also offers resonant philosophical reflections in the final poem from *the girl who then feared to sleep*, 'song of the aged' (80), which exists in perfect counterpoint to the opening poem, 'song of a fertility doll' (11). Aside from both being subtitled 'song[s],' they are con-nected in another way: they enunciate the two poles of existence: life and death. The poem enu-merates scenes of non-being, as experienced by an elderly person:

> where i used to live, i live no more
> dreams i used to dream, i dream no more

> friends i used to share with are no more
> stars i used to look up to are all gone (1–4)

The next six stanzas continue in a similar vein, chanting about all the lacks and losses that define the speaker's life. But the final stanza radically refocuses the poem's meaning:

> i've got nothing left now;
> but a bright star i hear far, far … .
> within. (25–27)

While the stanza starts with a negative summation, the next two lines foreground hope, as epitomized by the bright star. This suggests that amid all the scenes of loss and negation, there is energy that can offer hope and reactualize meaning. Within the inevitability of death, there is the potential force of life, and the certainty of rebirth, even if in a different form.

Nyezwa, in his ecstatic lyricism and ecological worldview, is consistently determined to depict the reality of society, and Dladla's humane and spiritually enmeshed critique of society, in different yet related ways, offers a vision of possibility. Each envisions an alternative way of living, bringing together the various, allegedly disparate, elements that comprise human-ecological life, which include the spiritual and the physical aspects of existence. Their poetry insists that crises such as we face now are acknowledged and understood, not as sudden troughs between waves, or ruptures and outbursts in a state of normality. Rather, we should understand them as the broader symptoms of the daily violence caused by dominating late-capitalist ideologies that ignore the actuality of things. Their aesthetics recognize that human beings are part of the broader organic world, even though we live under an illusion of self-sufficiency that is fostered by romantic capitalism. These complex connections are nothing to be afraid of; they bring a deeper rootedness to the very nature of being in the here and now, marked as it is by wounding and risk. From this awareness of the actuality of things, being cognizant of the power of words, that allows writers such as Nyezwa and Dladla not only to see the world as it is, but at the same time to reactualize it, to imagine new futures and prospects. In times of continuous disaster, such as our present, we need both.

Note

1   All references to Angifi Dladla's poems are from *The Girl Who Then Feared to Sleep* (2001). Nearly all references to Mxolisi Nyezwa's work are from *Malikhanye* (2011), barring a few that are specifically mentioned as being from *Song Trials* (2000) or *New Country* (2008).

Works Cited

Allan, Kyle. 'Editorial'. *New Coin* 56(1), 2020: 5.

Allan, Kyle. 'Tribute to Angifi Dladla'. *New Coin* 56(2), 2020: 102–9.

Allan, Kyle. 'Witness to Everything: Representations of Precarity in Selected Works of Four South African Poets'. MA thesis. U of KwaZulu-Natal, 2019.

Avert. 'HIV and AIDS in South Africa'.15 Apr. 2020. *Avert.* https://www.avert.org/professionals/hiv-around-world/sub-saharan-africa/south-africa. Accessed on 25 February 2021.

Bila, Vonani and Olufemi Abodunrin. 'Angifi Dladla (1950–2020): An Embodiment of *Ku Femba* as a Poetry Teaching Philosophy for Renewal'. *Education as Change* 24, 2020: 1–21.

Berlant, Lauren. *Cruel Optimism*. Durham, NC. Duke UP. 2011.

Cohen, Jeffrey Jerome. 'Undead (a Zombie Oriented Ontology)'. *Journal of the Fantastic in the Arts* 23(3), 2012: 397–412.

Dladla, Angifi. *The Girl Who Then Feared To Sleep, and Other Poems*. Cape Town: Deep South Publishing, 2001.

Dladla, Angifi. *Lament for Kofifi Macu*. Grahamstown: Deep South Publishing, 2018.

Dladla, Angifi. Interview by Joan Metelerkamp. *New Coin* 37(2), 2011: 62–75.

Fisher, Mark. *Capitalist Realism: Is There No Alternative?* Winchester: Zero Books, 2009.

Frumkin, Rebekah. 'How to Draw the Coronavirus'. 18 May 2020. *The Paris Review*. https://www.theparisreview.org/blog/2020/05/18/how-to-draw-the-coronavirus/. Accessed on 14 January 2021.

Havranek, Bohumil. 'Aktualisace'. *Dictionary of Standard Czech*. Prague: Nakladatelství české Akademie věd, 1960: 19.

Johnson, Cedric. 'The Panthers Can't Save Us Now'. *Catalyst* 1(1), 2017: 57–87.

Lorusso, Silvio. 'A Hauntology of Precarity'. 21 Feb. 2017. *Institute of Network Cultures*. https://networkcultures.org/entreprecariat. Accessed on 2 February 2021.

Mbembe, Achille. *Necropolitics*. Durham, NC: Duke UP, 2019.

National Institute of Communicable Diseases. 'World TB Day 2029'.13 Mar. 2019. *National Institute of Communicable Diseases*. https://www.nicd.ac.za/world-tb-day-2019/. Accessed on 14 February 2021.

Nixon, Rob. *Slow Violence and the Environmentalism of the Poor*. Cambridge, MA: Harvard UP, 2011.

Nyezwa, Mxolisi. *Malikhanye*. Grahamstown: Deep South, 2011.

Nyezwa, Mxolisi. Message to Tom Penfold. 2015.

Nyezwa, Mxolisi. Interview by Gary Cummiskey. 'Mxolisi Nyezwa: A New Dawn for Poetry'. 7 Jan. 2012. *The Dye Hard Interviews*. http://dyehardinterviews.blogspot.com/2012/01/mxolisi-nyezwa-new-dawn-for-poetry.html. Accessed on 14 January 2021.

Nyezwa, Mxolisi. *New Country*. Pietermaritzburg: UKZN P, 2008.

Nyezwa, Mxolisi. *Song Trials*. Pietermaritzburg: University of Natal Press, 2000.

Penfold, Tom. 'Black Consciousness and the Politics of Writing the Nation in South Africa'. Diss. U of Birmingham, 2013.

Penfold, Tom. 'Mxolisi Nyezwa's Poetry of No Sure Place'. *Social Dynamics: A Journal of African Studies* 42(3), 2015: 504–29.

Ramakuela, Ndahve. 'Stepping with Seitlhamo Motsapi: Direction for South African Poetry'. *English Studies in Africa* 40(2), 33–41.

Slasha, Unathi. 'Much with the Dead & Mum with the Dying, or: Rigidities of Rationalism, Camaraderie Criticism & Contemporary South African Literature'. 27 Jan. 2018. *Black Ghost Books*. http://blackghostbooks.co.za. Accessed on 11 January 2021.

Warren, Calvin. *Ontological Terror: Blackness, Nihilism and Emancipation*. Durham, NC: Duke UP, 2018.

Žižek, Slavoj. Welcome to the Desert of The Real!: Five Essays on September 11 and Related Dates. London: Verso, 2002.

Appendix of Poems

Due to the need for brevity and flow, I could not quote some of the poems in my essay at the length they deserve. The poems and key excerpts from selected poems appear here in the order they were discussed in this article.

Excerpt from 'from sunrise' (Dladla 1–13)

> at the malls
> eastgate, westgate,
> northgate, southgate, and
> all the gates,
> even imposing ones
> with glass complexes
> caved into mazy bunkers
> where escalators show
> phantasmagoria – whites
> of all ages in all seasons
> from sunrise to sunrise
> with their apprentices
> eat and eat and eat …

Excerpts from 'images from mamyang-chaza's tavern'

> there at the tavern,
> men and women
> of exotic status
> and nasal english
> relax in prides
> as if they are lions (31–36)

> there at the tavern,
> thorough and clear;
> on their knees, bellies
> and backs - a classic
> conquest and humiliation
> as if they are africa (79–84)

Excerpts from 'in this world' (Dladla 59–68)

> you'll see them
> with your own eyes
> walking tall on the red;
> …
> you'll hear them
> with your own ears

sloshing on the red
carpet of blood;
but never, never
will you meet them.

'the dead' (Dladla 1–10)

raggedly brown
and pitifully dry;
the dead, exhumed
for reburial, are not
a curiosity.
i say this in passing:
our city has a daring collection.
ours hunt, eat, drink and
ask extempore - but the mayor
buries them from the visitors

Excerpt from 'the sleepless world' (Nyezwa 70–78)

i know i must wait for you
under a red star
inside a green house
like a frightened man

but here there are only butterflies
only poles
which lack elasticity
skies
with bloodstains

Excerpt from 'Malikhanye' (Nyezwa 4–16)

listen, for once from a distance
this blue earth sings its guilt to a silent storm
this guilty earth resounds its depleted conscience
to the raging eye of the desert

i want to remember you forever
and not desire more happiness
than this simple outline of a star
which coalesces love

i want to know how the sea flows
how the winds blow
and how love is abandoned
why things have to happen like this
oh! so over and over again.

COVID-19 and African Postage Stamps

Damian Shaw 🆔

This paper investigates how African nations have portrayed the COVID-19 pandemic in their postage stamps. After an introduction, a timeline offering short descriptions of global editions of this theme from its inception until March 2021 will be established. The timeline will consider most issues to the above date, with the caveat that additional examples might still be found, and that more will no doubt be produced after the publication of this paper, as the pandemic persists. Major design types will then be determined based on the preceding information. Then various publications related to Africa will be discussed. These primarily concern the so-called 'Stamperijia' issues, produced in Lithuania, and then bogus stamps produced in the name of various African countries. Apart from the 'Stamperijia' and similar issues, it is noted that only two African nations have produced a COVID-19-themed stamp on the continent itself up to 20 March 2021. The implications of this will be discussed in the conclusion, with suggestions for future action.

It has been well established by writers in a number of academic disciplines that postage stamps are used to convey official messaging by national governments.[1] In particular, postage stamps have functioned as 'paper ambassadors' (Altman) and have been used to promote 'national identity and the objectives of the state' (Brunn 19). Such was indeed the case up to about a decade ago. The situation, particularly relating to Africa, has become more complex since then. In 2004, Agbenyega Adzedze could claim with confidence that 'the issuing of postage stamps remains the monopoly of the central government in every country in Africa' (1). By 2020, however, various African nations had outsourced their stamp production to a company in Lithuania. These particular issues will be discussed later. Bogus or illegal issues purported to have been issued by various countries but actually have nothing to do with those countries have also come to light and will be considered separately.

When not merely used to generate funds from tourists or collectors, as in so-called 'Cinder-ella' publications, postage stamps still generally reflect anything relating to a particular nation from historical anniversaries to current events, especially if they are deemed of sufficient impor-tance to be noticed. Even though stamps are not as ubiquitous as they were a few decades ago, most countries take great care when designing their stamps,[2] and there is still a substantial global collectors' market that ensures that these objects are disseminated worldwide. Postage stamps, therefore, can still be considered in general as potent vectors of government ideology, though especial care needs to be taken now concerning their provenance.

In the context of a global pandemic, we can expect that postage stamps will not merely rep-resent individual national concerns, but that there will be a great deal of interaction between the output of differing countries. Stamp designers do pay close attention to the philatelic output of other nations. Choosing to follow or not to follow a particular design trend is, therefore, a way of aligning themselves or not aligning themselves with broader global political affiliations.

This paper will consider the legitimate stamp issues concerning COVID-19 by African nations in 2020 and early 2021, followed by the quasi-legitimate outsourced issues, and then the bogus stamps. When analyzing the messaging of these texts, it is important to arrange them in strict chronological order of dissemination as the designs do influence subsequent pub-lications. It is also necessary to consider previous models used for representing pandemics to determine the extent of innovation in the message that an individual country wishes to portray. In the following paragraph, a very brief discussion of disease on postage stamps will be given, followed by a consideration of the SARS pandemic on stamps. A timeline and typol-ogy of COVID-19 postage stamps will then be established. After this, the various issues by, or seemingly by, African nations to date will be considered.

Historically, there has been a strong thematic connection between medicine and postage stamps.[3] During the Spanish flu pandemic of 1918–1920, however, there were no stamps specifi-cally depicting this event, so the Spanish flu does not act as an iconic model for later pandemics. Rather, the Spanish flu was subsumed under the Red Cross. The Red Cross (and the Red Cres-cent) became of major interest to stamp collectors, and so-called semi-postal issues have been used pervasively to generate funds for these charities.[4] Another disease of considerable interest has been tuberculosis. Its icon is the Cross of Lorraine. It is only since the SARS epidemic of 2003, however, that an icon for the coronavirus was developed, when China issued its miniature sheet entitled 'United as One in Fighting SARS' on 19 May 2003. This sheet contains the name 'SARS' covered by the red 'No' symbol alongside a masked face. As P. Wright noted in 2004, 'the face mask is destined to become the symbol of SARS' (305). Wright's remark has proved prescient, but the 'No' symbol has also persisted, as well as the symbol of the clenched fist that appeared on the cover of the Chinese presentation pack. The Swine flu (H1N1) outbreak of 2009 was not depicted on any stamps.

A Timeline and Typology for Issues of COVID-19 Stamps

In this timeline, I will only describe issues that have been seen to either set or follow trends in depictions of the virus. The reader may view Vojtech Jankovič's website to access images of many of the stamps discussed below. The first country to issue a stamp depicting the COVID-19 pandemic was Iran, on 17 March 2020.[5] This was part of Iran's 'national heroes' series and was entitled 'Frontline Fighters of the Coronavirus'. In the foreground, dominating the image, is a masked medical worker giving a 'V' for victory sign. To our right and behind this figure are a further two masked medical workers in protective gear. To our left a figure in a gas mask carrying a machine gun appears, which probably indicates the government's willingness to involve the military in its attempts to halt the spread of the pandemic. Three depictions of the coronavirus itself appear (in green). In the foreground there is the now familiar image of two spiky viruses. In the background a larger virus has a jagged fracture line through the middle, probably indicating its desired defeat. This issue, therefore, served to re-establish the image of the masked medical worker as a symbol of the coronavirus, but adds a military threat, which is a new element.

In the middle of March, Liechtenstein produced a non-official stamp, which nevertheless had postal validity, to show solidarity with China. This was followed shortly by the first probably bogus issue to emerge, attributed to Sri Lanka.[6] In this issue, a global map in different shades of red is given, showing the pandemic hot spots to be in China, Iran, Europe and North America (the deepest shades of red). The depiction of such date-specific information makes it unlikely that the design emerged from any official source. On 31 March, Vietnam issued a pair. In the first, the clenched fist is used, along with two masked scientists. In the second, several masked or suited members of society appear: civilians, healthcare professionals, and members of the police force and army (who are, however, not carrying weapons). The virus in the background is in red. On 7 April, China announced an issue, the release of which was delayed until 11 May. I will discuss it here, however, as it is linked to the Iran and Vietnam issues. The eventual issue (containing two stamps, one on the right and one on the left) depicts a masked figure and a 'No' symbol over 'COVID-19' on the right-hand stamp, a direct echo of the SARS stamp. The masked figure here, however, has a clenched fist, a borrowing from the Vietnam issue. On the left-hand stamp are masked healthcare professionals, a scientist looking at a laptop computer (a microscope in the withdrawn design) and members of the military. Though fourteen important changes were made to the original design,[7] the most striking in my view is that a small figure of a soldier carrying a machine gun was removed, showing sensitivity relating to issues of quarantine enforcement. The Iran/Vietnam/China type may be characterized, then, by a combination of assorted masked figures, including the military (either with or without weapons), clenched fists, the 'No' symbol, and visualizations of the virus in green, red or black.

A second, important, trend-setting type was published by Switzerland on 6 April. This issue features a red circle (which could be the Earth or the Sun) overlaid by a white cross that cleverly imitates the Swiss national flag, as well as being a reference to the Red Cross. Surrounding the circle are abstract human figures. The circle can be seen as a symbol of the Earth, but also, in a somewhat sinister fashion, as a depiction of the coronavirus itself with the human figures becoming the spikes that give the coronavirus its distinctive shape. Besides a reference to the Swiss (a country famous for its neutrality) the design demonstrates global egalitarianism, whereas the types above have national concerns.

In April, New Zealand issued a 'bear hunt' series, appealing to children, in support of the Red Cross. One of the teddy bears is masked. In June, Luxembourg issued stamps featuring drawings by children, as did Guernsey and Alderney in July.

On 4 May the Isle of Man issued eight stamps that depict ordinary civilians, healthcare workers and scientists. When viewed alongside stamps discussed earlier, those from Iran, Vietnam and China, it is noticeable that the military are absent. What will 'carry us through' according to these stamps is 'love,' 'faith,' 'care,' 'compassion,' 'work,' 'community,' 'words' and 'science'.

The first official African issue was from Morocco on 7 May. This was of the Iran/Vietnam/ China type showing various masked and suited figures including military personnel. The virus in the background is in green, with a map of Morocco in red. It is important to note that the military personnel are not carrying visible weapons. A similar issue from the United Arab Emirates (10 May) called 'Thank You Heroes' shows the typical masked and suited figures. Military personnel are not carrying weapons, but, strangely, one of the doctors in not wearing a mask. Uruguay (13 May): these stamps depict masked civilians with the virus in the background. Ukraine (29 May): these depict a masked face with the left half that of a health worker and the right half that of a soldier. May also saw issues from the Central African Republic, Guinea-Bissau, Sierra Leone, Djibouti and Togo, which will be discussed later.

On 3 June, Monaco issued an image of Prince Albert II holding the globe, as if protecting it magically (much like the Swiss type). The Czech Republic's 24 June issue depicted six colourful facemasks, each with designs alluding to a different aspect of society such as the Red Cross for health services and the post horn for postal services. The upper-centre mask has a camouflage design, obviously alluding to the military. Gabon's 24 June issue will be discussed later. Macao (24 June) produced stamps, sheets and related materials showing a masked woman with a clenched fist. All 200 000 stamps and 150 000 miniature sheets were sold by December 2020, giving some indication of how populated this collectors' market is.[8] Oman (June 2020) issued two stamps in a sheet showing the COVID-19 symbol and masked civilian and military figures. Of interest on the sheet is a figure of a medical worker, like Atlas, bearing the map of Oman on his shoulders. This is a good example of a local, rather than an international, tribute. Greece (June 2020): two personalized but official miniature sheets depict mostly unmasked figures except for one masked doctor. This is perhaps not surprising as the logo on one sheet reads: 'We stayed home and won'. This optimism was premature.

Brazil (8 July) issued a miniature sheet containing six stamps. 'No' symbols and masked figures are prominent. All the essential workers on the leftmost stamp are unmasked. This stamp also depicts military personnel, though they are not carrying weapons. A scientist looking into a microscope features prominently. Lebanon's July (probably bogus) issue depicts a globe with a clenched first thrusting out of it. Taiwan's 21 July issue shows masked figures, no military or police, with clenched fist in the label between two stamps. The masked figures in the left stamp stand in front of a stylized globe. Mali's 24 July issue is bogus and will be discussed later. Tajikistan's July issue is dominated by masked figures: 6 pairs, with some military personnel not clearly visible in the 'I' and 'T' pair of 'UNITED'. July also saw a very interesting issue involving Tajikistan, South Sudan, Niger, Djibouti, São Tomé et Príncipe, Central African Republic and Senegal, to be discussed later.

Singapore's 7 August issue shows cartoon drawings on five stamps, all masked figures. This is the first issue to incorporate comic elements into the stamp design, but military jets in formation betray enforcement mechanisms. The United Nations' 11 August miniature sheet is dominated by a masked figure. The sheet contains six stamps that are coloured circles (like the Swiss design), each containing different designs including a cross. There is no reference to the military or the police. This issue seems to be a hybrid design embracing both the Swiss and the Iran/Vietnam/China types. Thailand, on 14 August, issued two stamps, both with masked healthcare workers and civilians and no military or police. Slovakia (21 August): this issue depicts that face of young woman with a transparent mask in front of a bisected oval, possibly representing the virus or the globe. This issue is unusual as it is predominantly black and grey, suggesting death and mortality.

Columbia (7 September): here, the issue depicts a typewriter underneath a circle containing the map of Columbia. The circle is inscribed with the phrase 'reescribe su historia' or 're-write its history,' clearly referring to domestic problems surrounding the record of the pandemic in that country. Vatican City (10 September): in this, the virus, representing the globe, is injected (the Swiss type). October saw a comic stamp by Austria representing social distancing measurements, with an ant and elephant used as points of reference for distance. It was printed on toilet paper. On 9 October, the Sri Lankan post office also issued a stamp featuring the globe as coronavirus (like the Swiss type) in front of various masked figures, both civilian and military, though there are no weapons shown. On the same day, Portugal issued a set of five stamps highlighting support services in the pandemic, featuring mostly masked individuals. On Christmas Day 2020, India issued a set of four 'Salute to COVID-19 Warriors,' with masked civilian and military characters. No weapons are visible, and the 'V' symbol is used instead of a clenched fist. A drone is prominent on the first-day cover.

This list is fairly complete up to the end of February 2021, though it is possible that many more issues will be published in the forthcoming months after this writing. We can see that the two major types to have emerged are the Iran/China type showing masked figures (some civilian, some military, or a mixture of both, representations of the virus and often clenched fists), and the Swiss type, which highlights the globe as a virus. A variety of idiosyncratic issues have also come to light, from the sombre to the light-hearted. The emergence of two dominant types, however, demonstrates that there is, indeed, an ongoing 'intertextual' conversation taking place at an international level concerning the depiction of this virus. Future analysts and historians may reflect on how these types serve to align various countries into power blocs, whether in terms of aspiration or fact. For instance, India uses the Iran/China type, as many Asian nations have chosen to do. From this we are prompted to ask the following: does the use of the 'V' symbol, rather than the clenched fist and the absence of guns, have anything to tell us about India's attitude towards Iran and China? Questions like these require exhaustive analyses of the visual texts, which we do not have space to conduct here. One might also analyze these stamps in terms of tropes such as the depiction of the military, the presence or absence of weapons, and the general iconography of 'fighting,' 'war' and 'struggle' (militarized tropes), which have already received considerable academic attention concerning the 'wars' against terror, drugs and various other diseases.[9] This article, however, is chiefly concerned with attempting to establish the extent African nations partake in the international 'intertextual' conversation on stamps about COVID-19, and then to consider the implications of our findings. We will now consider the African issues in greater detail.

The African Issues – Morocco and Tunisia

The Moroccan issue of 7 May 2020 is entitled 'Morocco United against COVID-19'.[10] The stamp pays tribute to 'each institution involved in the battle, including doctors, medical staff, police officers, civil protection agents, and janitors'. All individuals are masked, which represents a strict national policy. The stamp stresses a local fight against the virus, yet the type of design also shows solidarity with a broader international effort linked with the Iran/China type, rather than the Swiss type. The inclusion of the Moroccan flag gives the stamp a distinctively African national character, however. The stamp was sold with a surcharge, with all profits being donated to a special fund for COVID-19 management and relief. The Moroccan post office also viewed this issue as part of their philatelic cultural heritage:

Barid al-Maghrib emphasized the new postage stamp enriches the Moroccan philatelic heritage, highlighting previous special releases it issued to raise awareness, including 'The world united against malaria' in 1962, 'Moroccan league for the fight against cardiovascular diseases' in 1980, 'World AIDS Day' in 1991 and in 2006, 'AIDS campaign' in 2011 and 'First National Cancer Day' in 2008.

It can be argued that this stamp issue has a practical economic function, plays a role in nation building and national solidarity, is part of Morocco's philatelic cultural heritage, and also positions Morocco in a particular way within a global community fighting the pandemic. If a postage stamp does indeed fulfil all these functions, as this one seems to do, then it seems strange that this is only one of two locally produced African COVID-19 stamps to date.

Morocco's neighbour, Tunisia, produced its COVID-19 stamp on 17 December 2020. This stamp, designed by Yassine Ghorbel, is titled 'The fight against the COVID-19 Virus "Tunisia still standing"'. It features eight masked figures, including police and postal workers and various preventative measures taken against the virus. The group of people in the centre seems to be in a bubble. The design belongs to the Iran/China type (especially with the 'No' symbol over the virus used as a cancellation on the first-day cover), but a red coronavirus, which seems to be setting like a sun behind a blue wave (Tunisia's tourism industry was severely impacted) seems to allude to the Swiss type. Of particular interest is the inclusion of aerial and ground drones. These, 'equipped with thermal cameras' were responsible for checking lockdown compliance, particularly in Tunis (Contesse). Like the Moroccan stamp, therefore, the stamp depicts a local reality as well as international solidarity.

The 'African' Issues – Stamperija

The reason I placed 'African' in inverted commas above is because, in recent years, 22 African countries have outsourced the production of their stamps to a company based in Vilnius, Lithuania, called Stamperija.[11] These issues are designed and produced by Stamperija, but officially authorized by the contracting countries. They are not officially for sale in the countries from which they purport to come, however, so they are in a somewhat murky philatelic zone. Many of the issues are so-called joint issues, which depict thematic subjects that have little specifically to do with the contracting countries, such as international fungi, dinosaurs or papal visits. Given that the COVID-19 pandemic is a politically sensitive issue, though, the pattern changed somewhat, with only eleven countries authorizing the early Stamperija issues, namely Central African Republic, Chad, Djibouti, Guinea, Guinea-Bissau, Liberia, Mozambique, Niger, São Tomé et Príncipe, Sierra Leone and Togo. Even so, departing from normal practice, not all these countries have authorized all the issues, and some countries have commissioned issues unique to themselves, which demonstrates that individual governments are still exercising some control over the messaging sent out in this medium.

Most astonishing of all the Stamperija issues, the bulk of which emerged in May 2020, is that of Djibouti (DJB200119c).[12] The set consists of four stamps: the first shows the Diamond Princess Cruise Ship as a vector of the virus out of China; the second shows Dr. Li Wenliang, the Chinese whistle-blower doctor; the third a map of China in red with vector lines radiating from it, one of them towards a representation of the virus, also in red; and the fourth an ambulance with the Red Cross and Red Crescent as well as the stars of the Chinese flag, representing the virus, in the background. There is also a miniature sheet, which is a combination of stamps two and three. This issue makes it clear that the virus originated in China and spread to the rest of the world from China, a narrative (that of the 'China virus' in the US) that the rest of the world has refused to portray on its stamps. No other countries authorized this issue, and it is possible that Djibouti did so before recognizing how politically sensitive this portrayal would prove to be.

The next issue, a popular one, authorized by the Central African Republic, Sierra Leone, Liberia, Niger, São Tomé et Príncipe, Guinea-Bissau, Djibouti and Togo is entitled 'The Penny Black against COVID-19' (CA200313, SRL200321, LIB200318, NIG200225, ST200417, GB200317, DJB200323, G200258). The issue is a miniature sheet of six penny black stamps with Queen Victoria wearing a variety of facemasks. There are slight differences between these issues: the facemasks are coloured differently for each country; there are two small national flags at the bottom of the sheet; and the issues from Francophone countries are in French rather than English. Otherwise, they are essentially the same. Even though this issue could be viewed as light-hearted, it could be interpreted in more serious ways. On the one hand, Africa could be seen to be protecting (or masking) itself against an external (colonial or viral) threat, or, by showing that mask-wearing is important, it could be a message to the rest of the world (represented by Queen Victoria) to wear masks. Unfortunately, there is very little in this design to link these sheets to Africa, besides the obvious names of the two countries and their national flags at the bottom of the sheet. The facemasks, for example, could have incorporated distinctively African designs, but they do not. The joke of masking cultural icons is continued by Guinea-Bissau, Chad and Niger (September/October) in 'famous monuments of the world in quarantine,' which depict statues, like the David by Michelangelo, wearing facemasks (GB200322a, TCH200306a, NIG200229). There are no African monuments in these issues.

The third Stamperija issue was a joint issue of the Central African Republic, Guinea-Bissau, Chad, Liberia, Niger and Tajikistan (CA200312, GB200316, TCH200301, LIB200317, NIG200224). There are two similar souvenir sheets that emphasize the Red Cross (not the Red Crescent, which is inappropriate in the case of Tajikistan), the United Nations, and several 'No' symbols over representations of the virus. In the background is a stylized map of the world with Africa on the left, Russia in the centre and Australia on the right (the Americas are not visible). There is a random grid of lines over this map, possibly representing the idea of viral propagation in the abstract. Both Europe and China are red 'hotspots,' with Africa being coloured relatively green. The shading gives only a very rough impression of the actual infection rates in various countries at the time. Togo borrows the main elements of this design (October), except that the sheet is dominated by a white man wearing a facemask.

A further issue from Togo (May/June 2020) shows a 'No' symbol over a representation of the virus, which contains a pair of lungs inside it (TG200257). Guinea-Bissau also issued a silk sheet in May showing a schematic grid-like map of the world functioning as a 'No' symbol over the virus (GB200318). Sierra Leone (October) brought out two issues celebrating Anthony Fauci (SRL200450). It seems that this theme sold well, as Stamperija continued to produce multiple issues. The Central African Republic (October) issued four stamps celebrating the Red Cross and Red Crescent (CA200311). On the only stamp depicting healthcare workers there are no black Africans. A similar issue by Chad celebrating healthcare workers shows no black Africans and also the American flag (TCH200304)!

Yet another joint issue from October is a sheet containing sixteen stamps issued by Chad, Guinea-Bissau, Liberia, Niger, São Tomé et Príncipe and Sierra Leone (TCH200305, BG200321, LIB200319, NIG200226, ST200416, SRL200448). All these stamps portray members of the public and healthcare workers. Astonishingly, not a single black person is shown in the over-forty depictions of people. Sierra Leone also issued six designs (October) that are heavily influenced by the Isle of Man Issue of 4 May (see above) (SRL200447). The figures on these stamps, almost twenty of them, are all white.

Though Stamperija has produced a large volume of stamps on the theme of COVID-19, we can see that these designs are not being imitated. They are not influencing representation of the pandemic in non-Stamperija countries. The sheer number of these issues, however, suggests that they are selling very well and will form an important part of the material cultural record of this pandemic. Most importantly, though, almost all their designs have no connection with Africa whatsoever, besides a few national flags. These stamps are being designed by Europeans in Lithuania for various African countries and fail to represent a uniquely African response to the pandemic. Is this a missed opportunity for Africa to represent itself? I will return to this discussion in the conclusion.

Stamperijia is not the only company designing stamps for African nations. On 7 August, a sheet of four stamps titled 'A Tribute to those on the Front Line' was issued by The Gambia. This was produced and designed by the Inter-Governmental Philatelic Corporation (IGPC), a private company based in the US that has operated since 1957. Its business model is similar to Stamperijia's in that its productions must be authorized by local governments. Its client list consists mostly of African countries and small-island nations. It produces many stamps containing icons of pop culture and is licensed to reproduce Disney cartoon figures. Like Stamperijia, the issues usually have nothing to do with the country to which they are attributed. The IGPC had only issued sixteen COVID-19-related stamps by 15 February 2021, and only one from Africa. The Gambia issue shows what appear to be white medical workers and security personnel. There is nothing on the stamp, besides the name 'The Gambia,' which appears to relate the stamp directly to that country. Similar issues in the series, or omnibus, have also been produced for Guyana, The Marshall Islands, Palau, Tuvalu, Grenada, Grenada Grenadines, Saint Vincent and the Grenadines, Nevis, Dominica, and Antigua and Barbuda. The stamp can be said to portray international solidarity on behalf of the Gambian government, but it has little or nothing else to do with that country. The IGPC has been accused of 'cultural imperialism' for its 'mass issue of stamps featuring images from American pop culture' ('IPGC', *Wikipedia*). If African countries continue to allow companies like the IPGC and Stamperijia to design, produce and distribute their stamps for them, then it is difficult to see how this 'cultural imperialism,' or at least cultural bias, can be countered.

Bogus or Potentially Bogus African Issues

A philatelic forgery is an illegal copy of a stamp legitimately issued or authorized by a country. A bogus issue, in contrast, is a design printed without the permission or authorization of any given country, though using its name. These may be produced for propaganda purposes, but, in the case of COVID-19, they seem to have been produced purely for profit, and do not seem to be critical or malicious. It is sometimes difficult to establish whether an issue is bogus, as many African countries do not comment on new issues on their official post office websites, nor do they respond to enquiries. One such issue may be a joint issue first produced in the name of South Sudan. The issue, at first, seems legitimate. There is a description of it, for instance, on a *Wikipedia* page for the postal history of South Sudan, which reads as follows:

On 21 July 2020 South Sudan released a new stamp issue commemorating the health
workers assisting in the fight against the COVID-19 pandemic. The new stamp series
titled 'Struggle against COVID-19 Pandemic: Tribute to healthcare personnel' is a
joint issue with a number of other African postal services based on a common design
depicting a medical crew surrounding planet Earth as a protective layer. The whole
form suggests the coronavirus shape. The South Sudan issue was designed by the
South Sudan Stamp Committee under the chairmanship of the South Sudan designer
Mr. Stanislaus Tombe Felix, using some design features of that joint theme. The set
has six face values: 50, 100, 200, 300, 500 and 1000 SSP and one souvenir sheet with
face value 1000 SSP. For both the set as well as the souvenir sheet an official FDC
has been made available for the first time. ('Postal History and Postage Stamps of
South Sudan', *Wikipedia*)

Rather than an official website, this information is based on a blog for an auction of these stamps,
which claims that they will be very expensive as there were only 300 copies of the souvenir sheet
produced.[13] It is very unlikely that any country would produce such limited numbers. Furthermore, this design is said to be part of a joint issue with similar versions being produced in the
name of Senegal, Niger, Djibouti, São Tomé et Príncipe and the Central African Republic.
This should give us reason for caution as these are all countries that contract to Stamperija,
but these are definitely not Stamperija issues. As one commentator noted, many of these
issues do not contain any African figures, and the depiction of a masked soldier carrying a
machine gun in front of Milan cathedral is also highly dubious.[14] Another unusual circumstance
is that all these stamps were originally on sale only from an Ebay store based in Algeria. In
addition, South Sudan has still not been able to establish international mail delivery owing to
political problems.

The South Sudan design itself is based on the Swiss model, with cartoonish stick-figures
surrounding the globe. A few of these figures are visibly black, which suggests an African presence in a global context, though there are no obviously black images in some of the other country
issues. It is also strange that the South Sudan issue is the only one that features a map of Africa
prominently on the globe. The others all centre on the Atlantic Ocean. Though I cannot prove
definitively that these stamps are bogus, it is astonishing that the South Sudan issue in this
cluster is the only one to date that focuses specifically on Africa in the map. This further suggests
that these issues are bogus, and do not represent a coordinated response to the pandemic by the
included nations.

Jankovič lists an issue from Gabon from June 2020. These are two miniature sheets that
depict three people whose faces are clearly visible, but none of them are black Africans,
which makes this issue dubious in my opinion. Another bogus issue that emerged around July
2020 in the name of Mali shows a globe centred on the Atlantic Ocean, as well as three
masked characters and one in a hazmat suit. The three characters with visible faces are all
white, which makes the issue suspect. Fortunately, in this case, the Mali post office lodged an
official warning with the Universal Postal Union on 6 July 2020 'strongly denounc[ing] and
condemn[ing]' these stamps issued in its name, so we know that it was fraudulent. After establishing the illegality of the issue, Mali post made the following comments:

Consequently, La Poste du Mali calls for the cooperation and support of all member
countries of the Union and its bodies to prohibit the sale and circulation of this fraudulent

issue, in accordance with their own regulations, as well as the provisions of the Universal Postal Convention.

> The continued production and sale of illegal issues are dangerous activities which not only harm philately and the reputation of the country concerned, but are detrimental to all countries and the wider postal sector.[15]

It is true that fraudulent issues might occasion some financial losses to all members of the Universal Postal Union if these issues are affixed to letters (and countries will not tolerate this just as they cannot afford to tolerate counterfeit currency), but this is usually not the case as they are almost exclusively bought by collectors online specifically for their own collections and not actually attached to postal items and sent through the mail. That fraudulent issues actually harm philately is also a moot point, as many people do collect, and are interested in fraudulent items or fakes in their own right. What I think is most important in this missive from Mali concerns the issue of representation. Mali, as a sovereign nation, reserves the right to represent itself on its postage stamps. Representations of any country that purport to be 'truthful' may indeed cause great harm to the reputation of that country if they are believed to be accurate when, in fact, they are not.

Conclusion

The Mali Post Office makes it clear that postage stamps are still intimately connected with the 'reputation' of individual countries, even if stamps are not as pervasively used as they once were. This issue of representation is, I would argue, of particular concern to African nations, especially because it has often been the case that European nations assumed the right to represent the continent during the period of colonialism, thereby producing a highly biased vision of Africa. In the post-colonial era, many African nations have stressed the importance of self-representation in literature, film, poetry, art, academic output and educational syllabi. This laudable effort of Africa to represent itself to the world (and also to itself) should be extended to postage stamps. One might argue, with some justification, that in countries where the postal system is operating at minimal levels, postage stamps would have very limited impact on national messaging, especially internally, as they would have restricted internal circulation, but this is an issue that individual countries could address.

More importantly, postage stamps, as part of material cultural history specifically linked to the nation state, become part of the artefactual historical record relating to these countries. In the modern world, they survive both as objects and as images in various media, particularly on the internet. Stamps, therefore, rather than just languishing in collections as they did previously, have a visible presence on the internet, where they can be viewed by many. Academic researchers, artists, ordinary people, now and in the future, who are interested in Africa, will encounter these images, and draw conclusions from them. The purpose they serve is similar to much other artistic production, telling the story both of the continent and the people who produced them. If the issues are bogus, or not directly produced by the individual countries themselves, they risk providing a misleading record.

I embarked on this project with an open mind, and certainly did not expect what I uncovered. It seems that only two African countries, Morocco and Tunisia, have produced COVID-19-themed postage stamps *in situ*. Africa's major economies, such as South Africa, Nigeria,

Egypt, Kenya and so forth, have not joined in the global production of these issues, at least as of March 2021. Future enquiry may reveal why so few African nations have chosen to represent this pandemic philatelically, but that is beyond the scope of this essay, and would be better conducted once the pandemic is over.

Three points seem important in conclusion here. First, failure to represent COVID-19 theme-based stamps by African nations seems to have opened the window for fraudsters who have potentially misrepresented several of these nations. Second, if the representation of African Nations by Africans themselves is at all important, then it seems that the outsourcing of philatelic output might be reconsidered. Finally, it is hoped that this investigation might stimulate Africans from the entire continent to participate in the several suggestion schemes that exist in individual nations across the continent and suggest COVID-19 designs that would portray the uniqueness of African responses to this pandemic within a global context. Postage stamps can still function as generators of funding for charitable relief, as shown by the Moroccan example, as well as serve as important media for the representation of national identities and the building of global cooperation. African nations still have the opportunity to join the global, 'intertextual' conversation on this topic, doing so on their own terms and with their own voices, if they so desire.

Notes

1   See Shaw 67.
2   See Jochim, 'New Issues' for a translation of the official China Post press release.
3   For full-length treatment of this theme, see Furukawa.
4   Gazay gives a good overview of how these stamps were marketed. In the case of diabetes, see Schuessler.
5   This timeline has been largely established by Jankovič and Jochim ('Truth, Lies'), though some uncertainty over exact dating still exists. Further technical information, though no analysis, on issues until May 2020 can be found in Cioruţa, Pop and Coman.
6   A bogus issue for Sri Lanka emerged in March 2020. See Jochim.
7   See Jochim, 'New Issues'.
8   See https://philately.ctt.gov.mo/XVersion/ProductList.aspx?admcode=MAC&emicode=202009&lang=en-us. Accessed on 2 December 2020.
9   See, for instance, Susan Sontag, 97–98.
10 These references are all taken from an article of 8 May in the *Morocco World News* by Taha Mebtoul.
11 These countries are Angola, Benin, Botswana, Burundi, Cape Verde, Central African Republic, Chad, Comoros, Djibouti, Ethiopia, Gabon, Guinea, Guinea-Bissau, Ivory Coast, Liberia, Mozambique, Namibia, São Tomé et Príncipe, Sierra Leone, Togo and Uganda. The bulk of this company's business comes from Africa, as they contract out to only eight other countries worldwide.
12 For all of these sets, I give the Stamperija catalogue numbers.
13 See http://commonwealthstampsopinion.blogspot.com/2020/07/1706-south-sudans-COVID-19-stamps.html. Accessed on 17 November 2020.
14 See http://commonwealthstampsopinion.blogspot.com/2020/07/1697-new-stamps-soon-from-south-sudan.html for more of this debate. Accessed on 10 November 2020.
15 See http://golowesstamps.com/reference/Illegal%20Stamps/Mali%20Illegal%20Stamps/Circular2020_94_upu_circular_en_Mali.pdf. Accessed on 4 December 2020.

ORCID

Damian Shaw ⓘ http://orcid.org/0000-0002-4162-1079

Works Cited

Adedze, Agbenyega. 'Commemorating the Chief: The Politics of Postage Stamps in West Africa'. *African Arts* 37(2), 2004: 1–17.

Altman, Dennis. *Paper Ambassadors: The Politics of Stamps*. North Ryde, NSW: Angus & Robinson, 1991.

Brunn, Stanley D. 'Stamps as Messengers of Political Transition'. *The Geographical Review* 101 (1), 2011: 19–36.

Cioruţa, Bogdan-Vasile, Alexandru Leonard Pop, and Mirela Coman. 'COVID-19 Stamps – A New Collecting Theme Vs Philatelic Promotion of Care for Affected Community and Environment'. *Asian Journal of Education and Social Sciences* 9(2), 2020: 25–37.

Contesse, Eric. 'Mon Blog Timbré'. 24 January 2021. https://timbredujura.blogspot.com/2021/01/stamp-and-souvenir-sheet-fight-against.html. Accessed on 1 February 2021.

Furukawa, Akira. *Medical History Through Postage Stamps*. Ishiyaku: EuroAmerica, 1994.

Gazay, M. 'Postage Stamps – A Reflexion of the Red Cross'. *International Review of the Red Cross* 9 (95), 1969: 109–10.

'Inter-Governmental Philatelic Organization.' *Wikipedia*. https://en.wikipedia.org/wiki/Inter-Governmental_Philatelic_Corporation. Accessed on 15 January 2021.

Jankovič, Vojtech. 'Thematic Philately: Tribute to the First Line Warriors – Corona Virus COVID-19 Pandemic and Philately'. https://www.postoveznamky.sk/tribute-to-first-line-warriors-coronavirus-COVID-19-pandemic-and-philately. Accessed on 18 July 2020.

Jochim, Mark Joseph. 'New Issues 2020: People's Republic of China (Fight the Pandemic)'. https://www.philatelicpursuits.com/2020/04/01/new-issues-2020-peoples-republic-of-china-fight-the-pandemic/. Accessed on 9 November 2020.

Jochim, Mark Joseph. 'The Philately of Covid19: Truth, Lies and Rumours'. https://www.philatelicpursuits.com/2020/04/12/the-philately-of-COVID-19-truths-lies-and-rumors/. Accessed on 8 October 2020.

Mebtoul, Tahra. 'Moroccan Post Issues New "Morocco United Against COVID-19" Stamp'. *Morocco World News*. 8 May 2020. https://www.moroccoworldnews.com/2020/05/301978/moroccan-post-issues-new-morocco-united-against-COVID-19-stamp/. Accessed on 9 December 2020.

'Postal History and Postage Stamps of South Sudan'. *Wikipedia*. https://en.wikipedia.org/wiki/Postage_stamps_and_postal_history_of_South_Sudan. Accessed on 17 November 2020.

Schuessler, Raymond. 'Stamping out Diabetes'. *Diabetes Forecast* 47(12), 1994: 1–3.

Shaw, Damian. 'Subtle Messengers: Literary Myth and National Identities in the Postage Stamps of Macao'. In *Macao – Cultural Interaction and Literary Representations*. Edited by Katrine K. Wong and C. X. George Wei. Oxford: Routledge, 2014. 67–88.

Sontag, Susan. *Illness as Metaphor and Aids and its Metaphors*. New York: Anchor, 1990.

Stamperija. https://stamperija.eu. Accessed on 27 October 2020.

Wright, P. 'Stamping out SARS'. *Journal of Hospital Infections* 55(4), 2003: 305.

Green Dream

Maren Bodenstein

Pangolin
Unfurls its belly
Opens one eye
Sees bat and wanders
From the forest
To the marketplace
Crawls into a boiling pot
Dissolves to feed a million supplicants
Who pass the broth from lip to lip
Hide inside their houses
And dream of drowning
Turn silent

The streets are empty now
The forest dreams
Of pangolin

Sonification and Music: Science meets Art

Chatradari 'Chats' Devroop and Michael Titlestad

The opposites, science and the arts, have always enjoyed a relationship. Recently, this relationship has been expressed in sonification, a branch of science seeking to add sound to data, giving data music-like intelligibility. Scientists believe that our aural capabilities are a potentially rich source of data that could assist in problem solving. In 2020, a sonic realization of the coronavirus was generated using its spike protein data. This sonification endeavoured to probe the coronavirus aurally. However, the creators of this sonified scientific probe are now claiming that their experiment is also a music composition. We examine this claim. This paper is underpinned by the conviction that not all sound is music. Music cannot represent anything other than itself because our understanding of music is always via allegory. Therefore, the efforts of Buehler, it is argued, are misdirected and trivial when placed in the stressed socio-political context of COVID-19.

New Music composer, Roman Haubenstock-Ramati, once remarked that pianist David Tudor 'could play the raisins in a slice of fruitcake' (Cox 38). Haubenstock-Ramati refers here to Tudor's ability to interpret indeterminate music scores.[1] No doubt, Tudor had been practising this skill on John Cage's music compositions, which, at that time, had something of the randomly distributed quality of fruitcake ingredients. In 2020, a bioengineer Markus J. Buehler and a group of scientists at the Massachusetts Institute of Technology (MIT) seized the headlines by converting the SARS-CoV-2 coronavirus protein data to music. Artificial intelligence generated an almost two-hour composition called the *Viral Counterpoint of the Coronavirus Spike Protein (2019-nCoV)*. The choice of tempo and instrumentation is ironically reminiscent of Brian Eno's *Ambient 1: Music for Airports* (1978) since airports were initially a primary vector of the global spread of coronavirus.

Buehler's project is not new in combining scientific research and sound. Efforts predating his mapping of particle data to sound include *The Climate Symphony and Other Sonification of Ice Core, Radar, DNA, Seismic and Solar Wind Data* (Quinn), *Higgs Boson* (Asquith), and Wayne Grim's *233rd Day, Before and After Totality, for Kronos Quartet and Computer Sonification*. Most data-mapping sonic experiments use an electronic sound source, such as a Musical Instrument Digital Interface (MIDI), or samples. However, in Grim's case, he used a live ensemble, the Kronos Quartet, to turn light data into sound (Grim 2018). What is significant, however, is that all of these 'compositions' are efforts to realize the 'sound' of data, a process called 'sonification'.

Present day researchers agree that the Geiger counter,[2] invented around 1908, was probably the earliest application of sonification. Sonification refers to the

> use of nonspeech audio to convey information. More specifically, sonification is transforming data relations into perceived relations in an acoustic signal to facilitate communication or interpretation. (Kramer 3)

The process of sonification translates data into an auditory representation for the purposes of analysis. This process is accomplished through a technique called 'parameter mapping' in which aspects of data are mapped onto elements of music (such as pitch, duration, variation, and brilliance). The rationale for sonification is that our senses pick up patterns differently: hearing, for instance, registers data differently from seeing. By using different senses for data apprehension, we may help the recipient to achieve a different outlook on the data – something like looking at a painting as opposed to someone orally describing that painting. If we analyze the ways in which our different senses receive and process data, it is hoped that we might stumble upon something intelligible and useful.[3]

Returning to the sonification of the coronavirus, *Viral Counterpoint of the Coronavirus Spike Protein*, Buehler asserts that 'the structural complexity translates into musical complexity,' and adds that '[t]here are many, many melodies layered into each other. It has a balance of order and disorder'(ISC 2020). Buehler further claims that

> the resulting music is a highly complex piece because we have many different melodies weaving into another, creating what we call 'counterpoint'. Counterpoint is a concept introduced and used very heavily by Johann Sebastian Bach, for instance, a couple of hundred years ago.

Musicologists agree that 'counterpoint' reached its height with J S Bach's *The Well-Tempered Clavier* (1722) during the Baroque period and the Enlightenment – a time in human history that also saw great scientific and artistic advances by Galileo, Newton, Leibniz and Caravaggio. It is apparent that Buehler sees his sonification of the coronavirus as a version of 'classical music'. His assertion is supported by the author of the article 'The sound of science – the SARS-CoV-2 virus as a piece of classical music' (ISC 2020), by claims that the 'composition' is 'protein music,' and that it transforms 'a source of anguish into something hypnotic and beautiful' (Roberts 2020).

We would argue that Buehler's proposition that his research is both an instrument of scientific enquiry and a musical composition is false because not all sound is music. Music cannot represent anything besides itself unless one counts scattered exceptions. We maintain that a human's understanding of music is always via allegory (other arts, historical periods, prevailing ideas, the market, and so on). Music is never literal and cannot be translated into another medium and thus does not lend itself to any direct interpretation. We further argue that what is unknown and worth finding out about the coronavirus is not in the virus itself, which like all viruses, is a dead-dumb-mindless chemical replicator. Rather, its nature (its 'meaning' even) exists in the hundreds of stress effects and instabilities that a pandemic creates. Our disorientation cannot be represented or resolved by making the structure of the virus available to sensory apprehensions through art.

Our argument unfolds using as a template Karlheinz Stockhausen's composition *Mikrophonie I* (1964) (*mikro* = microphone + *phonie* = symphony). In this composition, Stockhausen sets out to probe sound below our threshold of hearing using various objects and a microphone. Following in Stockhausen's path, we explore Buehler's claim that his scientific experiment has aesthetic value.

Is Buehler's viral counterpoint composition a heuristic device? To answer this question, we need to consider what it is in which heurism consists. John Ziman (1996) explores the usefulness of using sophisticated toys in enquiries and explanations in physics. He uses toys with an internal complexity, such as the Rubik's cube, that allow people to probe an idea or certain relations speculatively. They allow him to test hypotheses before formulating inclusive theories. Ziman speaks of the limitations forced on physicists' imaginations by standard notations, which in their case are mathematical. Even brief descriptions of the experimental or observational procedure are inadequate (42). Ziman's peer, Richard Feynman, remarked that the Feynman diagrams[4] (Brown), which represent critical aspects of the quantum electrodynamics process, could not be assimilated by common sense. Human intuitions cannot devise cognitive analogies corresponding to the intricacies of the logics of quantum processes.

The use of hallucinogens and their influence on great thinkers in science is well documented. Hallucinogens allow their users to go beyond reality; to see, hear and feel sensations that seem real, but do not exist. David Kaiser's book, *How the Hippies Saved Physics: Science, Counterculture, and the Quantum Revival* (2011), muses on the fact that taking Lysergic Acid Diethylamide (LSD) might be a way of emancipating physicists' capacities for visualization. Kaiser's musings indicate a gap between what scientists take to be a reality and the systems devised for communicating, capturing, probing or speculating on that reality. They 'see' and communicate their perceptions in systems of representation that are limited and limiting, and these very soon circulate and become entrenched in culture, textbooks and the protocols of the discipline. Is it possible to represent truths through sonification? People often assume that sonification, using complex computational methods, permits the representation of reality beyond that which can be conventionally represented in scientific and mathematical symbols and language. We need, though, to acknowledge that sonification is not, by any means, a novel method of translating abstraction into the domain of perception. Speech itself is just a version of sonification in which thought processes are translated into utterances.

We cannot know what sonification is without understanding de-sonification. The de-sonification of speech, its representation by the alphabet, not only permits the abstraction and dissemination of meaning, but also the translation of one spoken language into another. The Phoenicians used logic to develop a code, an abstract alphabet, as a no-man's-land between languages so that merchants could communicate with one another and with their customers. There are 'wide divergences of opinion' as to the origins of the Phoenician alphabet (Luckenbill 27), but it is agreed that it is, unlike other alphabets, purely 'symbolic' in the sense that letters are

not logically connected to create words, and they do not correspond to either phonetic or semantic elements. They neither designate a sound, nor are they used in recurrent predictable combinations. The Phoenician alphabet functions, then, as a storehouse or weigh station of meaning.
One language can be transposed into the alphabet, which in turn, can be translated into another.
The alphabet, in this instance, served a similar purpose to a modern tape recorder, enabling the
capture of sound shapes from a language, which are stored for 're-creation' in a different context,
in which it is rendered meaningful for listeners. Sound shapes, as is known from phonology,
have no meaning in themselves (Stebbing 1935). They acquire meaning only through a
process of combination in a specific order and subsequently being enunciated.

Mathematics is the signal instrument for conveying claims made by physicists. If sonification is to comprise a verifiable hypothesis, its results would have to be communicable in mathematical symbols, which also constitute a code of signifiers – a language. Mathematical
signifiers (symbols) obviously mean nothing in themselves. They signify only in specific combinations. Mathematics is a schematic of relationships used to model and explore reality.

Does sonification perform a similar function? Does it translate reality into a different,
abstract language of sound that communicates meaning to the listener? Even if sonification is
translation into an abstract language of purely acoustic signifiers, can their decoding by a listener
create meaning that is inherent in the sequence of sounds? To be more specific, if we turn to *Viral
Counterpoint of the Coronavirus Spike Protein*, can we translate it from abstracted, representational sounds into physical reality and coherent and cogent meaning? This is the primary
requirement of a functional abstraction – it can be decoded by the recipient, and the sonic
'message' can be translated into a natural language which enriches or redirects perception
and deepens our understanding. If we are to speak of 'mapping' reality using sound, we are
assuming that the map can be read and that it is both a meaningful representation of topography
and orientates our understanding of the world. Yet maps are also functional – through interpreting them we can find our way through real-world landscapes. It is this use-value that makes their
representation of reality plausible and coherent. Can sound be a map in this sense?

In the 1920s, the Russian formalists (Roman Jakobson, Viktor Shklovsky and Boris Eikhen-
baum) proposed an account of aesthetic perception in literature and poetry as the outcome of the
deliberate misuse of signs (Erlich 1981). This disruption of conventional signification results in
'defamiliarization' *(ostranenie)*, which enables us to perceive the world obliquely, as if we are
seeing it for the first time. If, in other words, we disturb the conventions of representation (tear
the veil of familiarity and habit from the world) we might register reality differently and thus
comprehend alternative, 'new' (at least hitherto unsignified) realities. Abstract codes both articulate meaning and, since their conventions also familiarize us with conventional representations
and interpretations, obscure the world from us.

Buehler's MIT research group claims, in effect, that *Viral Counterpoint of the Coronavirus
Spike Protein* 'defamiliarizes' our perception of the virus and thus permits a novel apprehension
that abets our comprehension, that it effects a perceptual jolt that changes (and deepens) our way
of seeing it. This assumes that sound – like the Phoenician alphabet – functions as a storehouse of
meaning, which, while listening, is translated into defamiliarized perception and, hence enriches
meaning. The work is held to extend our comprehension of the virus beyond the abstract
languages of science and mathematics.

The how, where, what and why of the coronavirus are also expressed in the languages of
molecular biology, virology, chemistry and evolutionary theory. Does sonification create an

encounter with a reality of the virus that is different from, even deeper than, these systems of representation?

'Coronavirus' does not refer to anything that is visible with the naked eye. The optical rendering of the virus, which the *Viral Counterpoint of the Coronavirus Spike Protein* supposedly describes (or scribes), begins well beyond the threshold of what photons, the units of energy in seeing, can resolve. It is only manifest under the bombardment and reflection of much smaller particles, electrons within an electron microscope. Hence the viral shape is a meta-optical image that can never enter the realm of unaided sight.

The characterization of the coronavirus is based on the spectra emitted by various molecules and elements, which add up to its characteristic unique sequence. The idea that a sequence, such as DNA or RNA, may designate a type of organism is derived from a comprehensive set of theories characterizing heredity, molecular noise or mutation, and evolution at the border of the inert and the living. Yet coronavirus does not generally appear to us microscopically but through its manifestation as a potentially deadly infection and because of its social, economic, cultural and political effects. Its meaning is not, in any significant sense, encapsulated in its appearance (or, more accurately, its topology). Mediating its topology in sound does nothing to represent its significance, its meaning, which inheres in the vague and uneasy accommodations between individual pathology, culture, knowledge and technology.

Is sonification something like the education of the wine taster, who at first may be unable to discern more than broad similarities between wines when tasting them but, after coaching and encouragement, is able to express more accurately in words what taste and bouquet they are registering (Latour and Deighton 2019)?[5] Wine tasters come to distinguish wines very accurately by type, cultivars, region, and fermentation and aging processes. Is it possible that sonification is like a sip of wine? It is accepted that the senses are not fixed but can be significantly altered by framing and prompting, and even more permanently by exercises in discrimination guided by a map of what they can discern. Just as the wine taster or the art expert whose opinion is sought in telling originals apart from fakes refines her judgements by a constant revisiting of the documented examples, could sonifying scientists improve their discrimination of features of their objects by being better coached in music?

To a trained musician, *Viral Counterpoint of the Coronavirus Spike Protein* sounds like the work of a naïve musical autodidact unaware of compositional possibilities and musical history. If one claims – as do Buehler and his team – that the sequence of sounds is music, it is important to acknowledge that this exalts naiveté and disregards questions of formalism and provenance. It endorses the Romantic conviction that naiveté (childlike innocence that translates into aesthetic primitivism) permits access to a truth obscured by sophistication, cultivation and immersion in the tradition. If Buehler and his associates claimed simply that the sonification amounts to a sequence of mathematically derived sounds based on microscopic characterization of the virus, that would be one thing. The claim to 'musicality' is quite another. The aestheticization of the found or rudimentary seeks to validate uncreative works by wilfully inserting them into a history of expression in which they do not belong.

The transposition of a visual modelling into a sonic one is not transposition in the musical sense. When Modest Mussorgsky's sketches were appropriated and re-mediated by Nikolai Rimsky-Korsakov and Maurice Ravel's orchestrations,[6] theirs was an act of musical interpretation and creative re-expression. Buehler's 'composition' (which does not really warrant the name) is neither a dialogue with other musicians nor does it entail anything like the arrangements of parts or dialogue among musicians. It is *sui generis* in the sense that it arose in isolation, without any reference to compositional tradition, practice or possibility.

Asserting the musicality of *Viral Counterpoint of the Coronavirus Spike Protein* is at once a meaningless claim and a claim that opens itself to ethical challenge, for the aestheticization of the virus (any notion that it is beautiful in itself) undercuts the catastrophe of its effects. To do so is – whatever else it is – also quaint, presumptuous, rarefied and misguided.

Musicians have always conceived of music as the source from which other music derives. Music was thus able to dispense with content as one of its necessary conditions. The discursive equivalent would be a radical intertextuality. Sonification is the practice of *all* musicians. They go about sonification either when reading a score or converting thoughts and ideas into sound using voice or instrumentation. Each musician engages their vernacular in this process. Their sonification process is accomplished by using a particular set of sounds and sound relations with which they are familiar. This allows musicians to extrapolate, to infer the following note and dig into deep structures, either through improvisation or when composing. It may even be possible to move beyond the habitual vernacular sonification by deliberately using new systems of notation, new kinds of sonority, or new kinds of instruments, which force the rethinking of the sonic vernacular. These are processes of educating the senses and the inferences that bind together the experiences of the senses and provide individuals with an acoustic world.

Music has long exploited the strategy of deliberately changing one or another aspect of the vernacular by introducing new instruments or by pursuing the transcription of pieces written for one instrument for different ones. Johann Sebastian Bach exploited this process extensively. But so did Luciano Berio and Franz Liszt and all of those who transcribed a symphony or opera for performance on piano in the 19th century. The contrary is also true: Ravel transcribed pieces he had conceived and refined at the piano into the idiom of the orchestra (Goddard 1925). Berio believed that transcription was one of the most significant sources of creativity in music, and of course, transcription in music is simply a form of alternative sonification. Hence, musicians have known for a long time that sonification can yield, if not always entirely novel results, new perspectives, new clues or ways of apprehending or new inferences.

Contrary to its perceived richness and varieties, music consists of sparse, almost impoverished materials. Most readers would accept that arithmetic with its four operations on a number line of addition, subtraction, multiplication and division, are a simple enough reality to be grasped in childhood along with shapes such as squares and triangles and their properties. Compared to musical materials, arithmetic is rich and complex, while musical operations correspond to a specific, restricted form of arithmetic known as Presburger arithmetic (Presburger 1931). Ultimately, any musician performing music or formulating a phrase, passage or entire composition constantly comes up against the intrinsic limits of the musical system, which is far more restrictive than the simplest games and their rules.[7] Therefore, musicians have sought for a long time to refresh the basic materials of music, the notes, intervals, scales and sonorities, which either come from natural resonance, available technology, metallurgy or the capacity to master the physical structure of sounding bodies or instruments. They also come from our understanding of overtones or hearing our physiology. But all these materials are fossils that have travelled incredible distances through cultures and times. They may seem laborious to learn because we know them in the context of developed musical styles and numerous conventions. The elements of music remain alarmingly simple and are quickly exhausted. John Stuart Mill speculated in his *Autobiography* that he was 'seriously tormented by the thought of the exhaustibility of musical combinations' (1873), suggesting that the day may come when all of the melodic combinations have been exhausted. It would then be impossible to produce any new melodies. Stravinsky is alleged to have countered this by saying that many fine symphonies are still waiting to be written in C major (Craft 2011).

Sonification, as a kind of mimicry, has previously been in vogue. In 1964 Karlheinz Stockhausen decided to use a tam-tam (gong)[8] as an acoustic source of white noise in his composition *Mikrophonie 1* (1964). This acoustic source distributes noise equally and randomly across the entire audible spectrum. The tam-tam, a carefully made instrument, is a tribe of metallurgy, and it has strange resonant characteristics. It does not respond in a linear way to an increase in excitation. Stockhausen noticed that the tam-tam seemed to resonate with a wide range of ambient sound. This sound can be heard when your put your ear very close to it. He conceived of a way of investigating the tam-tam with a microphone as if the latter were also a kind of instrument, a probe. Stockhausen then set about inquiring into other ways of exciting the different resonances which are latent in the tam-tam. This involved the use of several household objects, kitchen appliances, boxes, cardboard tubes, chalk scrapers and resin bows, to introduce different forms of an impulse of energy into the tam-tam in the hope of exciting the various possibilities of resonance within its physical structure. These sonorities, in turn, would be detected, transformed, amplified, and shaped with filters into something that has the typical characteristics of musical materials.

Like most modern music, *Mikrophonie I* is understood best through understanding its strategy of making, its process of derivation. We could take Stockhausen's *Mikrophonie I* as an early form of sonification because it is not simply a sonification of a tam-tam's properties. Instead, it explores the interaction between the tam-tam and a somewhat bizarre variety of methods and objects used to excite it. In other words, it is an investigation of the encounter between found objects and the tam-tam.

More recently, sonification as mimesis has become a standard idiom for anyone equipped with music production software tools that allow patterns or shapes to be given a sonic equivalent. Usually, these patterns or shapes are drawn from peculiarities of the number line. There is a certain charm in being able to sonify these characteristics. Still, it should be kept in mind that any sonification of numbers simply duplicates the numerical sequences. It is neither transposition in any meaningful sense and certainly not interpretation. It is possible that the addition of sound to these sequences might help us hear new connections and relations, but this should not be confused with musical composition since it entails simply repetition in a different medium.

When we add sound to numbers we are like radio astronomers who add colours to the information about galactic structures that they receive through their antennae. It should be kept in mind that these antennae are not in any sense optical; they are not telescopes. They register radiation. This radiation is then woven together according to specific fixed properties into approximations of galactic objects. The galactic objects are then presented in pictures simply because humans are able to assimilate information from images. These pictures are further enhanced by an arbitrary application of colours which is as random as our use of colours on a map.

Sonification should, therefore, be understood as an arbitrary metalanguage, imposition or over-coding of a reality that is already adequately coded. There is no sense in which the scientists investigating the coronavirus are reaching towards a more profound or immediate property of the virus by sonifying it. They are simply assigning it an arbitrary and, for them at least, an aesthetically pleasing sequence that is already established by the theory that allowed them to sequence amino acids in the first place and to characterize that sequence as the coronavirus.

In *Noise: The Political Economy of Music* (1985), Jacques Attali drew a conclusion about a new mode of music in which everyone effectively becomes a producer of music and a consumer. Attali was speculating about the rapid advance of domestic computing and software that would automate many of the functions and materials established and explored by western music since the beginning of the Baroque. He welcomed this period as a fundamental shift in the relationship between maker and consumer. Yet, he fails to take account of the relative disempowerment of the computer composer, who, like the amateur photographer, is limited to specific conventions and registers and, within these, to the production of clichés. It is true that most professional users of MIDI-based and even algorithmic open architecture synthesizer-based music production tools spend their time attempting to introduce variety, some type of novel inflexion. They seek to insert a sense of control or agency into the electronically sourced libraries to which they have access and to which they can add sampling. This allows collaging and management and the careful placement of notes sampled from acoustic instruments played in natural environments. This is the electronic editing that MIDI-based music production systems make available. But the endeavour of electronic music composition is constantly to avoid dull repetition by seeking new uses of the memory capacity of machines and developing new programs.

There is something fundamentally disappointing in sounding out a virus that is a deadly, rapidly mutating replicator, in serene, tradition-bound, clichéd and unvarying music that is of no particular aesthetic value. Once a listener has heard its basic assumptions from the musical propositional point of view, it is quite possible to switch off *Viral Counterpoint of the Coronavirus Spike Protein* and rejoin it half an hour later, only to realize that one has missed nothing. Buehler and his MIT group suggest that the rationale for this composition is that they are sonifying to better identify small changes or inflexions in the sequence of this virus's genetic expression. Every musician who uses repetitive devices such as stretti or ostinato, faces the same problem. Musicians, of course, solve this problem by providing shifts of accents or by releasing rhythm from timbre so that phrases can float above an unvarying set of proportions. At other times, proportions can seem to float above an unvarying repeated phrase. This practice was well known to Frédéric Chopin and Igor Stravinsky as well as other pianists who faced the formidable task of injecting life into existing piano sonatas. These creative techniques are stapled in twentieth-century music and are extensively practised in jazz. The very notion of swing, the idea of retardation of a phrase and accenting different notes within the rhythmic proportional structure, contributes much to our ability to highlight and make certain parts in jazz stand out.

It would not have been difficult, given new algorithms, to design rhythmic systems to transform the overly literal *Viral Counterpoint of the Coronavirus Spike Protein* into a work that engages and shifts listeners' attention. But the MIT sonifiers are limited by the existing approach contained within music software. There is little doubt that a greater familiarity with compositional and improvisational techniques would have allowed Buehler to express the dynamism of the mutating virus, as well as its multiplication and spread. Their 'composition' does not progress by shifts and variations, has no sense of various time signatures or shifting emphasis (it would be particularly enriched by syncopation or 'swung time' (Ermarth 1992), but is homogeneous, and thus at odds with its signified (the virus's changing topology as well as the vectors of its transmission). There is little doubt that the MIT project would have been not only enriched, but rendered more significant had they collaborated with a musician. A jazz musician would have been best.

The problem with the work *Viral Counterpoint of the Coronavirus Spike Protein* goes beyond the limits of the sonifiers and the software they used. The sonic mapping of an object entails its reduction to a mathematical line and then its translation into sound. Although painstaking, this process is mundanely literal. And the representational valence is further reduced by the fact that a mathematically complex (and changing) topology is mapped onto a simple system of tonal differences. The loss this entails, combined with the limitations of the sonifiers and the software, means that the sonification is highly unlikely to reveal anything of significance about the virus.

Why does *Viral Counterpoint of the Coronavirus Spike Protein* capture the imagination? A micro-version of 'the music of the spheres,' it suggests that we can sound out the world – shift sense modalities – and, in this case, listen to something that can only be seen and photographed under an electron microscope. This is a question of scale: we are invited to hear that which is too small to see with the naked eye, but which we know is an invidious and deadly presence all around us. There is obvious appeal in this access, and further charm in the apparent (but meaningless) harmony of this small omnipresent entity. What is the point of arguing that the sonification is misguided, dull and pointless? As we have seen, sonification is ubiquitous and fundamental to all musical practice. If one is to render an object as sound in a way that is productive of meaning (through defamiliarization), which creates new apprehensions and cognitive possibilities, it is necessary to consider far more carefully the interface of mathematics and music so as not to devalue both. Heurism entails the recognition of meaningful failure, which is the most apposite evaluation of the MIT sonification.

Notes

1   This refers to a music notation/text in which the interpretation of the text is left to chance or open to the interpreter's choice.
2   An electronic device used for detecting radiation. The device has an electronic circuitry that that generates 'clicks' as the quantity of radiation entering its components increases.
3   See YouTube data on how a blind astronomer found a way to 'hear' the stars.
4   Richard Feynman's diagrams are image-based representations showing the magnitude of a process or processes that can occur in multiple ways.
5   For a contextual discussion on sensation and the making of a nose refer to Bruno Latour's *How to Talk About the Body*.
6   For examples of such sketches refer to the reworkings of Modest Mussorgsky's *Pictures at an Exhibition* (1874).
7   In Chapter 3 of Eco's *The Role of the Reader* (1979), he explains how a language composed initially of simple elements rapidly evolves from basic expressions to highly complex ones.
8   For individuals unfamiliar with the tam-tam or gong, view the opening of any Rank film. Rank Organizations films are introduced with a scene of the company's trademark Gongman.

Works Cited

Asquith, Lily. 'Listening to Data from the Larger Hadron Collider'. Zurich, 9 December 2013. YouTube TedX https://www.youtube.com/watch?v=iQiPytKHEwY. Accessed on 20 February 2021.

Attali, Jacques. *Noise: The Political Economy of Music*. Manchester: Manchester University Press, 1985.

Brown, Laurie M. *Feynman's Thesis: A New Approach to Quantum Theory*. Hackensack, NY: World Scientific Publishing, 2005.

Buehler, Markus J. *Viral Conterpoint of the Coronavirus Spike Protein 2019-nCoV*. 13 March 2020.   https://soundcloud.com/user-275864738/viral-counterpoint-of-the-coronavirus-spike-protein-2019-ncov. Accessed 20 February 2021.

Buehler, Markus. J. 'Turning Sound into Matter'. Boston, MA, 9 September 2020. YouTube TEDxMIT https://www.youtube.com/watch?v=jHiGFCkXN1k&t=19s. Accessed on 23 February 2021.

Cox, Christopher. 'The Jerrybuilt Future: The Sonic Arts Union, Once Group and Mev's Live Electronics.' In Rob Young (ed). *Under-Currents. The Hidden Wiring of Modern Music*. New York, NY: Continuum, 2011: 35–44.

Craft, Robert. *Conversations with Igor Stravinsky*. London: Faber, 2011.

Diaz-Merced, Wanda. 'How a Blind Astronomer Found a Way to Hear the Stars.' 13 July 2016. TED https://www.youtube.com/watch?v=-hY9QSdaReY. Accessed on 12 March 2021.

Eco, Umberto. *The Role of the Reader*. Bloomington: Indian University Press, 1979.

Eno, Brian. *Ambient 1: Music for Airports*. London: Polydor Records. Record/Vinyl. PVC 7908 (AMB 001), 1978.

Erlich, Victor. 'Russian Formalism'. *Journal of the History of Ideas*. 34(4), 1973: 627–638.

Ermarth, Elizabeth. *Sequel to History: Postmodernism and the Crisis of Representational Crime*. Princeton: Princeton University Press, 1992.

Goddard, Scott. 'Maurice Ravel: Some Notes on His Orchestral Method'. *Music and Letters*. 1925: 291–303.

Kaiser, David. *How the Hippies Saved Physics: Science, Counterculture, and the Quantum Revival*. New York: Norton, 2012.

Kramer, Gregory, Bruce Walker, Terri Bonebright, Perry Cook, and John H. Flowers. *Sonification Report: Status of the Field and Research Agenda*. Report. Lincoln, Nebraska: International Community for Auditory Display, 2010.

Grim, Wayne. *233rd Day, Before and After Totality, for Kronos Quartet and Computer Sonification*.   2018.   https://waynegrim.com/233rd-day-before-and-after-totality-for-kronos-quartet-and-computer-sonification. Accessed 12 February 2021.

International Science Council (ISC). 'The Sound of Science - the SARS-CoV-2 Virus as a Piece of Classical Music'. 17 April 2020. https://council.science/current/news/thesound-of-science-the-sars-cov-2-virus-as-a-piece of-classical-music. Accessed 12 February 2021.

Kaiser, David. *How the Hippies Saved Physics: Science, Counterculture, and the Quantum Revival*. New York: Norton, 2011.

Kittler, Friedrich A. *The Truth of the Technological World*. Stanford: Stanford University Press, 2013.

Kittler, Friedrich A., and Susanne Holl. *Music und Mathematik I: Hellas 1/1, 1/2: Aphrodite/ Eros*. Paderborn: Brill/ Wilhelm Fink, 2020/2021.

Krahmalkov, Charles R. *A Phoenician Punic Grammar*. Leiden: Brill, 2001.

Latour, Bruno. 'How to Talk about the Body? The Normative Dimension of Science Studies. *Body & Society*.10(2–3), 2004: 205–29.

Latour, Kathryn A., and John A. Deighton. 'Learning to Become a Taste Expert.' *Journal of Consumer Research*. 26(1), 2019: 1–19.

Luckenbill, Daniel. D. 'Possible Babylonian Contributions to the So-Called Phoenician Alphabet'. *The American Journal of Semitic Languages and Literature*. 36(1), 1919: 27– 39

Mill, John Stuart. *Autobiography*. London: Longmans, 1873.

Mussorgsky, Modest. *Pictures at an Exhibition*. Mainz: Schott Music, (1874), 2011.

Northrup, Cynthia A (ed). 'Alphabet, Phoenician'. *Encyclopaedia of World Trade: From Ancient Times to the Present: From Ancient Times to the Present, Volumes 1–4*. London: Routledge. 2005: 24–26.

Presburger, Mojžesz. 'Ueber die Vollstaendigkeit eines gewissen Systems der Arithmetik ganzer Zahlen, in welchem die Addition als einzige Operation hervortritt. *Comptes Rendus du I congrés de Mathématiciens des Pays Slaves*. Warsaw: Sklad Gowny 1931: 92–101.

Quinn, Marty. 'Research Set to Music: The Climate Symphony and other Sonifications of Ice Core, Radar, DNA, Seismic and Solar Wind Data.' *Proceedings of the 2001 International Conference on Auditory Display*. Ed. International Conference on Auditory Display. Espoo, Finland: ICAD, 2001: 56–61.

Roberts, Andy. 'Francis Crick, DNA & LSD: Psychedelic History in the Age of Science.' 4 May 2015. https://psychedelicpress.co.uk/blogs/psychedelic-press-blog/23736769-francis-crick-dna-lsd-psychedelic-history-in-the-age-of-science. Accessed 12 February 2021.

Roberts, Maddy S. 'Scientists are Making Music from the Structure of Coronavirus'. https://www.classicfm.com/music-news/coronavirus/scientists-turn-spike-protein-into-music. 08 April 2020. Accessed 01 March 2021.

Service, Tom. 'A Guide to Luciano Berio's music.' *The Guardian*. https://www.theguardian.com/music/tomserviceblog/2012/dec/10/contemporary-music-guide-luciano-berio, 10 December 2012. Accessed on 12 February 2021.

Stebbing, Lizzie S. 'The Inaugural Address: Sound Shapes and Words'. *Proceedings of the Aristotelian Society, Supplementary Volumes 14, Science, History, and Theology* Oxford: Oxford University Press. 1935: 1–21.

Stockhausen, Karlheinz. *Mikrophonie I*. Vienna: Universal Edition, 1964.

Stravinsky, Igor. *The Rite of Spring*. Perf. London Symphony Orchestra. Eugene Goossens Classic Records, 2013.

Ziman, John. *Reliable Knowledge. An Exploration of the Grounds for Belief in Science*. Cambridge: Cambridge University Press, 1996.

Memory Book as a New Genre of Illness Writing: How a Ugandan Farming Mother Wrote about HIV

Machiko Oike

Abstract

A memory book is a therapeutic document and personal testament – a workbook written, most commonly, by a HIV-positive caregiver or parent for their child, about the family's background and the parent's life experiences, to guide the child in the parent's absence. In Uganda, memory projects first emerged in 1998 as public health outreach for people with HIV. They encourage writers, often agrarian widows with limited literacy, to deliver their messages to their children and the world. While reports have focused on the psychosocial support the projects provide to the beneficiaries, the content, and modes of representation in individual books, have received little attention. This article undertakes a close textual analysis of the words and images in one memory book, written in English by a subsistence farmer with seven years' schooling. Using the frameworks of narrative therapy and illness writing, it examines how this reticent writer represents, obliquely, through textual gaps and contradictions, her painful memories of her child's abuse by her husband and her co-wife and the difficult experience of living with HIV. This article argues that memory books as a new genre of illness writing can help less literate, less heard people with HIV write their stories in their own words and can help us, the readers, understand their experiences and lifeworlds from their perspectives.

The memory book is a therapeutic document and personal testament – a workbook written as part of public health outreach by a parent or guardian, usually an HIV-positive widowed mother, for her child. It discusses the family's background and the parent's life experience, to guide the child in the future absence of the parent.

This article offers a literary analysis of one memory book, based on my six fieldwork visits to Uganda (mostly Tororo District, Eastern Uganda) between 2008 and 2016. During these visits, I studied thirty memory books and interviewed their authors, the authors' family members, a trained writing assistant, NGO workers and community group leaders. Plan Uganda, the project organizer, supported the first three visits, and Community Vision, the local implementing NGO, supported the other three. I am a literary critic, and I first learned about memory book projects while engaged in research using literary methods to investigate social activism around HIV. Excited to read their memory books, guided by NGO fieldworkers, I approached the writers. The writers shared their precious books with me and taught me about their lives, their writing and their books. This article discusses the writers using their real names, which they themselves preferred, though the names of other people and locations referred to in memory books are redacted or replaced with single letters for privacy reasons. Minor grammatical errors in memory book excerpts are unmarked unless problematic.

Having originated in the UK in 1991 for the use of HIV-affected families of African origin (Smith 26–27), memory book projects appeared in Uganda in 1998 (Biryetega 30), before spreading to other African counties in 2004 (Dunn and Ward; Ward). Similar narrative interventions have been made in South Africa, such as oral memory work by the University of KwaZulu-Natal from 2000 (Denis) and visual-oriented memory works by the University of Cape Town from 2001 (AIDS and Society; Grünkemeier 180–86; Morgan and Bambanani). In Uganda, memory projects were most active from the early 2000s to the early 2010s. Their decline was most likely due to an HIV funding shift from psychosocial support to medical service provision, as Charles Lubega, a project manager for Community Vision, indicated (Interview, Kampala, 26 August 2013). However, at least one recent case report, on a 2018 workshop, can be found on a website (*Memory Book for Africa*).[1]

Memory book projects vary in structure, workshop content, workbook format and writing procedure depending on location and sponsoring organization. In Uganda, the aspiring memory book writers usually attended a five-day workshop on memory book writing, egalitarian parenting, child-centred future planning and more (Healthlink). After completing the course, the participants used their own time to write in the workbook of approximately thirty pages with topic headings such as 'Our Family Home,' 'Special To Me' (meaning the writer-parent) and 'Your Birth' (meaning the reader-child's). While some participants wrote in their first language, others wrote in English.[2] Less literate writers dictated their narratives to more literate relatives, friends, counsellors, trained writing assistants and/or others, who transcribed their narratives (often in English translation).

It was observed that the writers had in mind a wider secondary readership for their memory books than just their family circle, the primary readers. Several times, the writers in Tororo who wrote in English, including those who used transcribers, expressed their preference for writing in English because 'visitors can read' their stories if they are written in English. One facilitator, Raymond Ekwaro, explained that the facilitators sometimes encouraged English writing, because 'English can go far' (Interview, Tororo, 23 August 2014). Ayoo Rose made her book a quasi-official publication by adding pages for a table of contents and acknowledgements, and ended the latter page with an activistic message to the world: 'We the clients of Tororo District programe fully welcome ARVs [antiretroviral]-services to our district as a means of increasing household health and as per our recommandation. My the struggle continues. By Ayoo Rose client repres018ntative A and B sub counties. [Signature]'. While I, as a literary critic, believe in writing in one's first language and acknowledge the need to foster literate cultures in local languages, I also appreciate these writers' efforts to cater to a wider readership, and take it to be my responsibility to help their stories be heard in the world.

Reports and evaluations, questionnaires and interviews with beneficiaries and NGO workers have focused on the psychosocial support offered to HIV-affected families, which is the overt aim of the memory projects (Horizons Program; Witter; Witter and Were). However, memory books can be analyzed not only as a therapeutic tool but also as works of literature – as life writing, or more particularly illness writing – and close textual analysis can illumine the lifeworlds, sentiments and experiences of those living with HIV. The writers I met were usually widowed mothers, mostly small-scale farmers, traders and artisans with agrarian backgrounds and limited schooling – usually several years of primary education, sometimes a few more. Some writers detailed family customs and history dating back to colonial times, while others narrated their own life stories and philosophies, especially as they related to HIV. Some described their daily life of farming, social gatherings, church-going and workshops, while others expressed gratitude to their friends and NGO workers, and addressed their messages to their children and to society. Some wrote about their illness – symptoms, testing and treatments. In short, memory books can stand as a family chronology, essay, diary, personal letter, testimony and illness record. They are, then, uniquely hybrid texts written by people with HIV that have great potential as an emerging genre of life and illness writing.

Arthur W. Frank and Anne Hunsaker Hawkins emphasize the formation of a new self through reflection and narration of one's experience of illness in autobiographical illness writings.[3] Frank argues that a wounded storyteller reclaims their own voice, 'a personal voice telling what illness has imposed on [them] and seeking to define for [themselves] a new place in the world' (*Wounded Storyteller* 7). This is a counter-narrative to 'medicine's reduction of their suffering to its general unifying view' (*Wounded Storyteller* 11). Hawkins explains in a similar vein, 'Pathography restores the person ignored or canceled out in the medical enterprise, and it places that person at the very center. Moreover, it gives that ill person a voice' (12).

Read through such a lens (individualistic Euro-American illness writings), writers of memory book narratives may seem reticent about presenting their stories of living with HIV – they seem rarely to go beyond campaign narratives of positive living. One of the reasons for their apparent reticence may be because memory books are more about family than personal illness, as they are written primarily for the writers' children. Annet Biryetega, a former coordinator of the National Community of Women Living with HIV/AIDS (NACWOLA), a group that pioneered memory book projects, describes their nature: 'The book contains information about the parents and the early life of each child, about beliefs, traditions, hopes for the future etc. The focus is not on death and disaster but on helping children understand who they are and giving them the right information to make the best of the future' (31).

However, memory books do represent the writers' experience of HIV in their own voices, in their own ways. This article is about one such memory book, written in English by Christine Helda Athieno (November 1957–January 2020), an HIV-positive subsistence farmer of the Teso people (with seven years of primary education) from eastern Uganda, addressed to her younger child, her only son, who was born in 1979. I interpret her life story, as it is expressed in her own words and pictures in her memory book. My interpretation was assisted by interviews that I conducted with the author. I trace her elaborate steps toward narrativizing her life with HIV through a close textual analysis of her memory book and establish the potential of memory books as a medium for people to represent their lives with HIV.

In Uganda, life stories of people with HIV are often featured in HIV sensitization campaigns. An HIV-positive popstar, Philly Lutaaya, campaigned around the country, and his posthumous 1990 documentary film was shown on TV and in outreach programmes nationwide (Frank 152–55). At community-level, drama groups, most of whose members are living with HIV, were formed to perform message songs, educational drama sketches and folk dances, and to offer testimonies of their experience of living with HIV (Barz; Barz and Cohen; Mangeni). Many memory book writers wrote about their participation in such community presentations, and as Judah M. Cohen says, '[by 2004 in Uganda], drama groups had become a prominent part of the AIDS-related landscape' (312). In contrast, autobiographical stories written by people living with HIV are rare. Noerin Kaleeba, a co-founder of The AIDS Support Organisation (TASO), a pioneering local support group, who lost her husband to AIDS, published a collection of essays (Kaleeba and Ray) and an autobiography (Kaleeba), but she herself is not living with HIV. The Uganda Women Writers Association (FEMRITE) published an anthology of creative non-fiction life stories of TASO female clients based on interviews conducted by FEMRITE-trained writers (Kiguli and Barungi), which are, strictly speaking, not written by people with HIV. Memory books thus provided people with HIV a unique medium in which to write down their life stories and an answer to the problems experienced in disclosing their status, particularly to their loved ones.

Below, I introduce Athieno's life history in the first section. The second part comprises a discussion of two of her central preoccupations: the abuse of her son by her husband (the child's father) and her co-wife, and Athieno's own experience of HIV. There is now no way to clarify certain details, since Athieno is no longer with us. This limitation, however, does not constrain our analysis, since our purpose here is to understand her lifeworld from her perspective, as represented in her memory book. I conclude with a discussion of the memory book as a literary tool for writers with HIV – how writing one's experience of illness in a memory book can help the writers navigate living with the illness and, further, how it can assist readers in touching some of their muted or unheard sentiments, lifeworlds, worldviews and experiences of living with HIV.

Christine Helda Athieno: A Biography

Born in 1957, one of fourteen children, her father a clan leader and her mother his fourth wife among six, Athieno started her primary education at the age of five and progressed to seventh grade before working as a nursery-school teacher for two years. She attended a tailoring course and worked as a sales assistant but lived primarily by subsistence farming throughout her life. Efficient and diligent, she described her busy social life in her memory book: actively engaging in NGO training courses, church welfare committees and community projects as a leading member of various associations.

After finishing school, Athieno was married to a man fourteen years her senior and had a daughter and a son (it was for her son that she later wrote her memory book). According to her memory book, her marriage became unstable because her husband mistreated her and brought two more women into their relationship. To escape from these family troubles, she writes, her beloved son stayed with Athieno's mother-in-law. Finally, in 1993, Athieno's husband sent her away, while keeping their son with his other wife. Abused by his stepmother, the boy later joined his mother.

Athieno was tested for HIV in 1997, 1998 and 1999, when tests were being encouraged in the area. She contracted HIV in 1998 or 1999 (she tested positive in 1999) through a relationship with a man other than her husband (Interview, Tororo, 29 April 2016). In 2002, she returned to her husband as his caregiver since he was critically ill with HIV and she started to write her memory book in that year. Athieno began ARV treatment in 2003, but her husband refused treatment and passed away in 2005. His second wife also passed away and the third wife left the family. Athieno passed away in January 2020 from throat cancer (Charles Lubega, Manager of Community Vision, E-mail correspondence, 14 September 2020).

Protesting the Abuse of the Addressee Child

In her memory book, Athieno describes the facts of her life without much emotion, even when she writes about HIV. However, she exhibits her pent-up emotions most poignantly when she talks about the suffering of her son, the addressee. The page titled 'My Favorite Memories Of You' (18; see Image 1),[4] starts peacefully with lovely memories of the boy, then turns to protest, in an understated way, against his treatment.

Athieno starts the passage describing her 'favorite memories' of the boy, admiring his diligence both at school and at home. However, she cannot maintain her composure as she reminisces about the boy's life. The word 'Except' marks her turn to relating the suffering he endured. The forest, designated a national forest reserve and stretching for 25 square kilometres, is not a place where a teenage boy should sleep at night. The boy covered 40 kilometres unaccompanied, across the backcountry from his father's compound to his mother's. However, instead of including affective passages, for instance deploring her son's suffering, or analyzing the situation and identifying what and who to blame, Athieno describes what happened, in three short, simple sentences written consecutively without conjunctions, as if breathlessly ('Except your father mistreated you in * you came footing from * up to ** you even slept in the forest ***'). After thus – if only partially – releasing her feelings, without a paragraph break, she shifts her narrative and turns to advising her son directly to 'forgive your father for what ever he has done to you' and 'just put everything before God'. Her incipient bitterness and indignation are thus suppressed and replaced by forgiveness and submission to God.

Athieno's laconic words can be supplemented with the attached picture (see Image 1). According to her (Interview, Tororo, 5 May 2016), the picture was taken on Christmas Day a few years after the boy came to live with Athieno at her mother's compound. The boy poses for the picture, dressed up, probably in his Christmas clothes, showing his splendid, shining watch, probably to elicit the viewer's admiration. The closing words, 'this is the only son of mine and the last born of mine,' set the boy in a special position in his proud mother's heart. It expresses Athieno's hope that the love and care he has received from his mother's family will cure him of the pain inflicted by his father and consign the bitter memory of abuse to the past.

Athieno writes about the abuse of the boy again in 'Growing Up' (22). This time, she describes the situation in more detail, but the passage is rather detached, free of emotion. From the explanation given here, we learn that it was one of his stepmothers (the father's third wife) to whom the father had entrusted the boy, who abused him, though the father was also partly to blame – it was he who was ultimately responsible for the whole family. Athieno confirmed that, at the time, the father was staying with his second wife in C town, working as a clerk (Interview, Tororo, 29 April 2016).

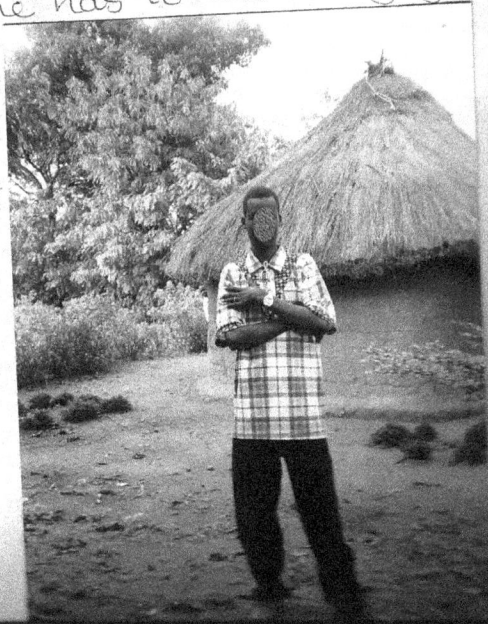

-My Favourite Memories-
Of You

You were crawling one leg infront, And first time you went to school you were doing very well And also you are hard working at home digging. You have a talent of growing crops.
Except your father mistreated you in ▓▓▓ ▓▓ you came footing from ▓▓▓▓▓▓▓ up to ▓▓▓ you even slept in the forest ▓▓▓▓▓▓, My son forgive your father for what ever he has done to you. You just put everything before God. May the lord bless you and have the strong heart. God has blessed you because what ever small thing you do he has to answer by giving you something.

This is the only son of mine and the last born of mine.

Image 1. "My Favorite Memories of You".

> Growing up was just a struggle, your father didn't even buy for you clothes and nappies You grew up in your [paternal] grandmothers hands *Because* your father wanted to fight me everyday. *So* I dicided to leave him and he married. *One time* he even took you to stay with his third wife, *but* the woman mistreated you *until* the neigbours told him. *That's when* he learned about it *and* he brought you back to me. Those days he was staying in C but he was working with Education's Office. (emphasis added)[5]

Instead of engaging the reader by protesting the abuse using direct address, as in the previous section, Athieno here, in a detached, composed manner, explains the situation using several linking words, and thus delineates the memory objectively.

The difference in the manner of presentation between the two passages relating to the child abuse shows the cathartic or therapeutic effect of writing for Athieno. From the perspective of narrative therapy, narrating one's problems helps the narrator 'externalize' and 're-author' (White and Epston 16, 41; White).[6] More specifically, from a scriptotherapy perspective, writing one's trauma 'may promote the formation of a structured narrative out of previously unstructured sensory fragments … [which] should lead to the cognitive assimilation of traumatic memories and subsequent biological alterations' (Smyth and Greenberg 153).[7] That is what Athieno achieves here. Even though she sounds restrained in expressing her inner turmoil in both passages, she engages her son in her narrative as she releases emotion in the first passage by creating an evocative picture. As a result, in the second passage, she manages to gain distance from the past and describe the experience objectively, in a sequential order.

Detouring around HIV, Pointing to a Troubled Marriage

Athieno is reticent about narrating her own HIV-related suffering compared to her reserved yet touching words describing the suffering of her son. 'My Health' (12) consists in two pages: the heading page (Image 2) and the reverse page including three captioned pictures, the last of which I will discuss later. This section most commonly discusses a writer's HIV experience. Athieno, in contrast, focuses on her troubled marriage and family-related suffering. In this passage, she refers to TASO, a local NGO, and the Centers for Disease Control and Prevention (CDC), Uganda, a local affiliate of the US CDC, which was managing a water sanitation project in the area.

The first paragraph, which is rather long for Athieno, discusses her marriage problems and contracting HIV. However, there is a gap in her life story, between the third and fourth sentences, before 'Now I am Positive'. In the first three sentences, she reminisces about her marriage, which was peaceful in the early days but then turned sour – when her husband added two wives. This was followed by her rejection by most of the family members. Here again, Athieno uses 'except' to introduce the cause of her subsequent troubles: her husband's polygamy. Leading with one 'Except,' she narrates her troubled life story in two grammatically convulsive sentences containing repetitions and another 'except'. ('Except when he married two women it's when he started mistreating me. And all the family members refused me; except your grandmother was **** was the Only one supporting me.') Then, suddenly, she jumps to her present condition in the stark fourth sentence: 'Now I am Positive'. After this declaration, she states philosophically, 'that is how the world goes' and gives her son simple advice: to 'stick on what you are doing' and to 'be near the lord all the time by praying'.

-My Health-

My health was not bad during those days when I was with your father ▓▓▓ ▓▓▓ Except when he married two women its when he started mistreating me. And all the family members refused me; except your grandmother was ▓▓▓ ▓▓▓ was the only one supporting me. Now I am Positive, dont get scared or worried, that is how the world goes So my son stick on what you are doing, dont put your mind in this world's things be near the lord all the time by praying.
I Joined Taso in 1999. In 2000 we were select to join CDC. So please know your status when you have not broken down or weak.
Here when I was still enjoying Life. I was in the Barrocks the place was called ▓▓▓
— I started ARUs in sep 2003 up to now I am doing well.
— I have planned for my children's future.
— Joining Taso when you are still strong is good Because you will not break down

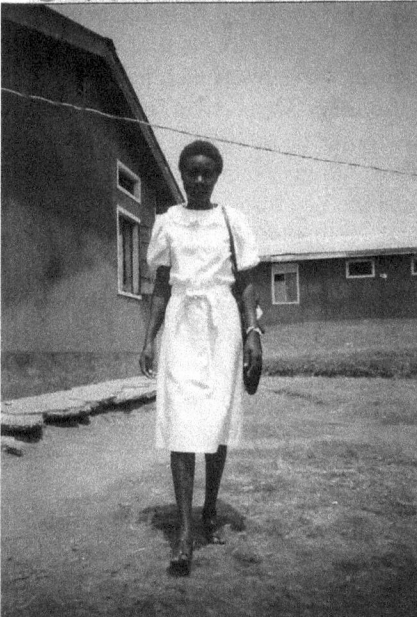

Image 2: "My Health".

From the second paragraph on, referring to her own experiences of treatment, Athieno starts to list concrete measures for prevention and management of HIV: get tested, know your status and start treatment in time.[8]

The whole passage foregrounds the stage Athieno has reached – positive living with the virus under control – but one may wonder what happened in the gap, and how she came to her present stage of positive living, after her husband's infidelity, her HIV diagnosis and the advent of her sickness. Although she does not give any clarification anywhere in her memory book (a possible practical reason is to avoid talking about sexual matters to her child), a draft sheet for her self-introduction, which I found stored between its pages, reveals what happened in the gap.[9] According to the draft, she tested negative three times in 1997 and once in 1998 yet positive in 1999. She then joined TASO to receive antibiotics, became involved in the CDC water sanitation project and later began to access ARV services.

Although this gap is significant, we should not focus on what Athieno did not write but on what she did if we are to understand her experience from her perspective. Although she contracted HIV from another man while staying away from her husband (which is omitted from her memory book narrative), the ultimate reason she was infected, from her perspective, was her troubled marriage. In other words, when she reflected upon her life and considered what had brought the calamity of HIV into her life, she seems to have perceived the 'real' cause, indicating it with the pivotal word 'Except': 'Except when he married two women it's when he started mistreating me'. Her insight reflects that what is important is not the clinical cause of infection but its interpersonal and social background. Athieno's reasoning, stated in 2002 or 2003, is highly perceptive and shows her lived knowledge of the virus, considering that the first UNAIDS review on HIV/AIDS programmes that considered gender was only issued in 1999 (Whelan). The first major book-length analysis of AIDS in Africa from the perspective of gender and sexuality was only published in 2000 (Baylies and Bujra).

Thus, we can understand why Athieno is most eloquent when describing the abuse of her son. Her bitter, abusive relationship with her husband, from her perspective, led to her illness and the maltreatment of her child. This may be part of why she chose her son as the addressee of her memory book and wrote down her bitter memories – to give him guidance to help him survive.[10] With the word 'except,' she braces herself and the boy to face the realities of child abuse (in 'My Favorite Memory Of You') and marital problems (in 'My Health') as best she could.

Another matter rarely discussed in Athieno's memory book is her deteriorating health. According to the above-mentioned draft page, her CD4 count (immunization indicator) had dropped as low as fifty by the time she started on ARVs, meaning that she was near death. It should be noted how strongly and repeatedly she emphasizes the need to 'know your status when you have not broken down or weak' ('My Health') to help her son not to repeat her misfortune. Throughout the memory book, however, she only briefly refers to her symptoms per se, and not in the main text but in the caption of a picture on the reverse page of 'My Health': 'my life started changing slowly. I was ever falling sick on and off' (Image 3). The picture does not clearly capture her poor health, though according to her interview remarks, she was critically ill at the time the picture was taken, around 2000, before she started ARVs (Tororo, 5 May 2016).

However, when we compare the image with the picture on the heading page of the same section (Image 2), taken 'when I was still enjoying Life,' we can certainly see a contrast. The heading page picture, taken around 1998 (according to Athieno, Interview, Tororo, May 5, 2016), captures her in a stylish white knee-length dress, with a bag over her shoulder, stepping forward and standing tall. The crisp white dress shining in the sun seems to emphasize her health and vitality, making her stand out from the background. She commented that she chose this picture to show herself healthy (Interview, 5 May 2016). In contrast, the picture on the reverse page, taken about two years later, when 'I was ever falling sick on and off,' shows her looking queasy in the direct sunshine while her relatives smile gently. Wearing a drab olive dress, she looks as if she is receding, experiencing discomfort and anxiety.

Musing on Living and Dying with AIDS

Even though the threat of HIV and death is not explicitly discussed, and thus barely kept in emotional abeyance in 'My Health,' it resurfaces in 'Thoughts On Life And Things I Believe In' (8), as Athieno ruminates over her life in general. The two paragraphs may sound unrelated, but they both begin with the phrase 'in my life' and muse about living.

> The thoughts in my life are with a wish that if I were normal like before, I would be doing a lot of productive developmental activities. But now that I am sick I am not able and I don't know how long my life time will be. And I dont know how my family will look like after me and after I have died?

> In my life I believe in the church and I am a christian, so you should do that. I believe in the children who are good mannered. You have to go for prayers and pray at night when going to bed. I am a Protestant and I was baptized by Rev. D.

In the first paragraph, writing about her 'Thoughts On Life,' Athieno unravels her anxiety about living with HIV. She wishes to invest in 'a lot of productive developmental activities' for the future but cannot. She regrets her past, wishing 'that … I were normal like before,' and she deplores her present: 'I am sick I am not able'. She then directly voices her insecurity about the

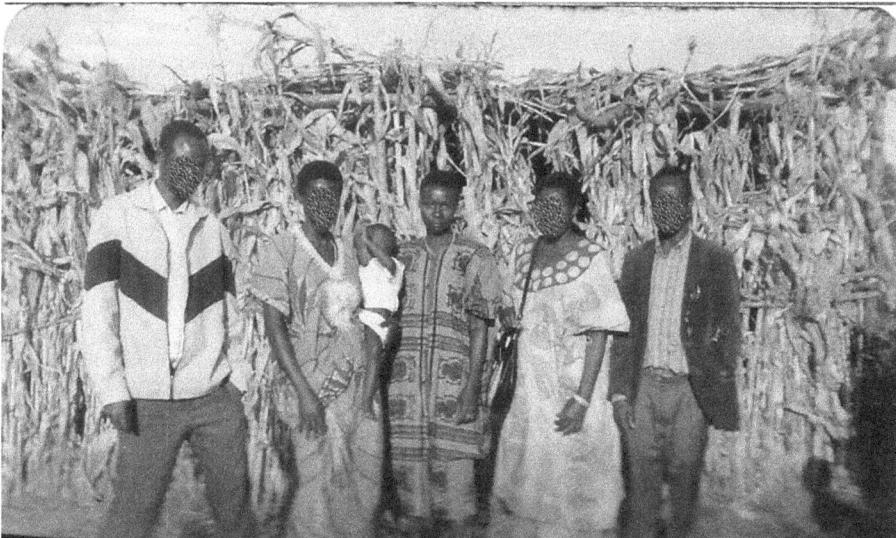

Image 3:   "I was ever falling sick on and off".

future: 'I don't know how long my life time will be'. The concluding declarative sentence ends anxiously with a question mark; she asks herself what it will be like for her family when she is gone. Such self-reflection, going backward and forward through her life, is rare in her narrative and poignantly reveals the deep anguish she was grappling with.

However, without seeking further words to convey what afflicts her mind or reconstructing her experience in a sequential narrative, Athieno starts the second paragraph concerning 'Things I Believe In,' emphasizing visiting church and engaging in prayer to deal with her distress and frustration at living with HIV. As past regret and anxiety about the future besiege her, she catches these moments in words in the first paragraph, but instead of further narrativizing them, she diverts them into prayer. This circumvention of life tragedy through orientating it towards faith or God is one tactic Athieno and other memory writers use to live positively with HIV.

Creating a Gap Between Pictures and Their Captions

The preceding discussion has shown that, most of the time, Athieno distances herself from exploring her troubles in words, but rather submerges them or accepts them as a part of life in order to live on. The accompanying images, however, can lead us to her unvoiced, suppressed anxieties. In most pictures, she looks healthy, but two pictures have captions that directly refer to the problems of HIV: one is in 'My Health' (12), (Image 3), and the other in 'Information About Your Mother' (3) (Image 4). We can interpret the selection of pictures and their captions as representing Athieno's deliberate or inadvertent perception of reality.

'Information About Your Mother' consists of two pages: the heading page contains basic information about Athieno, such as her birthdate, birthplace and the names of her grandparents and parents, while the reverse page (Image 4) includes two pictures with captions.

The right-hand photograph was taken, according to Athieno, in a local photo studio on Christmas 1999, the year she discovered her positive status (Interview, Tororo, 5 May 2016). Sitting on a chair with arms loosely folded, she looks straight ahead into the camera with a mild smile. Her bright yellow dress and the flower-print cloth hung in the background contribute to the cheerful atmosphere of the festive occasion. HIV-positive as she was, she said in an interview, she was maintaining her weight and had no health problems (5 May 2016).

However, the caption contradicts the atmosphere of the photo: 'Here when I have tested and I have known my zero status'. On the cusp of a new year, she returns to 'zero status,' a blank slate, where everything in her life has turned to nothing and she needs to start again from scratch. Looking merry and happy, inwardly she was probably desperate and apprehensive about what her new life status would bring.

The left-hand picture was taken in a workshop in 2002, a year before Athieno started ARVs. The caption is upbeat: 'Here I was in ***** for Agricultureskills and even it was Valatine day. That was how I enjoyed the day'. Another picture taken on the same occasion in 'Special Memories' (7) is captioned, 'The last day we came back from ***** with my gifts. Plan [NGO] was the one trained us'. The picture shows Athieno with several bags and a box, appreciating the happy occasion.

However, the atmosphere of the left-hand image again contradicts Athieno's verbal explanation. Its gloomy, serious mood is distinctly different from the photograph taken when she was

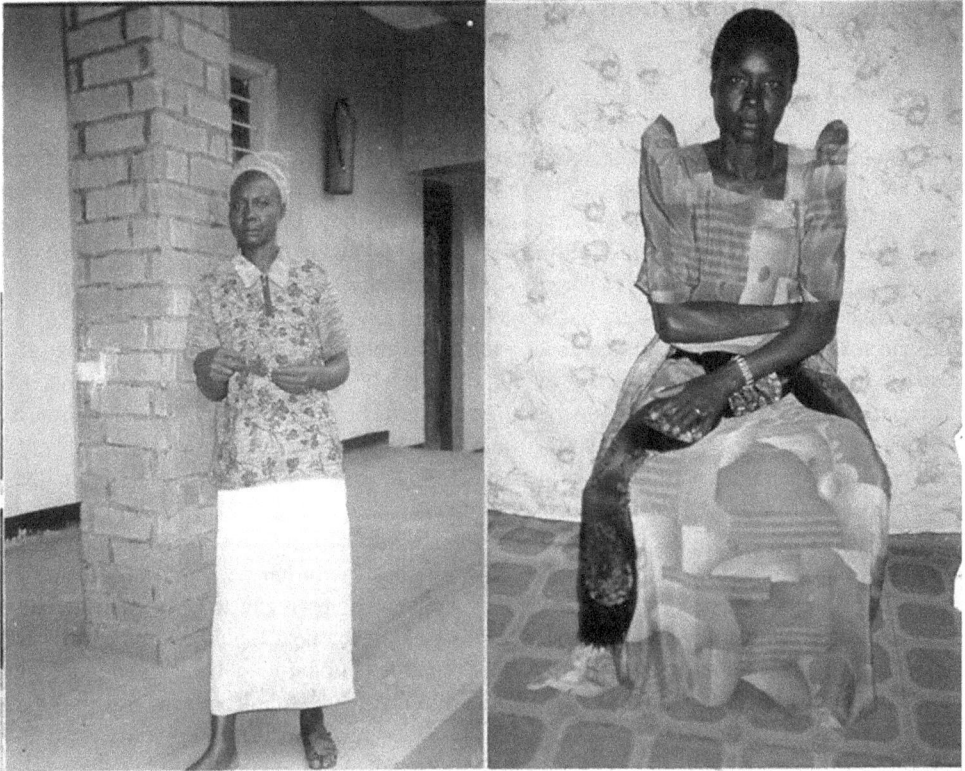

Here I was in ⬛⬛⬛⬛⬛ for
Agriculture skills and even it
was Valotine day. That
was how I enjoyed the
day.

Here when I have tested
and I have known my
Zero status.

Image 4:   "Information About Your Mother".

apparently healthy. Dressed in grey and white, she wrinkles her face and stares at the camera a little aslant, toying with the red Valentine's decoration in her hands. She looks withered compared with the picture on the right, taken two years and a few months earlier.[11] While celebrating Valentine's Day with her fellow participants, she seems to have been in deteriorating health. In the workshop, composed of two parts – succession planning and vocational training – Athieno learned how to prepare the family for her future death and how to write a memory book and a will. Her serious face conveys her determination to face any troubles leading up to her death – her life precarious without ARVs.

These pictures, with their contradictory captions, represent the gap not only between the picture and reality but also between Athieno's memory book narrative and her lived experience.

Possibilities and Limitations of the Memory Book as a Self-Story of Illness

As mentioned earlier, Frank discusses 'illness as a call for stories' (*Wounded Storyteller* 53). According to Frank, 'Stories have to *repair* the damage that illness has done to the ill person's sense of where she is in life and where she may be going. Stories are a way of redrawing maps and finding new destinations' (53). In terms of ways of 'repairing,' Frank defines three types of illness narratives. The restitution narrative tells how the ill person in physical and social misery restores comfort through medical interventions as in 'the television commercial for non-prescription drugs' (79): 'Yesterday, I was healthy, today I'm sick, but tomorrow I'll be healthy again' (77). The chaotic narrative '[denies] any possibility of restitution' (96); it is 'anti-narrative of time without sequence, telling without mediation, and speaking about oneself without being fully able to reflect on oneself' (98). Lastly, the quest narrative '[affirms] life beyond restitution' (96). It '[meets] sufferings head on' (115), and 'illness is the occasion of a journey that becomes a quest' (115) in the course of which the ill person '[believes] that something is to be gained' (115). The quest narrative 'speaks from the ill person's perspective and holds chaos at bay' (115).

Borrowing this classification of Euro-American illness writings, we can trace in Athieno's memory book, against the grain as it were, how she dealt with her deep and obfuscated pain caused by living with HIV. In fact, just when Athieno seems ready to give more details or explore her hurt, as we would anticipate, she proceeds to the next topic or turns to advise the addressee. In rare moments, her anxiety does emerge, but only to be submerged quickly under her usual, often didactic, narrative of positive living, which Frank calls the 'restitution narrative'. We should understand, however, that these elaborate circumspect steps detouring around HIV represent her efforts to live with HIV. At a moment, a crack appears in her daily coping tactics, her sense of anxiety and fear emerge, but it is soon plastered over so that she can go on with her life. This is her voice, neither loud nor vivid like chaos or quest narratives, just murmuring about living with HIV, managing her life.

Some may argue that considering the scarcity of words concerning HIV in Athieno's memory book, anthropological fieldwork and in-depth interviews might produce a richer, denser, more informative narrative. However, we should remember that the memory book should be regarded not as a mere record but as a literary work. Writers select details and organize their words and pictures on the pages, aesthetically and symbolically, as stories and messages to their readers – primarily their children, but ultimately anybody who reads their book. The writers thus actively design and weave the memory book verbally and photographically with pieces of their lives, such as facts, memories, messages, episodes, events, people and customs. Through these processes of active textualization and signification, writers, irrespective of their level of literacy, represent some of their experiences, and we, through careful interpretation, can hear something of their life stories.

Athieno, a rather laconic writer, works through blockage, deflection and reflection, filling and creating gaps in and between her words and pictures to represent an important part of her life story in her memory book: her troubled marriage, which led to the abuse of her beloved son and ultimately her own infection with HIV, the repercussions of which she experienced every day, and handled masterfully. In this process of signification, with reserved words and strategically placed pictures, she manages to express the regret and anxiety deep in her mind and affect, reconciling herself with her remorse for her son's treatment and presenting her determination to live and die positively. In this sense, the memory book works as an effective literary medium both for Athieno, in that she reorients her life towards her illness through the seemingly brief narrativization and representation of that illness, and for us, the readers, in that we can touch her life through interpretation.

Of course, there are limits to the interpretability of Athieno's experience through her memory book. The analysis conducted here required essential background information provided by interviews, which filled the gaps in the text and provided context for the pictures. These lacunae can be explained with reference to Athieno's primary reader, her son, with whom she had already shared much of this information. Although her memory book provides precious testimony to Athieno's sentiments and experiences, it will be most fruitful if supplementary research is conducted such as cultural-anthropological observations and in-depth interviews. Conducted exclusively, literary analysis has its limits, and it may become a foolhardy, almost impossible enterprise, particularly when applied to a work written by a less literate writer.

In Athieno's passage on storytelling, we may hear a resonant, Spivakian warning to us as literary critics to be aware of our limitation when trying to hear her story – the limitation that this article has tried to push against through the application of imaginative literary interpretation. The relevant section, 'What I Do In My Free Time' (11), comes just before 'My Health' (12):

> In my free time I sew my table clothes for sell. I chat with my children under the tree telling them stories. And hearing music and visiting my friends. In my compound I have a big tree for resting and chat with my children. Children will remember what stories I was telling them under that tree.

What did Athieno tell her children under her favourite tree, and what stories did she want her children to remember after she was gone? Does the passage mean that the stories she wanted her children to remember do not appear in her memory book? What stories does she tell and does she not tell there? Where do the stories she told under the tree reside? Are they kept in the children's minds and handed down to the next generation or are they lost? How do the children who listened to her stories and we – her readers – transmit her stories?

Notes

1   Precisely estimating the number of memory books written is difficult because they are distributed across various organizations with different completion rates. Community Vision (2004) counted 1 213 participants in their memory book workshops as of 2004, although not all the participants actually wrote books. Sophie Witter reported that 386 books had been completed in projects by NACWOLA as of 2004 with a completion rate of 75% of the books given out (10). As other organizations also included memory book writing in their activities, overall, perhaps several thousand memory books have been written in Uganda since the 1990s.

2   In Tororo, Beatrice Oyuki Acheinga, a writer and a community leader, explained that half of the writers in her group wrote in English and the other half in their own language, but that most of the completed books were in English (Interview, Tororo, 22 August 2014). Writers and readers in Tororo learned reading and writing in English at school (see Parry *Language*; Parry *Reading*) and found it easier to write in English, though they

emphasized their preference for, rather than reluctance toward, English writing, as will be discussed.

3   Hawkins calls nonfiction writing about illness 'pathography,' while Frank prefers terms such as 'illness narrative' ('Reclaiming') and 'illness story' (*Wounded Storyteller*). For his choice of terminology, see Frank, *Wounded Storyteller*, note 34 on p. 226–27.

4   The format Athieno uses has 28 headings; the parenthetical number after each heading in the article indicates the order of its appearance.

5   We cannot know exactly when the polygamous relationships started. We can infer from the statement here that Athieno left the matrimonial home before the husband married two more women. Another citation, however, indicates that he started these relationships while she was with him ('My Health' 12; see Section 3). We can guess that his relationships with other women and his mistreatment of Athieno may well have gone hand in hand while she was with him.

6   For a discussion on the memory book model and narrative therapy, see Morgan, then a memory project leader at the University of Cape Town.

7   Gladding and Drake mention memory books, in a broader context, as one of their scriptotherapy exercises (388).

8   It is most likely that Athieno added information about her ARV use on a separate occasion, judging from the different handwriting and chronology (she wrote the major part of her memory book in 2002, while she started on ARVs in September 2003).

9   Athieno could not remember why she wrote this draft (Interview, Tororo, 5 May 2016); possibly to introduce herself at a meeting involving people with HIV in her sub-county, since the sub-county name is written on top of the passage.

10   Athieno explained the reason she wrote for her boy and not the senior girl: 'the girl [had been] married' (Interview, Tororo, 22 August 2014). That likely means that the daughter lived independently with her husband, while the boy was still under Athieno's care. Athieno also explained that she started a second memory book, not for the daughter but for a son of her brother-in-law, whose mother had run away and whose father had mental problems. Obviously, her criterion was the perceived support need of the child, though his being a boy may have counted for something too, as her ethnic group is patrilineal.

11   Interestingly, the other picture taken in the same workshop included in 'Special Memories' (7) shows a different Athieno, with a round face, standing carefree, without expressing any particular emotion. The differences may unveil her tacit, probably subconscious will to highlight her anxiety with the picture of the serious and gloomy Athieno in 'Information About Your Mother' (3).

Works Cited

AIDS and Society Research Unit, Centre for Social Science Research. *Mapping Workshop Manual*. Cape Town: ASRU, CSSR, University of Cape Town, 2007.

Barz, Gregory. *Singing for Life: HIV/AIDS and Music in Uganda*. New York: Routledge, 2006.

Barz, Gregory and Judah M. Cohen (Eds.). *The Culture of AIDS in Africa: Hope and Healing in Music and the Arts*. New York: Oxford University Press, 2011.

Baylies, Carolyn, and Janet Bujra. *AIDS, Sexuality and Gender in Africa: Collective Strategies and Struggles in Tanzania and Zambia. Social Aspect of AIDS*. London: Routledge, 2000.

Biryetega, Annet. 'Origins (II): Experience of the National Community of Women Living with HIV and AIDS in Uganda (NACWOLA): The Memory Book Project in Uganda'. *Medicus Mundi Schweiz Bulletin*, 97(6), 2005: 30–33.

Community Vision Uganda. *End of Project Report on the AIM Sponsored Activities*. Tororo: Community Vision Uganda, 2004.

Denis, Phillippe (Ed.). *Never Too Small To Remember: Memory Work and Resilience in Times of AIDS*. Pietermaritzburg: Cluster, 2005.

Dunn, Alison, and Sarah Hammond Ward. *Inspiring Futures: Learning from Memory Work in Africa*. London: Healthlink Worldwide, 2009.

Frank, Arthur W. 'Reclaiming an Orphan Genre: The First-Person Narrative of Illness'. *Literature and Medicine* 13(1), 1994: 1–21.

Frank, Arthur W. (1995) *The Wounded Storyteller: Body, Illness an Ethics*. Second Edition. Chicago: University of Chicago Press, 2013.

Frank, Marion. *AIDS Education through Theatre: Case Studies from Uganda*. Bayreuth African Studies 35. Beyreuth: Bayreuth African Studies, 1995.

Gladding, Samuel T. and Melanie J. Drake Wallace. 2018. 'Scriptotherapy: Eighteen Writing Exercises to Promote Insight and Wellness'. *Journal of Creativity in Mental Health* 13 (4): 380–91.

Grünkemeier, Ellen. *Breaking the Silence: South African Representations of HIV/AIDS*. Woodbridge: James Currey, 2013.

Hawkins, Anne Hunsaker. *Reconstruction Illness: Studies in Pathography*. 1993. Second Edition. West Lafayette: Purdue University Press, 1999.

Healthlink Worldwide. *The Memory Work Trainer's Manual: Supporting Families Affected by HIV and AIDS*. London: Healthlink Worldwide, 2005.

Horizons Program, Makerere University Department of Sociology, and Plan Uganda. *Succession Planning in Uganda: Early Outreach for AIDS-Affected Children and Their Families*. Washington, DC: Population Council, 2004.

Kaleeba, Noerine and Sunanda Ray. *We Miss You All: Noerine Kaleeba: AIDS in the Family*. 1991. Harare: SAfAIDS, 2002.

Kaleeba, Noerine. *BENT but not BROKEN: My Story of Resilience*. 2019 [no publisher]

Kiguli, Susan N. and Violet Barungi (Eds.). *I Dare to Say: Five Testimonies by Ugandan Women Living Positively with HIV/AIDS*. Kampala: FEMRITE, 2007.

Lindsay Smith, Carol. 'Origins (I): London, 1991: The Memory Book—and Its Close Relations … '. *Medicus Mundi Schweiz Bulletin* 97(6), 2005: 26–29.

Mangeni, Patrick. 'Negotiating the Space: Challenges for Applied-Theatre Praxis with Local Non-Governmental/Community-Based Organizations in HIV/AIDS Contexts in Uganda'. *Matatu* 43, 2013: 3–30.

Memory Book for Africa. http://www.memorybookforafrica.org/. Accessed on 19 May 2021.

Morgan, Jonathan. 'Memory Work: Preparation for Death? Legacies for Orphans? Fighting for Life? One Size Fits All, or Time for Product Differentiation'. *AIDS Bulletin* 13(2), 2004. http://web.uct.ac.za/depts/cgc/Jonathan Aids%20Bulletin. Accessed on 21 July 2006.

Morgan, Jonathan, and The Bambanani Women's Group. *Long Life … : Positive HIV Stories*. Stories from the Pandemic 3. Melbourne: Spinifex; Cape Town: Double Storey, 2003.

Parry, Kate (Ed.). *Language and Literacy in Uganda: Towards a Sustainable Reading Culture*. Kampala: Fountain, 2000.

Parry, Kate (Ed.). *Reading in Africa, Beyond the School. Literacy for All in Africa, vol 2.* Kampala: Fountain, 2009.

Riordan, Richard J. 'Scriptotherapy: Therapeutic Writing as a Counseling Adjunct'. *Journal of Counseling and Development* 74, 1996: 263–69.

Smyth, Joshua M. and Melanie A. Greenberg. 'Scriptotherapy: The Effects of Writing About Traumatic Events'. In *Psychodynamic Perspectives on Sickness and Health*. Edited by Paul Raphael Duberstein and Joseph M. Masling. Alexandria, Va.: American Psychological Association, 2000. 121–63.

Ward, Nicola R. 'Scaling Up Memory Work: The Challenges'. *Medicus Mundi Schweiz Bulletin* 97(6), 2005: 34-39.

Whelan, Daniel. *Gender and HIV/AIDS: Taking Stock of Research and Programmes*. Geneva: UNAIDS, 1999.

White, Michael. *Maps of Narrative Practice*. New York: Norton, 2007.

White, Michael and David Epston. *Narrative Means to Therapeutic Ends*. New York: Norton, 1990.

Witter, Sophie. *Breaking the Silence: Memory Books and Succession Planning: The Experience of NACWOLA and Save the Children UK in Uganda*. London: Save the Children UK, 2004.

Witter, Sophie and Beatrice Were. 'Breaking the Silence: Using Memory Books as a Counselling and Succession-Planning Tool with AIDS-Affected Households in Uganda'. *African Journal of AIDS Research* 3(2), 2004: 139-43.

Two Poems

For my brother who beat COVID-19. For my family

Phelelani Makhanya

The Surname

My brother was the first to test
positive for COVID-19 on our side of the village
From that day the walls and the yard of our home
grew quills and spikes
I saw my brother sitting behind the house,
eroding and dissolving in the liquid sun
like a soluble pill
Ants already feasting on his shadow
like a starter dish.
I have carried many heavy stones
in the backpack of my eyes
but not this heavy.

There is a gravel road that passes near our home
but our neighbours have forged new detour pathways
that split like a Y;
Pathways that go deep into the woods

They will rather crisscross with black Mamba trails
than pass near our home
They look at our home with dangling eyes
To them we are walls and rafters
stuck between monster's jaws.

When women get married
they adopt a new surname
Our home got married to a virus
Our fence is a black diamond ring
that eats both flesh and ring finger bones
Our neighbours no longer call our home Kwa-Makhanya
They have given us a new surname; Kwa-Corona
They tell their children;
'Don't go near that yellow house, Kwa-Corona;
We don't want to bury you'

We are a home with a new surname; Kwa-Corona
A surname that has no clan name
A surname that claims every clan name
But to those who know how to weigh and taste
metal and steel in a syllable-
in pronouncing it;
they will know that in the bowels
of this new surname, simmers a family
that fought a ruthless organism and won.

One in the Chamber

Since he lost his job
due to COVID-19,
He spends his afternoons
sitting under the Avocado tree
behind the house
Summer flies provoke him
He swears at them in a raging voice

Flies can smell a lot of things
They can also smell defeat in a man.

He mumbles things
Avocado leaves are ears
He places his index finger
on his lips
His thumb on his chin
The other three folded fingers
hang like a deformed fist
This is a hand miming
the shape of a revolver.

Every day he argues
with the bullet in the chamber;
lusting after the folds of his brain.

Some Speculative Musings on COVID-19 Affectivity, Raymond Williams' 'Structure of Feeling' and Zadie Smith's *Intimations*

Ronit Frenkel

Abstract

Zadie Smith's *Intimations: Six Essays* (2020) is a partial history of affectivity of the present, which I am speculatively positioning as a type of transnational archive of privileged pandemic-circumscribed life. Raymond Williams' work on a 'structure of feeling' is useful here to understand new patterns of experience that have emerged during this pandemic. Williams uses the phrase a 'structure of feeling' to distinguish between formally held beliefs or ideologies, and meanings and values as they are lived and felt in relation to those beliefs or ideologies. Theories of emotion, atmosphere and feeling broadly correspond to Williams's correlation of material, social and affective structures. Smith can help us theorize emergent affectivity from inside a pandemic-strained world through the narration of the ambiguous operational logic that her essays describe. She has created a continuum made up of affective normativities and transformative affectivities on either end, with her essays tracing the rhythms of privileged life across locales, to help us understand pandemic inspired change.

In addition to pointing out the importance of the affective infrastructure of our everyday life, Williams also adds a few directives on how to analyze its manifestations. First, Williams intimates, we are generally not very good at analyzing cultural change. We recognize the facts of cultural life once they are established and institutionalized, but we tend to miss those moments when new patterns of experience emerge, when people start to think differently, when new sensibilities arise, when habits swerve. We should learn

> to think about cultural life as a present and unruly reality, and not only in the past tense,
> as that which eventually became the case. (Sharma and Tygstrup 12)

Sometimes, we are very aware when new patterns of experience emerge. The harder part is analyzing what those changes mean. It has been one year since the first case of COVID-19 was
detected in South Africa on 5 March 2020. What followed has been an extraordinary upheaval
of everyday life with lockdowns, movement restrictions, limited social interactions, changes in
work and schooling, within the framework of increased digital connectivity and decreased physical sociality. This emergent and emerging cultural change is, as Raymond Williams observed
decades ago, difficult to synthesize. Yet, in this particular case, we most certainly did not
miss the moment when things changed. COVID-19 life has alerted us to systemic change as
the globe has been immersed in this altered reality of pandemic induced shifts, where the unpredictable is now the everyday, even when we struggle to understand just what that change means.
Zadie Smith's *Intimations: Six Essays* (2020) is a partial history of affectivity of the present,
which I am speculatively positioning as a type of transnational archive of privileged pandemic-circumscribed life. Her essays, I believe, offer us a glimpse into how some are living
in this strange new world where there is a need 'to understand and theorize affects and affectivity, simply in order to understand what is happening around us – and to us – in a world where
politics, economy, and culture are becoming increasingly affect-driven' (Sharma and Tygstrup
11) – or in this case, simply in order to understand what is happening around us in terms of pandemic or COVID-19 affectivity.

Raymond Williams's work on a 'structure of feeling' is useful to understand new patterns of
experience that have emerged in the wake of this pandemic. Williams uses the term a 'structure
of feeling' to distinguish between formally held beliefs or ideologies, and meanings and values
as they are lived and felt in relation to those beliefs or ideologies – what he refers to as 'affective
elements of consciousness and relationships' that form elements made up of 'thought as felt' and
'feeling as thought' (Williams 23). He says:

> We are then defining these elements as a 'structure': as a set, with specific internal
> relations, at once interlocking and in tension. Yet we are also defining a social experience
> which is still in process ... Methodologically, then, a 'structure of feeling' is a cultural
> hypothesis actually derived from attempts to understand such elements and their connec-
> tions in a generation or period, and needing always to be returned, interactively, to such
> evidence. It is initially less simple than more formally structured hypotheses of the
> social, but it is more adequate to the actual range of cultural evidence ... . (Williams
> 23–24)

This 'cultural hypothesis,' or speculative investigation, can be traced through a history of affectivity in the present, to examine the shifts both emergent and emerging that the COVID-19 pandemic has wrought. Theories of emotion, atmosphere and feeling broadly correspond to
Williams's correlation of material, social, and affective structures (12) as the collection by
Devika Sharma and Frederick Tygstrup so eloquently lays out. Written at the start of 2020
during the first spate of restrictions that accompanied the pandemic, *Intimations* offers us an
affective cultural analysis of the structure of present feeling. Smith begins her collection:

> There will be many books written about the year 2020: historical, analytical, political, as
> well as comprehensive accounts. This is not any of those – the year isn't halfway done.

> What I have tried to do is organize some of the feelings and thoughts that events, so far,
> have provoked in me, in those scraps of time the year itself has allowed. (Smith xi)

Smith's collection offers what she promises – practical assistance in understanding the affectivity of life in this time. While Smith turned to Aurelius for help – '[t]hat the assistance Aurelius
offers is for the spirit makes it no less practical ... ' (Smith XI) — I have turned to Smith.

The first essay in *Intimations* is called 'Peonies' and captures the dissociative wistfulness
that accompanied the beginning of restricted pandemic life. Smith stands at the bars of a
garden looking at 'garish,' 'unsophisticated' tulips (Smith 1) with two middle-aged women,
wishing they were peonies, as they could be in imaginative retellings. These flowers symbolize
fertility and renewal (Smith 3), linking to the positionality of the middle-aged female viewers
who are approaching perimenopause, and the hope for renewal that the limbo of early pandemic
life induced. These two strands of the stages of gendered and pandemic life are woven together
by Smith to convey the affect of restrictions of various kinds and how we wish for them to be
different. The immediate and emergent collide with material and social structures, conveying the
affectivity of submission that accompanies both physical restrictions on movement and gendered
concepts of aging. Smith says:

> ... it's these dumb tulips that served as a tiny, early preview of what I now feel every
> moment of every day, that is the complex and ambivalent nature of 'submission.' ...
> This type of woman and that type of woman – just so many life rings thrown down to
> a drowning Heraclitus. Each one a different form of fiction. (7)

Submission to textualized aging and pandemic restrictions coalesce around issues of representation, the third strand that Smith introduces in this essay. For Smith, writing is control (6),
where tulips may become peonies and each novel read may provide the reader with a repertoire
of possible attitudes, unlike unruly experience that has no chapter headings or ellipses. What I
am calling 'dissociative wistfulness' is perhaps a reaction to the submission Smith sees as being
required in both female aging and contained pandemic life, for people who are used to choices
and the more expansive affectivity that accompanies choice. While submission implies a form of
stasis, the tulips and peonies imply growth and renewal, thereby forming something both dissociative in its ambivalence and wistful in its yearning for something other as it pulls conceptually
in different directions.

In 'The American Exception,' Smith uses one of the then-president Donald Trump's few
truthful comments to unravel concepts of death and the inherently democratic or egalitarian
notion of plagues – the irony of the title of the essay conveying the bombastic assertions of
Trump's exceptionalism. Trump's 'I wish we could have our old life back. We had the greatest
economy that we ever had, and we didn't have death' (Smith 11) is her starting point, as she
reveals that the phrase she considers to be truthful is 'we didn't have death'. Smith draws out
notions of culpability that circulate around death in American culture:

> Wrong place, wrong time. Wrong skin colour. Wrong Zip Code, wrong beliefs, wrong
> city. Wrong position of hands when asked to exit the vehicle. Wrong health insurance
> – or none ... Death absolute is the truth of our existence as a whole, of course, but
> America has rarely been philosophically inclined to consider existence as a whole, pre-
> ferring instead to attack death as a series of discrete problems. War on cancer, poverty,
> drugs and so on. (12–13)

Death is framed, not as an inevitable absolute for everyone, but rather as something that could have been avoided. This circulating narrative, that inserts individual complicities into the idea of unnatural death as some sort of avoidable event, is textualized by Smith to reveal the unequal underpinnings of both the narrative and the unnatural deaths inflicted on marginalized groups. COVID-19, like all plagues, is commonly understood as inherently egalitarian in that anyone anywhere may contract the virus. However, Smith reveals that COVID-19 deaths, unlike the virus itself, are not as egalitarian as we may presume, but highlight the effect of systemic inequalities. She says:

> A plague it is, but American hierarchies, hundreds of years in the making, are not so easily overturned … Black and Latino people are now dying at twice the rate of white and Asian people. More poor people are dying than rich … . Ultimately death has rarely been random in these United States … . For millions of Americans, it's always been a war. (15)

Smith forces us to reconsider ideas of natural death in this context, linking the killings of African Americans by the police to the disproportionate death toll of minorities during the pandemic. While death from a virus would usually be considered a natural death, Smith's trajectory repositions both 'natural' COVID-19 deaths and violent deaths as being unnatural given that they are directly related to systemic inequalities. So, the 'war on cancer, poverty, drugs and so on' is also a war on pandemics. COVID-19 mortality rates are then, in some ways, very familiar in their consolidation of the material, social and affective structures of inequality. The less than random nature of death is repositioned here as an unrelenting war against the poor and vulnerable.

The metaphorized link between war and the fight against COVID-19 has been utilized by Presidents around the world. Churchill, Smith reminds us, learned that even when people follow you into war and you fulfil your role as a great war-time president, that does not mean that they will want you to lead them into a new one or back into the old one after the war because '[w]ar transforms its participants' (Smith 15). Smith traces that transformation through the shift from Churchill to Attlee in Britain after the Second World War, and opens the question of what this might mean for the globe once the war on COVID-19 is over – what will we transform into? And it is with such deceptively simple connections that Smith reignites the notion of fecundity and renewal in a nebulous future, the affectivity signified by peonies and tulips with which this collection begins, which teases the line between stasis/submission and renewal.

Where 'The American Exception' blurs the line between natural and unnatural death in terms of inequalities, 'Something to Do' exhibits the privileged positioning of Smith (and others like myself) amid the uncertainties of pandemic life. The essay, as its title reflects, explores the affective quality of reduced movement and social interaction outside of the home. As someone who was not hampered by food scarcity or under-resourced living conditions, Smith articulates a restless languor that marked the COVID-19 affectivity of lockdown:

> Out of an expanse of time, you carve a little area – that nobody asked you to carve – and you do 'something'. But perhaps the difference between the kind of something that I am used to, and this new culture of doing something, is the moral anxiety that surrounds it. (20)

The moral anxiety that she describes pertains to time and how we fill it outside of work or school when homebound, with life 'served neat' (23), devoid of our routine practices. Things like banana bread baking, pet adoption and Minecraft challenges seemed to become ubiquitous in privileged enclaves across the globe. I found myself moving through recipes in a new cookbook for weekday dinners in a schedule that suddenly had time for more elaborate cooking, coupled with a desire to offer my family different tastes in a confined environment of sameness.

> Watching this manic desire to make or grow or do 'something,' that now seems to be consuming everybody, I do feel comforted to discover I'm not the only person on this earth who has no idea what life is for, nor what is to be done with all this time aside from filling it. (Smith 27)

Smith reveals an existential undercurrent that emerged in the early months of the pandemic when most countries entered a limbo state, reduced to the bare scaffolding that keeps societies in motion: home space, food access and time outside of work and school rhythms. My own desire to create something new in my home environment reflects the same existential impulse experienced by Smith on the other side of the globe, with her essays reminding me that I am not alone in my responses. This returns me to Raymond Williams. Smith does not miss the moment when new patterns of experience emerge or when new sensibilities arise. She articulates them here, infused with anxiety and privileged positionings, restlessness and languor; and once again the desire for renewal in making something grow. Smith's centralization of affect as both a critical object and perspective, to borrow the phrase from Clare Hemmings (548), facilitates an understanding of the social world and our place within it amid a pandemic.

Rob Nixon, in a different context, highlights the unpredictable dynamics of cross-cultural translation. He uses the example of Jamaica Kincaid rejecting any affinity with Henry James's writings, but forming a profound connection to Tsitsi Dangarembga's fictional character, Tambu:

> This recognition scene between an Antiguan-American essayist and a fictional Zimbab-wean character speaks to the politics of the unforeseeable imaginative connection, to the far-off, serendipitous chance find that becomes an exhortation. The scene speaks, more broadly, to the unpredictable dynamics of cross-cultural translation that attend the creative circuits of globalization from below, in literature and other cultural forms. We see this process at work in the way activists like Saro-Wiwa, Maathai, Chico Mendes, and Mahatma Gandhi have assumed an allegorical potency for geographically distant struggles. (Nixon 45)

Nixon's unpredictable connections resonate across spaces through an affective overlay for me here. The 'unforeseeable imaginative connection' of Smith's essay, 'Things to Do,' resonates across privileged locales, in which affectivity has been partially flattened by COVID-19. Yet, I am sure that there are many 'Henry James' perspectives circulating within this same affective critical object. As such, the different circulating currents of COVID-19 affectivity collide with the politics of both 'unforeseeable connection' and a lack of familiarity within this same critical object.

If 'Something to Do' creates a connection between privileged life and COVID-19 affectivity, 'Suffering like Mel Gibson' develops a different conversation about affect and suffering. Smith uses a meme of Gibson and an actor dressed as a bloodied Jesus with a crown of thorns, both sitting in director's chairs, as Gibson speaks. The caption reads 'Explaining to my friends with kids under six what it's been like isolating alone' (Smith 35). The relative but absolute nature of suffering is represented in humorous form, where 'what some other person seems to think is pain' (Smith 36) is humanized, revealing the impossibility of measuring who is suffering more – the lonely or those inundated with company. Mel Gibson as a public figure also signifies in this context as he has become associated with fundamentalist Christianity, conservativism and anti-Semitism in the wake of his 2004 film, *The Passion of the Christ*. The link here is to various forms of prejudice and their representation, which forms another strand in this essay: '[b]y comparing your relative privilege with that of others, you may be able to modify both your world and the worlds outside of your world – if the will is there to do it' (Smith 34). Gibson, through either lack of will or awareness, is not usually understood as being able to do this. The image of someone associated with extremism and prejudice, talking to a bleeding Jesus about his own suffering, compounds Smith's point as Jesus on the cross is the archetypal figure of 'real suffering'.

The essay starts with a beautifully written passage that captures the many faces of lockdown life, from the loneliness of living alone to suffocating in an overly full domestic space filled with children, a partner, work; the lonely dream of company and the married with children but '[e]verybody learns the irrelevance of these matters next to "real suffering"' (Smith 30). Smith teases out the relationship between suffering and privilege, revealing the subtle but crucial affective line between them:

> Just before the global shit hit the fan, we were in a long, involved cultural conversation about 'privilege'. We were teaching ourselves how to be more aware of the relative nature of various forms of privilege, and their dependence on intersections of class, race, gender and so on. As clarifying as this conversation often was, it strikes me that it cannot now be applied, without modification, to the category of suffering. The temptation to overlay the first discourse upon the second is strong: privilege and suffering have a lot in common. They both manifest as bubbles, containing a person and distorting their vision. But it is possible to penetrate the bubble of privilege and even pop it – but the suffering bubble is impermeable. (31)

Smith positions privilege as something that can be modified in the world but sees suffering as something that contains a person: 'Suffering has an absolute relation to the suffering individual – it cannot be easily mediated by a third term like "privilege"' (34).

This is a complex positioning that captures some of the internal questioning of things that has accompanied pandemic-constrained life for me. I recognize the suffering of my privileged children, cut off from real-life social activities of childhood. I also recognize the 'real suffering' of indigent people on the peripheries of my neighbourhood who scramble for food and shelter. I can talk to my children about the real suffering of others, which they understand, but does it help them to feel differently in their own suffering? As levels of depression and anxiety have skyrocketed globally during the pandemic, we can certainly say that suffering has increased, regardless of how or where we live. Yet, there is still a coherent concept of 'real suffering' for me that lurks outside of the privileged milieu that I inhabit. I am reminded here of conversations with my Holocaust survivor mother who spent her childhood in a concentration camp. She speaks of other Holocaust survivors as suffering more than she did, of surviving worse concentration camps than the one in which she was imprisoned, while simultaneously saying that she survived hell – suffering emerges as a murky construct that is hellish but was not as bad as the 'real suffering' of others. This is something that escapes expression in language or words, but not in terms of affect. Smith reveals the ambiguous affective economies that undergird suffering in ways that include both relative and absolute states or experiences. And thinking through these affects assists us in adapting to this new COVID-19 constrained world.

'When an unfamiliar world arrives, what does it reveal about the world that came before it'?) This is one of the questions used to describe what Smith is exploring in 'Screengrabs. (After Berger, before the virus)'. 'Screengrabs' comprises a series of short essay vignettes that capture pre-pandemic interactions with strangers or acquaintances. In some ways Smith articulates for me what has been lost in terms of casual human interaction during the pandemic, while also depicting the financial and affective toll of locked-down life on a broader scale. This final essay, made up of shorter ones, moves between portraying what has been lost in the pre-COVID-19 world and the pre-pandemic roots of violence that the pandemic exaggerated.

In 'A Man with Strong Hands,' Smith describes a nail salon that she frequents for chair massages a few times a week in Manhattan that is midway between work, school and her favourite bookstore – the vectors of space that made up her everyday world pre-pandemic. Smith describes how she does not like pedicures or long massages because she cannot read during the treatment and because of the amount of time they may take in her overly scheduled pre-pandemic life. The compression of activities into time slots is a familiar one, which marked pre-pandemic life for many of us. The shift from the compression of activities to the compression of time that the pandemic produced has a particular structure of feeling attached to it.

The contrast with what came before frames this essay from the start, as we already know that lockdown forced people to fill time as one of her previous essays described, as opposed to the lack of it in Smith's tightly managed pre-COVID-19 schedule. She will have a chair massage and read Berger; or mark student papers but cannot have a massage without filling that time with something productive. While she is a 'regular' at the nail salon, nobody there knows her name, but she is greeted with 'fond familiarity' (39). Her masseur is Ben, who also manages the place. They have established a symmetrical pattern of interaction where they speak of 'my boy' and 'your boy'.

> For reasons of convenience we have settled into this symmetrical pattern. It is not the only false symmetry. The fact that the school is closed for Ben's boy is a genuine emergency; for me it is an inconvenience only. I know Ben knows this, but out of what I interpret as his customary optimism and civility and desire to maintain symmetry, he allows me to complain with him, as if my husband or I cannot work from home, or lose a day's work, without disaster … . (40)

The spectre of COVID-19 restrictions hangs over this description, forming an overlay of anxiety through which to view the vignette of soon to disappear everyday life for both Smith and Ben. The constructed symmetry established in the everyday interaction of Smith and Ben allows for a type of casual connection between acquaintances who inhabit different social worlds; a connection that will soon fray, leaving an affective gap. The impact of these types of mundane interactions is really only felt once absent, with an inarticulate sense of loss inhabiting an affective space that I previously barely realized had a structure of feeling attached to it. I no longer have conversations with the car guard about life in the Democratic Republic of Congo on the street where I buy food, out of fear of COVID-19 exposure. I do not share my old detective paperbacks with him out of fear of exposing him to possible infection. Like Smith, I am presenting this interaction in terms of its fake symmetry – I view these interactions as an exchange of some kind but have no idea how he understands them. The gap here for me points to a loss of basic human understanding through this exchange of information about our world. It leaves an off-kilter experience behind that I can only articulate through a feeling of loss, of something made present by its absence. Williams captures the texture of this insight as being part of a need to find other terms for the undeniable experience of the present as a moving thing (28). He extends this idea as follows:

> We are talking about characteristic elements of impulse, restraint, and tone; specifically affective elements of consciousness and relationships: not feeling against thought, but thought as felt and feeling as thought: practical consciousness of a present kind, in a living and interrelating continuity. We are then defining these elements as a 'structure': as a set, with specific internal relations, at once interlocking and in tension. Yet we are also defining a social experience which is still in process … . (Williams 31)

The affective gap left behind when these interactions cease or shift is bewildering in various ways. What happens to social interactions if I lose my conversational skills through lack of use? How does my understanding of the world change when I can only learn through books and technology? How does a lack of interaction between people from different social worlds impact on us personally and globally? This 'living and interrelated continuity' of experience is still in process and I can only look at its affective residue to try to understand its resonance.

The next vignette in *Intimations,* 'A Character in a Wheelchair in the Vestibule,' is a snapshot of Smith running out of her home to draw cash from an ATM machine as her family prepares to leave NYC at the start of pandemic restrictions. Smith comes across Myron, a homeless, legless veteran in her neighbourhood whom she had previously converted into a character in one of her stories. The real Myron is shouting into his cell phone about people running like rats from the city fearing catching a cold: 'I'm not scared of this shit! … I'm staying right where I'm at. This is my city' (Smith 45). While Myron might exhibit some of the bluster that characterized parts of America over the year following this encounter (mask wearing was couched as an infringement of personal rights and lockdown as totalitarian), he is also intimately familiar with sentiment on a wider scale. Myron, in a more extreme form, mirrors my own initial reaction to COVID-19 in that I thought it was hysteria about a bad flu. This 'unforeseeable connection' of COVID-19 affectivity links me to a bombastic homeless man shouting into an enclosure near an ATM machine in Manhattan at the unimaginable start of the pandemic. The inherently byzantine nature of affect ' … shows that affect is a complex beast, not only attaching us to what we already know, or producing affects that capture us in the most familiar and routine of ways, but that also suture us to others in different, often surprising, ways' (Hemmings 155).

While Myron and I might inhabit different structures of feeling, Smith's narratives provide a source of insight into COVID-19 affectivity that has transformed the way I think of connectivity and rupture. While my everyday social interactions with people I barely know, like a car guard, have disappeared with COVID-19 circumscribed life, my affective connection to strangers like Myron, who I interact with through Smith's essays, have revealed an affective economy to me in different and surprising ways. There is a fascinating link between what is lost in terms of the casual social and what is gained in terms of the imagined affective affinity across worlds. Williams makes similar connections:

> Such changes can be defined as changes in structures of feeling. The term is difficult, but 'feeling' is chosen to emphasize a distinction from more formal concepts of 'world-view' or 'ideology'. It is not only that we must go beyond formally held and systematic beliefs, though of course we have always to include them. It is that we are concerned with meanings and values as they are actively lived and felt, and the relations between these and formal or systematic beliefs are in practice variable (including historically variable), over a range from formal assent with private dissent to the more nuanced interaction between selected and interpreted beliefs and acted and justified experiences. (Williams 31)

What this shift in affectivity will result in remains undetermined until a post-COVID-19 world reveals its secrets. For now, the peculiarities of the present place me in an affective loop with Myron while severing affective connections with familiar strangers in my local area. If this results in a loss of social skills and understanding or creates new and wonderful imagined communities based on affect rather than place or identity, will be clear only in reflective hindsight. What is certain is that the present is changing.

One of the unfortunate rhythms of pandemic-circumscribed life has been an increase in violence globally. The last three vignettes of Smith's *Intimations* focus on different forms of violence, specifically the quiet violence of curtailed youth, domestic violence and hate crimes. In 'A Hovering Young Man,' Smith talks about what life for someone in their twenties should be like – 'a thrilling time, an insecure time,' 'a season full of possibilities,' all now 'radically interrupted' (57) by the pandemic. The ordinary quiet rupture of early adulthood forms another strand of COVID-19 affectivity, while simultaneously posing the unanswerable question of what the effects of this rupture will be, after.

Lockdowns resulted in a global increase in domestic violence, which Smith includes here in its most everyday form – as part of a banal online conversation with her mother that forms the next vignette. She describes a somewhat circular conversation as her mother catches her up on people she may remember from her childhood. The conversation between mother and daughter is casual and familiar, with the ordinary horror story of a woman from her brother's year at school being murdered by her partner suddenly thrown into the mix (Smith 62). Smith's narrative technique is both subtle and extraordinarily forceful in that the form conveys how ubiquitous stories of domestic violence have become, but the fiery death that accompanied this one is jarring. The affective response induced in this narrative conveys both the horror of the story, along with the horror at the slight delay that accompanies the reader's reaction, because we get caught up in the form of the conversation portrayed in this essay as it resonates on a personal level. It is almost as if there is a pause when we synthesize what has just been conveyed in such a seemingly familiar form. There is something about this pause, this moment before recognition comes, that represents the affect of pandemic-circumscribed violence on a larger scale, where incomprehension and familiarity collide. Perhaps the implication is that violence has spread like a virus, increasing along with COVID-19 droplets in the air, and has become uncomfortably familiar.

In tracing these very different but related types of violence, Smith plays with notions of fake symmetry on a global level, as the first vignette heralds. She seems to be saying that there is no real symmetry due to structural inequalities which pandemic-constrained life has exacerbated. The privileged 'we' are on some level, always in conversation with Ben from the nail salon, while engaging in conversations of fake symmetry with people whose lives are far more constrained than our own. What does this fake symmetry mean for them? What is lost along with these mundane interactions? What will this affective gap do to all of us? Smith's essays make me aware of the gaps of the everyday that COVID-19 has exacerbated as I can only see from my side of the fake symmetry of unequal interactions. If this section articulates some of what was lost during COVID-19 restrictions in terms of the everyday rubbing along with strangers or acquaintances, which I have positioned as leaving an affective gap behind, this gap implies that something will fill it – a hope for renewal that trails behind these gaps waiting to be filled.

Smith' s *Intimations* allows us to see COVID-19 affectivity as a single frame in which multiple asymmetrical relations form an ambiguous structure of feeling. Or perhaps it is rather that structural issues combine with affect theory, muddied by imagined forms of liveability in the context of COVID-19, to produce a single frame for multiple histories. The main point then, in a structure of feeling, is to identify a configuration of elements that lays out the profile of its affectivity, where 'we are then defining these elements as a "structure": as a set, with specific internal relations, at once interlocking and in tension' (Williams132). Reading through Smith's essays reveals the elements of COVID-19 affectivity as what I have speculatively calling a type of dissociative wistfulness that pulls conceptually in different directions, a restless languor of the privileged which is accompanied by a moral anxiety about time and how we fill it, about the time after. The stasis of COVID-19 lockdowns results in a need to create something across locales. Further, COVID-19 affectivity has brought together unforeseeable connections as well as a lack of familiarity, in unusual ways. The ambiguous affective economies of suffering, as both relative and absolute, form another circuit in this unstable present loop, where violence is a different sort of virus that has increased as COVID-19 has travelled. These elements then form a structure that is both interlocking and in tension. Claire Hemmings positions affect similarly as 'it is precisely the critical attention to affect as a contested site of reproduction and disruption, and as a particular form of knowledge that requires methodological invention, that remains so compelling' (149).

These musings on COVID-19 affectivity through Zadie Smith's *Intimations* centre the work speculation 'does in enlarging our apprehension of the world and our possibilities for being in the world' (Macharia 17). Smith can help us to theorize emergent affectivity from inside a pandemic-strained world through the narration of the ambiguous operational logic that her essays describe. She has created a continuum made up of affective normativities and transformative affectivities on either end, with her essays tracing the rhythms of privileged life across locales, to help us understand the present.

Works Cited

Bachmann-Medick, Doris, Carl Horst, Wolfgang Hallet & Ansgar Nunning (Eds.) *Structures of Feeling: Concepts for the Study of Culture*. Boston: De Gruyter, 2015.

Hemmings, Clare. 'Invoking Affect. Cultural Theory and the Ontological Turn." *Cultural Studies* 19(5), 2005: 548–67.

Hemmings, Clare. 'Affect and Feminist Methodology, Or What Does It Mean to be Moved?' In *Structures of Feeling: Concepts for the Study of Culture*. Edited by Devika Sharma and Frederick Tygstrup. Boston: De Gruyter, 2015. 147–58.

Macharia, Keguro. *Frottage: Frictions of Intimacy across the Black Diaspora*. New York: New York University Press, 2019.

Nixon, Rob. *Slow Violence and the Environmentalism of the Poor*. Cambridge, Massachusetts: Harvard University Press, 2011.

Sharma, Devika & Frederick Tygstrup. 'Introduction.' In *Structures of Feeling: Concepts for the Study of Culture*. Edited by Devika Sharma and Frederik Tygstrup. Boston: De Gruyter, 2015. 1–19.

Smith, Zadie. *Intimations: Six Essays*. New York: Penguin, 2020.

Williams, Raymond. 'Structures of Feeling.' In *Structures of Feeling: Concepts for the Study of Culture*. Edited by Devika Sharma and Frederick Tygstrup. Boston: De Gruyter, 2015. 20–25.

No author. 'About Zadie Smith's *Intimations. Six Essays*' https://www.penguinrandomhouse.com/books/669582/intimations-by-zadie-smith. Accessed 20 July 2020.

Active Thumbs, Confined Bodies: Eluding the *'Insect'* in Times of the Plague

M. D. El Maarouf ⦿, Taieb Belghazi ⦿ and Ute Fendler ⦿

This paper examines games during the COVID-19 pandemic as ontological barriers or *barzakhs* (singular: *barzakh*). The traditional meaning of barrier as separation is coupled with the Greek meaning of play as *Poiesis* (which may also be understood as describing acts of creation). We expand the semantics of 'barrier' so as to describe pandemic phenomena that exist at the points at which opposites meet: synthetic game and the world of real game;[1] the infected and the healthy; the player and the character being played; life and death. Our perception of both home and the exterior world has changed significantly in the time of the plague. At-home gaming, far from signalling our modern confinement, enables moments in which we may challenge our imprisonment. To bring this idea home, we deploy *barzakh* as a moral imperative, a site of both necessary isolation and opportunities of engagement, proof of our need for both interaction and distance, a place for the enactment of our knowing and strategic waiting in relation to the pandemic. Through the term, we theorize the link between barrier and other similar categorical divides (distances, masks, gloves, borders and quarantines) which we activate during lockdown to work through our puzzlement, win the social game of civil goodness and to downplay, and ultimately survive, the pandemic of our times.

Introduction: Defining our Place

COVID-19 created a condition of horror, replete with safety directives that kept falling on people like meteorites from the sky, forcing them back to their epistemological 'caves,' while the outside world was full of risk. Consequently, the world turned to video games and on-rug entertainment to pass the time and interact with friends and family they could not see in person for the foreseeable future (Howley 2020). To be sure, play as performance is not accessible to all and thus cannot be studied as such (see figure 1). Places of play (henceforth *playces*), are influenced by the players' sex, class, race, religion and ethnic group. We cannot speak of a monolithic *playce*. Also, *playces* are mutable: places within and outside a game get transformed by the play's expanding conditions, such as its need to accommodate various trance states, mental transferability or imagination.[2] Generally speaking, when the plague reached its zenith, people, poor or rich, wanted to make sure that their morale, and that of their children, were maintained, despite being trapped at home, by seeking the safest and most affordable leisure practices possible. The home must be shared by all its occupants while waiting out the pandemic. Household spaces are re-organized by players in such a way that they turn into play ephemera. They become *playces*, recognized as such by adults and children alike. Such recognition is prompted by three factors: an intrinsic and instinctive desire for play; the presence of a potential player in every person; and the play potential in every moment, which thus renders every *playce* playable insofar as one's imagination would allow.

The shift to interior activities, gaming included, is determined by a change of epoch, in which love and care are expressed through distance rather than proximity, leaving us with the paradox that while social bonds are important – and the individual cannot survive away from the community – survival of self and other lies in keeping everyone else away.[3] In the context of disaster, this understanding of separation as a thinking and knowing position, and as a period of grace, has been further underscored by the proliferation of terms like borders, continents, masks, gloves, distance, quarantine and isolation, which have become part of the daily language with which we describe and seek to fix our predicament. In this

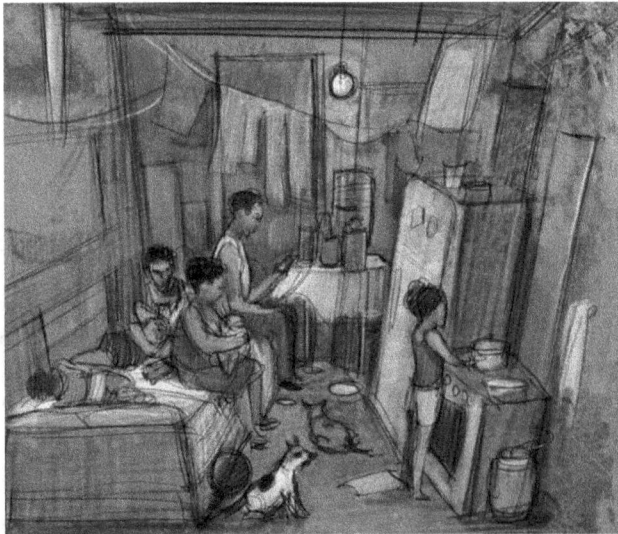

Figure 1:   Not in the same *Playce*. This Image (artist unknown) went viral during the outbreak of the pandemic in 2020 under the caption: "Work from home & submit your assignments online." Available at: https://globaledleadership.org/2020/12/16/education-around-the-world-a-few-of-our-favorite-photos-links-stories/. The copyright holder could not be established. If you are the copyright holder, please contact us.

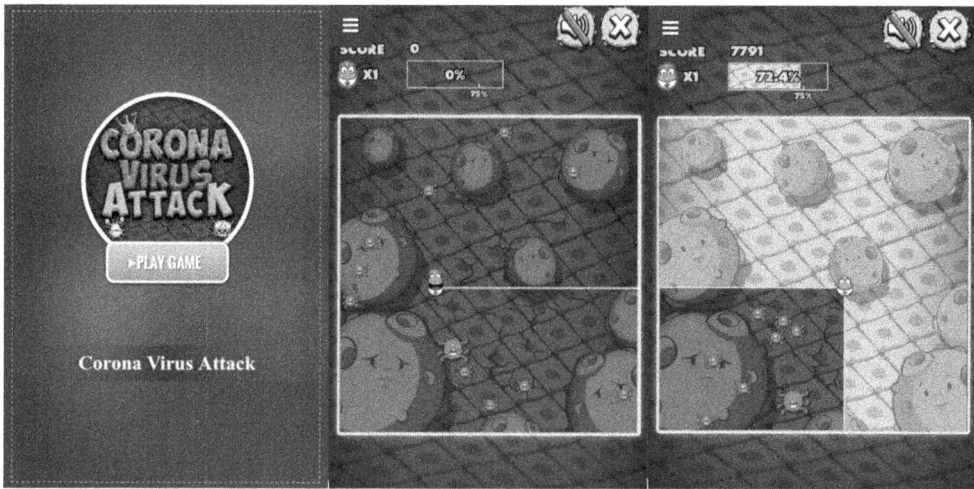

Figure 2: M(a)rking safe territories. "Corona Virus Attack" Publisher: HTML5 Arcade Game, by Code This Lab/Codecanyon Year: 2020.

paper, we analyze play as an extension of the poetics of separation (where separation may be thought of as the severance between home and the outside world, the infected and the healthy, play and seriousness, life and death, the playable and playing character), while reflecting on the way it intersects with the idea of border, which, by the same token, is also traversed by the moralities of the plague (particularly along the lines of collaboration, social responsibility, solidarity, patriotism, good citizenship).

To bring the idea of separation home, we use the term *barzakh* (barrier) as a metaphor to account for the way at-home entertainment is enacted in some sort of barrier zone. We seek to measure the extent to which disaster-centred confinement has allowed for spatially opposi-tional categories to merge in the house as the safest *playce* (the place to underplay the virus). The word *barzakh* offers a qualitative conceptual and semantic framework for a deeper under-standing of the lexicon of play during the coronavirus lockdown moment. *Barzakh* is a Persian word for 'limit' or 'barrier'. Etymologically, *barzakh* (plural: *barazikh*) denotes a divide between two things. In geography, it refers to a piece of land sandwiched between two seas con-necting two islands (example: the Suez Canal links Africa and Asia). Semantically, it signifies that which lies in the middle of two things. We use *barzakh* because it signals a non-static middle space that handles everything within itself and outside it as a third space (in Bhabhian thinking), where this third space is itself a *barzakh*, since 'every existent thing is a *barzakh*, since every-thing has its own niche between two other niches within the ontological hierarchy known as the cosmos' (Chittick 14). The term also flaunts a mystic dimension given, first, its Sufi meaning as a thinking and knowing position, and, second, its *Shi'ite* meaning as a period of grace (*imhal*). Concepts such as 'dual-globalization' and 'dual-spacization' (Ameli 1384; Ameli and Hassani 1391) are interesting for scholars who want to analyze the virtual space (as a new space of social life) and real space as conjoined twins. However, because such scholars recognize the virtual space as a new space, underlying, at the same time, the interplay between real and virtual spaces, this conceptual vocabulary falls short, as an individual between these spaces is

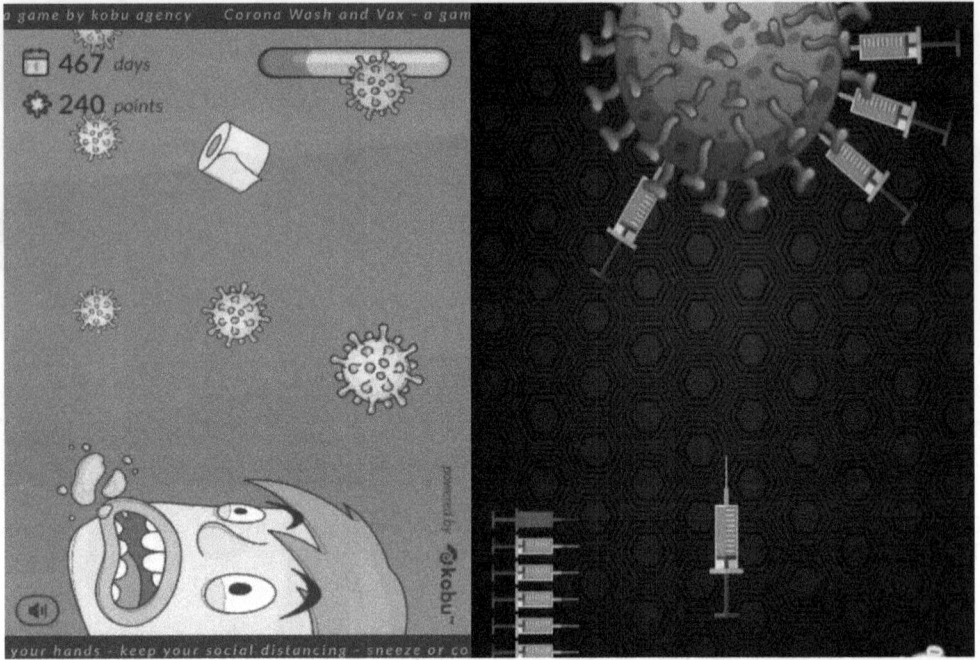

Figure 3:   Fighting the Deadly Enemy. "Corona Wash and Vax". Publisher: Kobu Agency. Year: 2020.

either in the real space or in the virtual space and never both simultaneously.[4] *Playce* as *barzakh* is closer to the blended space that Fauconnier (*Mappings*; *Mental Spaces*) calls a 'mental space,' in which virtual world and real world experiences blend, except that this blended space (of *playce* as *barzakh*) is administered through the players' knowledge of their presence in the barrier. It is the waiting space between here and there; it introduces the player into ways of knowing how to react to threat, intensifying emotions, multiplying facts (fake and real) and growing uncertainties. In fact, the player's presence in the game is enacted through the aware-ness of, and conscious movement across, the three forms of space that Espen Aarseth uses in reading games: the physical (simulated); the abstract (imaginary); and the social (conventional). The intersecting games at play (social games, ethical games, indoor manual or synthetic games) in the way they build and un-build, structure and de-structure, can be further understood along-side Kant's architectonics or 'the art of systems,' particularly in the way it allows for philosophy (knowledge) and architecture (building/unbuidling) to regulate one another. In this reading, the *barzakh* comprises an architectonics of play that permits the building of a philosophy of knowing around categories like distance, space and confinement.

    Playce should not be looked upon as a site for the enactment of a modern immoralism, in Heidegger's thinking (*Remarks on Art*; *Technology*), in which digital games can be criticized for promoting predetermined ends and preset value structures, which prevent players from design-ing their own goals. *Playce* is charged and recharged by the players' being in the world. It is also charged by the game as a *barzakh*, which allows the players and the playable character to be creative constructors of the game's topography: they may contribute to the world's folkloristic heritage.

To be sure, even the game is not entirely safe. There have been cases of reported outbreaks in games with no major plague themes. In late September 2005, an outbreak begun when the *World of Warcraft* video game invited a new creature with the power to cast 'corrupted blood' on his opponents, triggering a strong infection that causes them to die after a few seconds. Things got out of control when the dying characters infected close contacts who in turn spread the disease. Taken unawares by corrupted blood's viral effect, the administrators did not know how to treat this unplanned virtual scenario, especially after ill characters started teleporting to quarantined areas and non-infected places of the game world, causing the horror to take lethal shape (Balicer 260).

While the goals in the game may be predetermined, the poetics of play (imagination, dream, narrativization and affect) may expand upon the game's modest values. Similarly, we do not argue that the *barzakh* is meant to accommodate those who wish to flee into digitality, trading the real plague for the fake plague. Instead, we propose that it accommodates those who *wish* to play; those who *wish* are the ones who benefit from, and get sustained in, the barrier zone. The *barzakh*, besides, acts less as a hierarchical system, and more as a system that deploys hierarchical principles to encourage people to adopt safety measures to raise their chances of eluding the virus, hence saving the world. And while digital games may be accused of reinventing hierarchies in the way the player climbs up and advances through stages with increased difficulty to the top, achieving utmost knowledge and power, these hierarchies are also useful. They emulate the hierarchical modalities at play in the outer world (the healthy over the infected; safe over unsafe; alive over dead) in which the game of survival began as simple reports of a new plague in Wuhan before it escalated to shutting down borders and implementing hardcore measures of distancing. A similar kind of augmenting challenge occurs in video games, emulating the escalation of death rates and tragedy in the real world. *Playces* during the plague are therefore non-arbitrary sites of gaming that bear the player's enactment of his or her significance. That is, a *playce* is not an inconsistent world that exists parallel to the real one. A *playce* is a reasoned field of presence, a site of imagination that offers a compromise between two realities.

Imagination vs. the Plague

Imagination is an important and pivotal dimension when reflecting on play and gaming in relation to the plague. The purpose of introducing imagination here is to supplement our understanding of homes, which may be defined as clearly demarcated space where one dwells. The tools and themes of play are deeply influenced by the player's habitat (figure 1). In poor societies, for example, challenging circumstances allow for the emergence of *playces* that are dissimilar to those in affluent societies. Players in poor societies subvert their realities through the spectacle of play, using what James C. Scott calls the so-called weapons of the weak (laughter, imagination, trance, role playing and theatricality). Our games happen in different *playces*. These *playces* are nurtured by our imagination, a social practice (Appadurai 327). '[I]magination may function to preserve an order [thus] staging ... a process of identification that mirrors the order,' as Paul Ricoeur says (285). Yet it should also be pointed out that imagination can have 'a disruptive function; it may work as a breakthrough. Its image ... is productive, an imagining of something else, the elsewhere' (Ricoeur qtd. in Kearney 165). So, despite the different ways we conceive of *playce* or in which *playces* are lived, imagination informs the elsewhere they engage.

Although imagination is widely used in the humanities, it is most often suppressed on the grounds that it does not lend itself to scientific scrutiny. Humanities researchers think they are using concepts and coming up with good and valid truth claims but in fact are starting a whole series of optional metaphors. This is best shown in Derrida's problematization of the relation between metaphor and concept, on the one hand, and between dead and live metaphors, on the other. It is also evident in the way he manoeuvres certain words like retreat or '*retrait*,' in the 'Retrait of Metaphor,' into a position where they mean something radically different, something other than any sense attached to them in conventional theory. For Derrida, metaphor does not involve any relation between the signifier and the signified, since, in his interpretation, the signified does not exist. On the other hand, metaphor does involve some sort of grafting from one context to the next. This dismantling of the notion of origin in the case of metaphor implies that there can be no phenomenological basis by which we may explain its meaning. Moreover, for Derrida, the idea that metaphor gets worn out is a myth: even as a metaphor is literalized, it generates new meanings and gets absorbed into new conceptual chains. Any reflection on the category of metaphor will wind up deconstructing the category of metaphor because we have no reliable means of distinguishing metaphor from literal usage. We are denied the possibility of fixed or fixing meaning.

Our attempt at addressing play in times of utter seriousness may depart from this Derridian insight concerning the metaphoricity of language as well as from Arjun Appadurai's view of the centrality of the image and imagination. Following Appadurai, we think of game as imagination: far from being

> mere fantasy (opium for the masses whose real work is everywhere), ... simple escape (from a world defined principally by more concrete purposes and structures), ... elite past time (thus not relevant to the lives of ordinary people) ... or mere contemplation (irrelevant for new forms of desire and subjectivity), ... [It] has become an organized field of social practices, a form of work (both in the sense of labor and of culturally organized practice) and as a form of negotiation between sites of agency (individual) and globally defined fields of possibility. (327)

We do not claim that the plague at hand has triggered an unprecedented rise of newly imagined spaces. We also do not claim that players' differences globally are flattened, and all are equal candidates for infection. Rather, we contend that the confinement and its inevitable by-products (quarantine, social distancing, self-isolation) have allowed for the rise of *possible* equality, where individuals and their children, their pets, their machines and individuals alone are more likely to perform within the best *playce* possible on a common and flat platform. In the best *playce* possible, players meet as equals, unified by confinement and by their roles as players with equal chances for loss and victory.

These situations allow us to take our reading beyond the classic aesthetic arguments (Hunicke, LeBlanc and Zubek), narrative arguments (Rouse and Ogden; Schell) and counter-narrative arguments (Salen and Zimmermann) in game theory since our focus is on games in the *barzakh* we call *playce*, concepts that are fundamentally different to what theories have previously considered. We take our cue from Heidegger's phenomenology and his notion of being, which allows for a more holistic view of game as space (Hagström). In times of disaster, play allows for hermeneutics of relocation in which we keep reinterpreting ourselves alongside our ever-changing needs and goals (Hoy 1996) inside and outside the game. The hermeneutics of relocation help us see the different subject positions and roles we keep embodying outside and inside the game.

The current 'stay at home; save lives' motto of the gaming community happens within larger 'stay at home; save lives' games at the level of states. These scenarios of games-within-games happen through the constant relocation of the gamer, in the aforementioned Aarsethian orders, between the gamer's play missions, their social responsibilities and the general ethical considerations of *being* in the game. The *barzakh* helps us articulate the uncertainty of our being in the pandemic, which, for the most part, may be defined as a field of uncertainty (Bateman; Malaby; Caillois). Between the world and the game, the *barzakh* functions as a fluid barrier that is awash with traffic, informed by how much of the world of the game is allowed to escape into the world of the outer game and back. It is not a silent and stagnant separation; it is full of poetics (*poiesis* in Greek), especially if we think of poetics as a productive act (Hagström). Our being in the game is not divorced from 'This entity which each of us is himself and which includes inquiring as one of the possibilities of its Being, we shall denote by the term "Dasein"' (Heidegger, *Being and Time* 27). In times of the plague, categories like time and space, which are signs of our being, become so charged that the activities that unfold in them also intensify, most particularly because they are enacted at the verge of other categories like death, separation and trauma. This is reminiscent of Heidegger's understanding of play as a form of 'seeing that takes its departure from lived experience' (Dreyfus and Wrathall 9), without necessarily 'getting us outside of this world, rather only providing a different route into this one' (Hagström 7).

The world of the game and the world as we know it are merged through the *barzakh*'s capacity for enfoldment, allowing different worlds to meet through the game. In the Koran, *barzakh* refers to the line that makes a difference. It occurs in the following two verses: 1. 'It is He who let forth the two oceans, this one sweet, grateful to taste and this one salt and bitter to the tongue and He set between them a *barzakh* [partition] till the day they are raised up'; 2. 'He let forth the two oceans that meet together, between them a *barzakh* they do not overpass' (Murata 160). The general understanding of these two verses is that they allude to three worlds: the spirits, the imaginable things and the corporeal things. However, Ibn al-Arabi, the Sufi philosopher who was born in Andalusia and died in Syria and spent a long period of his life travelling across the Mediterranean, shows that *barazikh* do not offer mere syntheses of opposite forces. They do not homogenize difference or rise above conflicting forces. On the contrary, they keep heterogeneity in play while at the same time revealing homogenizing tendencies. We do not know whether this third element (barrier) is generated as a consequence of this meeting or whether it is a natural self-sufficient body (of water) between the two waterscapes. The same goes for games and disasters, the kind of chicken-or-egg uncertainty that this paper has no ambition of entertaining. What we know is that it constitutes the barrier that makes a difference, the space that permits the two seas to meet.

In this reading, games become the catalyst of the joining or meeting of two different worlds without transgression. The three layers of the plague's gaming reality (the game, the game's world and the real world) are not symptomatic of a disagreement, even if the partitioning occurring therein visually speaks of a corporeal dialysis. The *barzakh* does not revolve around the idea of disjunction; rather it is an example of how these seemingly connected layers, all appearing as familiar worlds (possibly liveable worlds in the game and reality),[5] are subject to a physics of particularity that enables them to 'meet,' to happen in adjacency to one another, without synthetically being swallowed by one another. These entities team up to form a triad that the *barzakh* ties into a complex network. The image of the *barzakh* as 'partition' standing in-between other entities, 'preventing that they overpass or overrun each other' (Koran 55:20), reveals the contradictory nature of borders and frontiers while simultaneously pointing to their nature as sites of possibility. Also, the relational positioning of opposite ends serves as a metaphor of relativist thought and allows an escape from the grip of homogenizing narratives (Graiouid 2007).

This form of existence in the *barzakh* of the game is not only cryptic, but also metaphysical. Although it tends to prevent different bodies from merging, it serves as a panorama that lies in between other narratives, a panorama in which the connection, though apparently sectorializing, is meant to help the two bodies retain their sense of autonomy, flaunting their particular physics (or distinct narratives). We might want to look at it as a sectorialization of two worlds by a barrier that forces them to interact while staying where/how/what they are. *Playce* then refers to borders, in-between spaces that fulfil the double function of linking and de-linking often referred to in Sufi literature as the world of imaginal existents; *playces* are entities that occupy an intermediate space between two opposite phenomena (the luminous and the dark, the spiritual and the corporeal, the subtle and the dense, the high and the low); they are 'both/and' instead of 'either/or'. In this reading, as Ibn al-Arabi points out, a 'barzakh is something that separates (*fasil*) two other things while never going to one side (*mutatarrif*) as, for example the line that separates shadow from sunlight' (Chittick 117).

The game of surviving disaster allows the confined player and playable character to gravitate towards the *playce*, a site for the enactment of the gaming situation in which the playing and playable character are linked and delinked (from the game) both in and out of play. Pandemics offer a reformulation of the game less as a fleeting moment and more as a chance to return to contradictory realities: our 'utopia' or our 'dystopia': our 'plague' or our 'vaccine': our 'union' or our 'separation'. Pandemics offer the chance to return from the game outside to the game inside and vice versa. This return is made more meaningful through an understanding of 'home' as the pandemic's 'safest' sanctuary, one that is made, by the same contradictory logic, more of a 'stable' place through confinement. The game that we call *barzakh* and the *barzakh* that we call game separate a 'known from an unknown, an existent from a non-existent, a negated from an affirmed, an intelligible from a non-intelligible' (Chittick 118). In other words, the *barzakh* does not homogenize difference; it rather constitutes a place for thinking that difference through.

Killing the Virus from Home: Expanding the Meaning of Home via Play

Disaster and confinement have expanded the meaning of home through the expansion of the ways home could replace or act on behalf of other places. During the plague, home has encapsulated other places like café, theatre, school, playground, gym and supermarket. It has been somehow charged with meanings that allow it to barter for and offer a replacement of other spatial and physical categories of locality. The way home has become proxy for public space under the pandemic is most interesting. The pandemic meant that certain activities, those normally designated to outside the home, were moved inside the home. This is an example of a conceptual restraint of locality by force of disaster: we are forced to be in our homes. It is this conceptual restraint, delimited as it were by the pressing demands of 'now,' our modern *Dringlichkeit* (urgency) and *Notfall* (emergency), that make the meaning of imprisonment (at home) during confinement different from the traditional meaning of confinement (in prison). While in the former it could symbolize opportunity, solution, morality, conscientiousness, law-abiding citizenship, solidarity or patriotism, it could, in the latter, also mean punishment, problem, lawlessness, discord or disloyalty. In the prison house of home, the game offers an interesting enfoldment that allows home to accommodate or *be* more of what it traditionally excludes. In its elastic world, the game allows for the internalization of external themes, concepts and actions in the same way the *barzakh* allows itself to be permeated with entities that it separates/links. The game played at home during the disaster does not speak of a fundamental incivility, that of playing while people are dying, but rather that play and life are homologous and correspondent, that they are characterized by poetics, which in Greek entails 'bringing something into being that did not exist before' (Polkinghorne 115). Everything is a game inasmuch as gaming is synonymous with doing or acting with the intention to make (something happen); play during confinement in Heidegger's reading is resistance, and it is resistance because it happens through the technology he praises for being the invention of men with 'a thinking hand'.

The eyes that see the problem in the game, and outside it, are linked with the thinking hand of the player, who through play seeks the best ways to think of a relief from the disaster of her time; play informs the way we laugh at disaster; it informs how we cling to life while people are dying; in the case of COVID-19, play, even better, informs the way we attack the virus.

Corona Virus Attack (CVA) and other online games like Corona Wash and Vax (CWV) and Kill the Virus (KV) are some of the many games that proliferated after the outbreak of COVID-19 and the passing of social distancing laws. In CVA, the player is told in the description that she has a new mission: 'to kill the coronavirus and its race, claiming … portions of screen weaving line, … while being … careful with the deadly viruses which will try to destroy you and your lines'. In this game, the player controls a small, blue, animated character who moves across a backdrop of sad-looking round beings (that we understand to be body cells). If the player succeeds in drawing a line and eluding the insect-looking virus at the same time, the infected zone gets quarantined, which is then divorced from the other infected area, hence happy cells.

In CWV, we are told that 'scientists are racing to come up with a vaccine against our ultimate enemy: CORONAVIRUS! Meanwhile we all must commit to two fundamental things: social distancing (stay home!) and washing up!' The player has to prevent the virus from touching the face of a young male, killing every virus individually by touching the screen. Touching the toilet paper rolls will give you extra points. In KV, the player is simply told 'to arm with a pack of syringes and kill the deadly coronavirus'.

In all these games, the virus comes in different cosmetics (skin colours, faces that look like Halloween pumpkins, or faces that look like insects with dangling trunk-like extensions). These games offer the hopeful scenario of a virus that can be seen, fought and killed. In reality, the virus can be fought and killed, but it cannot be seen with the naked eye. It is killed through measures of separation (CVA), through hygiene and constant washing up (CWV), while scientists are trying to find a vaccine (KV). Outside the game, in the real world, we are not sure whether we are killing the virus or if the virus is killing us, due to the virus's mechanism of invisibility and delayed medical diagnosis. In the game, the player and the virus are of the same size, as in CVA, which also disadvantages the fighter as an entity that is susceptible to attack. This is what is lacking in reality, at the time of writing, which the game symbolizes through its life bar, a computable testimony of mortality.

In the real world, however, people develop cleaning compulsions that slowly begin to disrupt their daily life, with no proof that they are eluding the 'insect'. Ritualization of cleaning through repetitive cleaning sessions cannot spare people the infection, because dodging the 'insect' is hard when it cannot be seen. This explains why several medical doctors and nurses caught it while in full protective gear. In the game, however, there is a chance of keeping clear of the visible virus without getting obsessive or irrationally compulsive. Trying to kill that which cannot be seen is absurd, especially in the midst of ever-changing and conflicting theories about the nature of the virus, the efficacy of masks and gloves, the number of feet needed in social distancing, and the length of time it can stay 'alive' on surfaces or in the air. The only certainty we have is our own uncertainty.

Confinement: Playing in *the Inside* of Something

During the pandemic, the internet witnessed spikes in users jumping online to play games ranging from Epic's Fortnite to Activision Blizzard's free-to-download Call of Duty: Warzone, thus influencing the dynamics of playlore worldwide. The latter saw thirty million players in just four days following its launch on 10 March (Herrick 2020). Daniel Howley describes this as a crush of players hitting the services of gaming networks, resulting in a massive surge in bandwidth usage in Italy from players signing up to play games like Fortnite, Doom Eternal, and Animal Crossing: New Horizon (2020).

Sometimes, however, the effects of this increased uptake have been sobering. The conception of play as an external activity has been replaced and encroached upon by games in which players play inside of something. Indeed, this has come as a reminder to players of *Plague Inc.* on the company's website:

> The coronavirus outbreak in China is deeply concerning and we've received a lot of questions from players and the media. *Plague Inc.* has been out for eight years now and whenever there is an outbreak of disease we see an increase in players, as people seek to find out more about how diseases spread and to understand the complexities of viral outbreaks. We specifically designed the game to be realistic and informative, while not sensationalising serious real-world issues. However, please remember that *Plague Inc.* is a game, not a scientific model and that the current coronavirus outbreak is a very real situation which is impacting a huge number of people. We would always recommend that players get their information directly from local and global health authorities. (2020)

For Lorenzo Servitje, '*Plague Inc.* participates in the reinscription of anxieties relating to a bioapocalypse and of the desire for the biogovermental process to control it' (86). It is interesting how intramural games, where players play in 'the inside,' constitute a paradigmatic shift in defining today's play geographies as places where knowledge on our predicament can be had. Players play 'in the inside' to get a better understanding of the anxieties caused by 'the outside,' counting on games as 'knowledge producing' outlets (Gerlach et al. 20). The current pandemic 're-stages' imagined narratives to a point where our hands get busy actively trying to search for solutions for the pandemic outside and inside of the game. The speed with which scientists are searching for and improving a vaccine outside, and the mirrored speed with which we try to test the limit of the plague's monstrosity in the game, points to how 'epidemics dramatize the need for regulation with "terrible urgency"' (Wald 17).

Prior to COVID-19, *Plague Inc.* used to give its players a sense of what could become real; today we resort to it for verification, mainly. We do so because '[its] narrative content and interactive functions hover somewhere between science fiction and science fact' (Servitje 86). In the game prior to the plague, 'the boundary between present reality and future potential' becomes uncertain (86). We are not tending towards any resolution to this uncertainty in the current pandemic; during the pandemic, we have inhabited the boundary itself (the *barzakh*) where the plague narrative has wholly engulfed us both in reality and in the simulated world of the game.

As we remain confined, we play again the games we played in the past, but games now grow hyper-real in the liveable spatial imaginaries of the virtual game. Using Lefebvre,

> this means taking into consideration representations of space not just as perceived rep-
> resentations of physical space, but also as conceived representations in relation to
> third spaces: culturally produced space, in which symmetrical and asymmetrical rep-
> resentations, together, constitute 'symbolic' space, which is lived. (Günzel 173)

The player, who is at the same time eluding the insect in the real game, finds the internal game useful, because in it, 'epidemiological mapping serves as real-time visual feedback for the player's biopolitical interventions in the form of pathogenic calibration. [This acts] as an inverse to Foucauldian regulatory biopolitics' (Servitje 87). Servitje uses Foucault's regulatory 'biopolitics,' where longevity, health, mortality/birth rates and wealth and its circulation are deployed to control the processes of a social body's life (Foucault qtd. in Servitje: 243, 249). Servitje argues that *Plague Inc.* and its likes formulate scenarios for the reversal of this order by rewarding players for empowering the apocalyptic plague, where 'death infects life … it slips into life, perpetually gnaw[ing] at it, diminish[ing] it' (Foucault qtd. in Servitje 87: 277). Plague-centered games like *Plague Inc.* experiment with the extreme inversion of infection plots: players, as the game time progresses, 'gain "DNA" points that they use, not to cure people, but to evolve the pathogen, making it more lethal, infectious, resilient or some combination of the three' (Servitje 87–88). In the same vein, Andri Gerber reminds us that 'video games – and games in general – quite literally celebrate ruin and destruction, explaining the steady need to destroy without the possibility to construct, this being a suitable spatial metaphor for Kant's deployment of architectonics' (139).

These gaming examples are part of a world endeavour to play with and cut into our understanding of *playce*. The visceral quality of modern games is symptomatic of a shift beyond the physical world, without altogether dismissing the idea of physicality. The promotion of digital games, such as those containing plague themes, is contingent on three premises (or sources of pleasure): the physical world can be explored or interrogated hopefully more efficiently via play; such efficient explorations, however replete with imminent danger, are quite safe; and players can play the same thing in different geographies. Besides, gamers who readily associate being at home with entertainment are already complying with the state's self-isolation objectives; gamers naturally comply to the state's ideas of good civic behaviour. Dozens of memes laughed about the gamers' change of status during the outbreak. Far from being looked upon as useless homestayers, they get accolades and congratulations from the state for their patriotic commitment to the Confinement.

Games could hence also be construed as instantiations of the sublime. The sublime is an indeterminate site for subverting modes of thinking that depend on orderly arrangements of events. It is a subversion of modernist temporal organization and an assertion of contingency, hence its association with drift rather than spontaneity, paralogy rather than invention. As David Carroll puts it, '[t]he sublime serves to push philosophy and politics into a reflexive, critical mode, to defer indefinitely the imposition of an end on the historical process' (182). It it through the sublime that we see the relationship between *playce* and *barzakh*. The sublime takes us beyond the arrest/the prison by opening up new horizons, new ways of seeing. Both *barzakh* and play can be seen as relational terms:

> When we consider the pairs of terms which denote the extremes as relative terms, then all of them apply to imagination, depending on the perspective. Imaginal things are subtle in relation to the corporeal world, but dense in relation to the spiritual spirits ... Ibn al'Arabi often employs expressions like "corporealization of the spirits" (*tajasud al arwah*) and "spiritualization of the corporeal bodies" (*tarawhun al ajsam*) to explain all sorts of events taking place in the imaginal realm ... or barzakh. (Chittick 15)

The principle of staying home coheres with the players' understanding of the meaning of entertainment (now more conditional than any time before). Gaming while isolating, and isolating while gaming, also configures the semantic register available to the player on the meaning of being 'human,' 'player,' 'citizen,' 'possible victim/survivor,' 'hero' and 'traitor'. 'By staying home, you save lives' is the motto that signals no detraction whatsoever from the surety of the idea of one being a saviour of lives.

Modern game industries rely on old games becoming obsolete so that new games may be produced, new content be made available. New games with pandemic content are heralding a new culture of consumption that binds game designers to confined gamers, where designers give and the confined gamers play and be heroes. It supports the triangular relationship of the mutual benefit between designer, player and hero. In the *barzakh* period of grace, the thinking-knowing period, the more knowledge you possess around the problem, the more likely you act along the codes of goodness, hence the more you can give to yourself and be given, beyond guilt.

This reading handles *playce* and gaming as instantiations of Foucault's disciplinary modality. This modality is reflected in the World Health Organization's efforts to encourage people to play video games during the pandemic, effectively also encouraging non-gamers to become gamers. The organization's ambassador for global strategy is reported as saying that 'games could be an important way for people to follow public health guidelines. He also thanked the gaming industry for their part in the new project'. WHO's ambassabor launched the game 'Play Apart Together' in partnership with eighteen organizations such as Riot Games, Zynga, Twitch, Unity, Technologies and YouTube Gaming.

It is a fact that we are not less disciplined (as used by Foucault) in the current situation of confinement than we used to be before confinement. Disciplines, or the techniques of the regulation of the body that existed before the lockdown, persist in ways that are more perceptible to us. When people talk about deconfinement as a movement away from restrictive modes of being, they forget that we will simply move back to the familiar mode of disciplinarity; we are talking here about the technology of power that regulates the moves and gestures of the body. Confinement is an instantiation of spatialization of power, the deployment of new techniques of management of the body and the production of subjectivity. An important insight of governmentality, according to Foucault, is that it is informed by a fundamentally productive modality that operates by shaping and mobilizing particular subjectivities:

> If power were never anything but repressive, if it never did anything but say no, do you really think one would be brought to obey it? What makes power hold good, what makes

it accepted, is simply the fact that it doesn't only weigh on us a force that says no; it also traverses and produces things, it induces pleasure, forms knowledge, produces discourse. It needs to be considered as a productive network that runs through the whole social body, much more than as a negative instance whose function is repression. (307)

Foucault is helpful here in understanding the architectural dimension of discipline under confinement. Before, we could speak of a relation of externality between the body and disciplinary institutions (the prison, the school, and so forth). The body has to move into these institutions to become docile. Now, bodies internalize the technologies of power. Gaming is an example of this.

Conclusion: On Death in our *Playces*

The majority of modern games are focused on the dichotomy of death and life. Modern gaming attaches the idea of the success of the self to the ability to keep the playable character alive. It is built around the concept of the game as a site of death, which can be circumvented through measures of play that showcase the player's skill at surviving a series of perils. Gratification in the game resides in wining (learning how to survive and become stronger) after enduring a set of failures (deaths, falls, crashes and so forth). The self plays within the awareness that success is contingent on the possibility to 'fail'. The addictive nature of play mostly happens in exploring and developing the skill necessary to save the playable character. Exploration of the game, in this sense, is not determined by a temporal factor (time spent), but by a technological exegesis; that is to say, by the self's interpretation of self in the game, through a translation of self into certain codes on the screen. The rendition of self into, and the consent to be portrayed as, a digital image on the screen captures an intricate act of fusion between the real and the synthetic. The game represents the construction of an ambivalent mirror situation, in which one's digital self-reproduction becomes an indication of our presence (life); the game's digital reproduction of self is such that our playable character becomes existentially bound to us. We no longer belong to anything but the game. The modern game singularizes us. It positions us operative on a digital platform, positions us as figures possessing features of singular heroism. The game does not necessarily signal the withdrawal of the player from his sense of original selfhood in the outside game; the games in the two worlds are interrelated. This speaks not only of a duplication of one's individuality and its projection on multiple game sites, but also of how this duplication is a moment when the self becomes both different and similar.

In this moment of play, the self becomes different because the player's reality is peculiarized in the game, where he experiences a moment of disunity with and within the real, replaced by a sense of unity with and within the unreal. The player's protagonistic endeavour inside the game is informed by a parting from, and at the same time unification with, self (one dies inside the game to survive the other game). Her protagonistic endeavour is informed also by an antagonization of the real self (the real self that hides, unlike in the game, from the virus), informed by a disaffection inside the platforms of the known, by a corporeal schism, an aesthetic rupture, a distraction of the idiosyncratic.

In the game, the self becomes similar because the self, at the moment of play, becomes one with the device (machine or state machine), forming a union in which the mind of the player is in total harmony with the logic of the epoch, with the dictates of the disaster at hand, with the conception of the game designer and the game's unfolding narratives and themes. These can be at odds with those of the lived world, yet the game cushions any possibility of estrangement within a prevailing sense of unceremonious familiarity, a false intimacy that builds up to restage the aloofness of the unreal within a new order of coherence. To be sure, similarity as we speak of it in this context signals a technological sagacity in the global age that coerces the player to assume a position inside the enterprise and therein undertake a fellowship.

The games (inside and out) offer peculiar scenarios of death and life that fall within all the bizarre realms of picturesque (in)justice. If one misses the virus and shoots a blood cell in the game or if one plays the wrong protocols of safety and destroys lives, where sneeze is bullet and cough is sword, then how just is our (social and digital) gaming? A gap exists between the occurrence of these acts of justice and an account of them, as Lyotard (in response to Jean-Loup Thébaud), in *Just Gaming*, also explains. Justice, in this reading, is not an object of the cognitive faculty, it is often deferred, hence its indeterminacy. In both games, one cannot be held accountable for causing a genocide in good faith. The occurrence of an act of justice is different to its transposition as a meaning:

> If you asked me why I am on that side [the question is of possible attack on an American computer in Heidelberg used to programme the bombing of Hanoi], I think that I do not have an answer to the question 'why' and that this is of the order of transcendence. That is, here I feel a prescription to oppose a given thing, and I think that is a just one. This is where I feel that I am indeed playing the game of the just. (Lyotard and Thébaud 69)

Caught unaware of the danger posed to their lives, they had no chance of survival. Vulnerable to the 'war machines' of the current global context, the victims of the game could not have predicted their tragic fate. As we try to elude the insect, it is right to think of the extent to which our responsibilities as gamers (within the codes of morality, ethics and entertainment), and how the turbulent uncertainties within the physics of our *playces*, help reorganize us physically and epistemologically in a different coordinate system, a system that embodies more adequate geometries of justice in which we kill the virus. Only.

Notes

1   This is a reference to how things are played out in the real world. Games borrow concepts and narratives from real-world situations. This is what we refer to as internalization of externals. It is also interesting to look at these worldly situations as games in their own right (involving players, playgrounds, tactics, gain and loss, triumph and defeat).
2   See Götz, especially his discussion on the relationship between reality and architecture in games.
3   See El Maarouf, Belghazi and El Maarouf.
4   See Kosari and Amoori.
5   See El Maarouf, Belghazi and El Maarouf.

ORCID

M. D. El Maarouf ⓘ http://orcid.org/0000-0002-7956-8218
Taieb Belghazi ⓘ http://orcid.org/0000-0002-5893-1524
Ute Fendler ⓘ http://orcid.org/0000-0001-5570-9568

Works Cited

Aarseth, Espen. 'Allegories of Space: The Question of Spatiality in Computer Games'. In *CyberText Yearbook 2000*. Edited by Markku Eskelinen and Raine Koskimaa. Saarijärvi: U of Jyväskylä, Research Centre for Contemporary Culture, 2001. 152–71.

Ameli, Saeid R. 'Do-Fazāyee Shodan-e Shahr: Shahr-e Majāzi, Zaroorat-e Bonyādin Barāy-e Kalānshahrhā-ye Iran. [in Persian: Dual Spacization of City: Virtual City, A Fundamental Necessity For Iranian Metropolitans]'. *Journal of Cultural Studies and Communication* 1(2–3), 1384 (2005 A.D): 117–34.

Ameli, Saeid R. and Hossein Hasani. 'Do-Fazāyee Shodan-e Asib-hā Va Nāhanjāri-hā-ye Fazā-ye Majāzi: Motāle'e-ye Tatbighi-e Siāsatgozāri-hā-ye Beinolmelali'. [in Persian: Dual Specialization of Deviances and Abnormalities of Virtual Space: A Comparative Study of International Policies]'. *Journal of Iranian Cultural Research* 5(1), 1391 (2012 A.D): 1–30.

Appadurai, Arjun. 'Disjuncture and Difference in the Global Cultural Economy'. *In Colonial Discouse and Postcolonial Theory: A Reader*. Edited by Patrick Williams and Laura Chrisman. London: Harvester and Wheatsheaf, 1993. 324–39.

Balicer, Ran, D. 'Modeling Infectious Diseases Dissemination through Online Role-playing Games'. *Epidemiology* 18(2), 2007: 260–61.

Bateman, Chris. 'Implicit Game Aesthetics'. *Games and Culture* 10, 2015: 389–411.

Caillois, Roger. *Les Jeux et les Hommes*. Paris: Galimard, 1958.

Carroll, David. *Paraesthetics Foucault Lyotard Derrida*. New York: Routledge, 1987.

Chittick, William C. *The Sufi Path of Knowledge: Ibn al-'Arabi's Metaphysics of Imagination*. Albany: State University of New York Press, 1989.

Derrida, Jacques. 'The Retrait of Metaphor'. *Enclic* 2(2), 1978: 6–33.

El Maarouf, Moulay Driss, Taieb Belghazi and Farouk El Maarouf. 'COVID-19: A Critical Ontology of the Present'. *Educational Philosophy and Theory* 53(1), 2021: 71–89.

Fauconnier, Gilles. *Mappings in Thought and Language*. Cambridge: Cambridge University Press, 1997.

Fauconnier, Gilles. *Mental Spaces: Aspects of Meaning Construction in Natural Language*. Cambridge: Cambridge University Press, 1994.

Foucault, Michel. *Society Must Be Defended: Lectures at the Collège De France, 1975–76*. Translated by David Macey. New York: Picador, 2003.

Gerber, Andri. 'The Architectonics of Game Spaces, Or, Why you Should Play and Design Video Games to Become a Better Architect'. In *Architectonics of Game Spaces: The Spatial Logic of the Virtual and its Meaning for the Real*. Edited by Andri Gerber and Ulrich Götz. Bielefeld: Architekturen, 2020: 135–52.

Gerlach, Neil, Sheryl N. Hamilton, Rebecca Sullivan and Priscilla L. Walton. *Becoming Biosubjects: Bodies, Systems, Technologies*. Toronto: University of Toronto Press, 2011.

Götz, Ulrich. 'From Asteroids to Architectoids: Close Encounters between Architecture and Game Design'. In *Architectonics of Game Spaces: The Spatial Logic of the Virtual and Its Meaning for the Real*. Edited by Andri Gerber and Ulrich Götz. Bielefeld: Architekturen, 2020: 201–14.

Graiouid, Said. 'From Post-Modernism to Post-Traditionalism: Rethinking Social Organization in a Post-Traditional Society'. *Reconstruction*. 7(4). 2007. http://reconstruction.digitalodu.com/Issues/074/graiouid.shtml. Accessed on 19 Aug. 2021.

Griffin, Andrew. 'Coronavirus: World Health Organisation Tells People to Stay at Home and Play Games.' *Independent*. 31 Mar. 2020. https://www.independent.co.uk/life-style/gadgets-and-tech/news/coronavirus-world-health-organisation-play-games-covid-19-advice-a9438916.html. Accessed on 19 Aug. 2021.

Günzel, Stephan. 'The Lived Space of Computer Games'. In *Architectonics of Game Spaces The Spatial Logic of the Virtual and Its Meaning for the Real*. Edited by Andri Gerber and Ulrich Götz. Bielefeld: Architekturen, 2020: 167–82.

Hagström, Anders. 'Poetically Man Dwells in Game Space: A Phenomenological Investigation of Video Games as Art'. Bachelor's Diss. Uppsala University, 2017.

Heidegger, Martin. *Being and Time*. Translated by John Macquarrie and Edward Robinson. Oxford: Blackwell, 2001.

Heidegger, Martin. *Remarks on Art – Sculpture – Space*. Switzerland: Erker Verlag, 1996.

Heidegger, Martin. 'The Questions Concerning Technology'. In *The Question Concerning Technology and Other Essays*. Translated by William Lovitt. New York: Harper & Row, 1977. 3–55.

Herrick, Justin. '15 Million Players Love "Call of Duty: Warzone" Already'. *PC Mag*. 15 Mar. 2020. https://www.pcmag.com/news/15-million-players-love-call-of-duty-warzone-already. Accessed on 18 Aug. 2021.

Howley, Daniel. 'The World is Turning to Video Games Amid Coronavirus Outbreak'. *Yahoo! Finance*. 18 Mar. 2020. https://finance.yahoo.com/news/coronavirus-world-turning-to-video-games-150704969.html. Accessed on 16 Aug. 2021.

Hoy, David Couzens. 'Heidegger and the Hermeneutic Turn'. In *The Cambridge Companion to Heidegger*. Edited by Charles B. Guignon. Cambridge: Cambridge UP, 2006. 177–201.

Hunicke, Robin, Marc LeBlanc and Rober Zubek. 'MDA: A Formal Approach to Game Design and Game Research'. 2004. http://www.cs.northwestern.edu/~hunicke/MDA.pdf. Accessed on 26 Mar. 2021.

Kant, Immanuel. *The Critique of Judgment*. Translated by James Creed Meredith. Oxford: Clarendon, 1998: 692–93.

Kearney, Richard. *Poetics of Imagining From Husserl to Lyotard*. London: Routledge, 1993.

Kosari, Masoud and Abbas Amoori. 'Thirdspace: The Trialectics of the Real, Virtual and Blended Spaces'. *Journal of Cyberspace Studies* 2(2), 2019: 163–85.

Lefebvre, Henri. *The Production of Space*. Oxford: Blackwell, 1991.

Lyotard, Jean François and Jean-Loup Thébaud. *Just Gaming*. Translated by Wlad Godzich. Vol. 20. Manchester: Manchester University Press, 1985.

Malaby, Thomas M. *Making Virtual World: Linden Lab and Second Life*. Ithaca, NY: Cornell University Press, 2009.

Murata, Sachiko. *The Tao of Islam: A Source Book on Gender Relationships in Islamic Thought*. State University of New York Press: Albany, 1992.

Plague Inc. 'Statement on the Current Coronavirus Outbreak'. *Ndemic Creations*. 23 Jan. 2020. https://www.ndemiccreations.com/en/news/172-statement-on-the-current-coronavirus-outbreak. Accessed on 18 Aug. 2021.

Polkinghorne, Donald. *Practice and the Human Sciences: The Case for a Judgment-based Practice of Care*. Albany, NY: State University of New York Press, 2004.

Ricoeur, Paul. *Lectures on Ideology and Utopia*. New York: Columbia UP, 1986.

Rouse, Richard and Steve Ogden. *Game Design: Theory and Practice*. Plano, TX: Wordware, 2005.

Salen, Katie and Eric Zimmerman. *Rules of Play: Game Design Fundamentals*. MIT P, 2003.

Schell, Jesse. *The Art of Game Design: A Book of Lenses*. Burlington, MA: Morgan Kaufmann Publishers, 2008.

Scott, James C. *Weapons of the Weak: Everyday Forms of Resistance*. New Haven: Yale University Press, 1985.

Servitje, Lorenzo. 'H5N1 for Angry Birds: Plague Inc., Mobile Games, and the Biopolitics of Outbreak Narratives'. *Science Fiction Studies, Digital Science Fiction* 43(1), 2016: 85–103.

Wald, Priscilla. *Contagious: Cultures, Carriers, and the Outbreak Narrative*. Durham, NC: Duke University Press, 2008.

COVID-19: Between Panic, Racism and Social Change

Omar Moumni ⓘ

Abstract

The emergence of the novel coronavirus has led to panic, vulnerability and racism all over the world. This paper traces the roots and routes of the different faces and facets of such responses and explores their impact on individual and collective behaviour. It focuses on the un/ethics of self-care and collective care and the impacts these responses have had on Moroccan society. It argues that the pandemic pushed individuals to behave 'globally' against local and cultural norms, demonstrating new societal behaviour that is based on avarice, self-interest and self-care.

Introduction

COVID-19 has uncovered different faces of both panic and un/ethics. Our social, personal, cultural and professional relationships have changed; people have started to think about their 'selves' and to ponder their own existence (Turner 1). The effects of the pandemic are certainly hazardous and the state of panic and emergency created uncertainty. Suddenly, everything changed, 'rulebooks were torn up, financial restrictions thrown out of the window, and liberties and freedoms that we all took for granted disappeared overnight' (Atkinson 327). This panic exacerbated people's sense of uncertainty. Fear, anxiety, frustration and other emotions created doubts about self-existence and pushed people towards an apocalyptic outlook; hope diminished as people felt uncertain about the future while they also expressed desire for a return to normalcy.

In this paper, I focus on the rise of the pandemic in Morocco and its effects on Moroccan society. I reflect on the scenes of panic, the different ethics and un/ethics of self-isolation, and the new forms of individual behaviour associated with the pandemic. The paper focuses on such behaviour between ethics and un/ethics of 'self,' collective care, and their impact on Moroccan society. It argues that the pandemic pushed individuals to behave 'globally' against local and cultural norms, demonstrating new societal behaviour based on avarice, self-interest and self-care.

When the pandemic first broke out in Wuhan, China in late 2019, the world watched the media reports with scorn and indifference. People ridiculed the pandemic and mocked its origin as being Asian, and particularly Chinese. These racist and xenophobic attitudes multiplied as the virus spread.

Racism during disease outbreaks is not new and did not emerge with COVID-19. At the beginning of the AIDS pandemic, public discourse was riddled with racist and exoticized stereo-types of Africans' sexuality, a sexuality that was framed as distinct from western and European cultural and social norms. The mode of writing about Africa and Africans was characterized by what Coetzee calls a 'repertoire of amazing facts' (Coetzee 13). Such writing, along with other academic, scientific and journalistic writings, has surely contributed to the spread of old stereo-types about Africans and Africa as mysterious entities. Eileen Stillwaggon notes that:

> Racial science and popular racial stereotypes stressed sexual differences between the races, and the representation of physiological differences in the portrayal of Africans in art was an important pillar maintaining the popular view of Africans as exotic, strange, and even disturbing. (814)

> The media also continue to perpetuate an unsubstantiated but potent image of a lusty, ancestral African careening headlong for doom because of sexual behaviour. (826)

In addition to the AIDS stigma against Africans, AIDS discourse functioned in terms of another paradigm in which sexual minorities were discriminated against, where that discourse capita-lized on these minorities' perceived sexual promiscuity as an explanation for HIV transmission: 'Despite increased visibility, acceptance, and recent sociopolitical advances, gay and bisexual men continue to live in a society that privileges heterosexuality while denigrating non-heterosex-ual relationships, behaviors, and identities' (Halkitis 5).

In many countries, there was intense and skewed media scrutiny of these and related issues and the press reported their findings with unfairly discriminatory headlines such as 'Alert over gay plague' and 'Gay plague may lead to blood ban on homosexuals,' all of which associated HIV with homosexuality and deemed it a 'gay disease' (Moyer and Igonya 1012). The already biased discourse against the queer community meant they were doubly discriminated against: as a minority group that already suffered oppressive social structures and inequalities, queer people were now faced with disease stigma. The nature of the unfair discrimination also functioned differently to other kinds of discrimination. While race and gender are susceptible to visible stigmas, sexual orientation and illnesses are prone to 'invisible stigmas' (Clair, Beatty and Maclean). As a result of this association of the transmission of a stigmatized disease with a sexual minority, 'the "gay" stereotype has survived through the years, even though evidence shows that the HIV epidemic among young adults in sub-Saharan Africa is mainly transmitted through risky heterosexual behaviors' (Nduna and Mendes 25). It is evident that HIV discourse was initially weaponized against Africans, queer and black communities in different parts of the world. Such minorities are 'often stigmatized as high-risk groups and thus discriminated against' (Yuen-man Siu 9).

Similar to AIDS, the outbreak of Ebola in 2014 attracted worldwide attention. Western media coverage of the Ebola disease conceptualized it as African, creating fear, panic and anxiety. Africans were homogenized, marginalized and constructed as a source of fear, threat and menace. With the repetition of such themes on news and social media, stereotypes were consolidated into a distorted truth. In such scenarios, Africa is othered and stigmatized. As Sarah Monson puts it:

> Often, 'the other' is not perceived as neutral or benign, but as a threat to what is perceived as normal. In the American media discourse of Ebola, Africa became the homogenized other, leading to the explicit discrimination and stigmatization of Africans currently living in the United States and those returning from West Africa, including non-Africans. Homogenization and otherization processes are not always obvious, unless made explicit as in the *New York Times* headline 'New York Doctor, Back from Africa, is Sick with Ebola'. (4)

Indeed, this Ebola narrative recalls old discriminatory discourse that was fuelled by classification and categorization, a discourse that allowed Europeans and Americans to justify their colonial projects. So, conceptualizing Ebola as African, and figuring Africa as a country, fostered a discourse of stigmatization against Africans not only in Africa, but against Africans the world over.

At the beginning of the spread of COVID-19 in Morocco, as in many other Arab countries, people within those areas trivialized the virus using humour and sarcasm. They decided that their own immune systems were resilient, and perceived countries with high hygiene standards as immune to the virus. They were so confident about their ability to resist the pandemic that they positioned themselves as spectators of the spread of COVID-19 as opposed to participants or actors. Indeed, 'the privilege of spectatorship marks people's abysmal (un)responsiveness to the horror happening on the ground in Wuhan' and elsewhere (El Maarouf, Belghazi and El Maarouf 72).

When the pandemic appeared in different corners of the world, experts expected the worst for Africa. With the high rate of poverty and informal settlements, the social distancing required to manage the spread of the virus seemed difficult or impossible to acheive in many parts of the continent. However, the fatality rates appeared relatively low (at least as far as data coming out of the continent showed). In response, western media reinforced stereotypes of Africa by framing it as exception to the rest of the world (Peters 757).

The pandemic excited the imagination, often in the worst possible ways, and perpetuated a discourse of illusory difference. In Morocco, like many other Arab and African countries, the situation was dire. Many hospitals were overwhelmed and many people died, a fact that forced many to reckon with a new reality that seemed at first like a dream. Now it was necessary to construct a new normal, a 'new form of our entire social life' (Žižek, Communism 2020).

Vulnerability and Racism in the COVID-19 Era: From Global to Local

The history of epidemics and pandemics, and how that history is told, are closely intertwined with our emotional responses to them. With each pandemic, different emotional responses are generated: anxiety, panic, fear, uncertainty, inequality, frustration, hope and others. COVID-19, like previous pandemics, generated different positive and negative emotional responses, either directly through personal or familial morbidity, or indirectly through the different biased discourses transmitted across media and everyday life. Understanding emotional dynamics more broadly will aid in understanding psychopathology and well-being more specifically (Wichers, Wigman and Myin-Germeys). Also, one's emotions and behaviours during pandemics and other challenging times offer insight into how one might deal with such circumstances in the future (Martín-Brufau, Suso-Ribera and Corbalán 2).

Positive emotions and responses such as caring about others, collaboration, cooperation and complying with rules and regulations fixed by civil society and the state are apparent all over the world. However, negative emotions and responses like anger, annoyance, panic, fear, hate and greed are equally present. They are shocking, trenchant and virulent as they fuel 'hate crimes, hoarding, protests, violence, and xenophobia' (Huang 9).

The pandemic cultivated a state of continuous societal risk, instigated, in part, by global interconnectivity and the relatively instantaneous flow of (mis)information. COVID-19 created a moment of total loss and unpredictability, pushing some people all over the world towards radicalism and irrational behaviour. As Demertzis and Eyerman mention, 'the pandemic generate[d] an emotional climate of uncertainty, not as in "we know that we don't know," but as in "we don't know what we don't know"' (Demertzis and Eyerman 430). Such behaviours are, in part, emotional, where 'emotions can distort risk estimates, risk perception, decision readiness, decision making, deliberation, thinking, judgment, and information acquisition' (Huang 7). The pandemic was a 'facilitator and accelerator of structural calibrations and cultural shifts' largely the effect of such blended emotions (Demertzis & Eyerman 445). It is clear that such emotions push people to act in a certain way to keep safe and to protect the self.

The spread of media misinformation about the pandemic only aided the spread of these negative emotions that ultimately endangered the entire world. Such misinformation or 'massive infodemic, interacts with risks of pandemic itself, creating a multilayered risk' (Krause et. al. 1).

Risky behaviours are perpetuated not only by misinformation but also by virulent scenes of racist acts. At the beginning of the pandemic, several racist media campaigns were launched against Chinese people and their culture. In Canada, for example, Chinese people faced intense racism to the extent that Prime Minister Justin Trudeau warned Canadians against racist acts, emphasizing the need to demonstrate solidarity. At a ceremony for the Chinese New Year, Trudeau said, '"there is no place in our country for discrimination that is fueled by fear and misinformation"' (Benslimane 2020). More than that, xenophobia affected even those not of Chinese descent. Roberto, Johnson and Rauhaus show that, in Canada during the time of the pandemic, 'a Vietnamese cultural center was vandalized, [and] two Korean men were stabbed' (370). These incidents were widespread amongst Asian individuals and communities across the world. France, too, witnessed scenes of racism towards Asians. French Media reported that students of Chinese origin were bullied in schools, with some Chinese students launching a counter-campaign on Twitter under the hashtag: 'I am not a virus' (Benslimane 2020). The French media intensified such racist acts by fostering similar attitudes not only in print media, where racist headlines were propagated, but also on TV, where racist discourse about the coronavirus targeted the Chinese and other nationalities (Benslimane 2020).

During a show aired on 2 April 2020 by LCI, a French television channel, two French doctors argued live that 'treatment for COVID-19 should be first tested on Africans' (*North Africa Post* 2020). One of the doctors was the president of the French Intensive Care Society, Jean-Paul Mira, and the other a research director at the French National Institute of Health and Medical Research (INSERM), Camille Locht (*The North Africa Post 2020*). Such openly racist attitudes enraged many people, especially those from former-French colonies, provoking many media debates denouncing such talk. These racist utterances reflected a colonial mentality. El Maarouf, Belghazi and El Maarouf, with reference to the work of T.L. Smith, argue that,

> the real apocalypse for the Indigenous peoples, with their fundamental pluralistic out-looks, histories, sexualities, spatialities, socialities, and traditions, is obviously not COVID-19, but rather colonialism. Colonialism has left them with the severe task of creating meaning out of the rubble caused by the colonial encounter, and of digging up, in what seems to be a tricky archeology, relics of their suppressed knowledges from under the stifling vestiges of a resilient coloniality. (75–76)

Racist speech in the present reflects a deep-rooted egoistic and essentialist 'self' that is bound by the narcissistic glories and victories of the colonial era. Targets of such racism must then resist both the COVID-19 pandemic and racist colonial discourse that exploits such human catastrophe to nullify those considered savage 'others'. The two doctors apologized for their racist utter-ances, and the Moroccan Lawyers Club decided to file a complaint with the public prosecutor in Paris against the two channel hosts for defamation and racism (*The North Africa Post 2020*). 'The lawyers club also launched an online campaign, "We are not laboratory rats," to denounce the comments' (*The North Africa Post 2020*). Amnesty International's media manager for Europe and Turkey, Stefan Simanowitz, tweeted that the comments were 'disgust-ing'. According to the *North Africa Post*,

> Several international football players, including Moroccan Medhi Banatia, Cameroonian Samuel Eto'o, Senegalese Demba Ba, Ghanaian Christian Atsu and Ivorian Didier Drogba have all posted messages denouncing the French doctors' 'serious, racist and contemptuous remarks' insisting that Africa is not a laboratory and that Africans are not guinea pigs. (2020)

COVID-19 continued to unveil antagonistic feelings towards people all over the globe. In France again, the French television channel Canal Plus mocked Italians by suggesting that the virus was, itself, Italian, doing so by broadcasting a mock advert that showed Corona Pizza, 'in which a coughing chef hacks green phlegm onto Italy's national dish' (*South China Morning Post 2020*). This mockery was strongly condemned by Italian authorities and the global community as being racist, forcing the French television station to apologize for the advertisement.

The Danish newspaper *Jyllands-Posten* published a satirical drawing depicting a picture of the Chinese flag with the image of the coronavirus in place of the five stars. This incident sparked tensions between China and Denmark. Chinese people launched a counter campaign on social media networks against Denmark, publishing Denmark's flag with Nazi skulls and slogans, while demanding an official apology. Despite the Chinese embassy's remarks about the immor-ality of the cartoon, the Danish Prime Minister refused to comply and insisted that the newspaper acted within the framework of freedom of expression (Oelze 2020). In Britain, teenage boys attacked a student from Singapore on Oxford Street on 24 February. The student was told, "'we don't want your coronavirus in our country'" (BBC News 2020). Indeed, such racist atti-tudes reflect different faces of epistemic violence and some 'inherited conceptual apparatuses and temporal frames' that fix the 'other' (Neilson 1).

In India, people originating from north-eastern states faced racially motivated attacks because of their appearance – they resemble the Chinese. According to Haokip, constructing an 'Indian face' which is highly diversified and an inclusive concept, Wouters and Subba argue 'that Mongoloid phenotypes ... have not found a place in common imaginaries of the Indian Face. Instead, Northeasterners are non-recognized and misrecognized, mirrored back by the wider Indian society as foreigners, hailing from such places as China, Nepal, Thailand, or Japan and on a visit to India, or as 'lesser Indians' rather than as equal citizens; and this withholding of equal recognition of 'Indianness' works to discriminate against and marginalize them. (4)

Indeed, people from north-eastern states are systemically discriminated against because they do not exhibit what are considered typical Indian physical characteristics and so are doubly victimized. Historically, India's north-east has witnessed frequent unrest, especially in the postcolonial Indian nation state, provoking strong secessionist movements (Bora 1). However, the state suppressed all these movements, reinforcing violence and discrimination against the north-eastern people. Such experiences become a 'problem without a name,' understood primarily in terms of cultural difference, which elides issues of racism, and where culture becomes a substitute for race' (Bora 2).

These acts of racism have transcended physical appearances and have been identified also in religious encounters. In the early days of the COVID-19 pandemic, a doctor in the Mathura area reportedly turned away Muslim patients saying, 'We will treat only Hindus, not Muslims'. A video shared widely on social media depicted the incident and increased tensions between the religious groups in India. Prejudice based on racial, cultural and religious differences articulates and revives separatist colonial principles, producing old hatred in new scenarios. In India, work towards solidarity with various marginalized groups, including Muslim groups, is long overdue (Haokip 16). These acts of racism present the Indian government with opportunities to build a strong framework against racial discrimination and reduce its effects, with the possible outcome that this would build a culture of trust and belonging among all Indian citizens.

Other areas in Africa and South America witnessed aggressive behaviours based on stigmatized traits. For example, online harassment targeting 'light skinned' foreigners has been reported in countries like Cameroon, Ethiopia, Kenya, Nigeria and South Africa (Roberto, Johnson and Rauhaus 370). In Brazil, a government official was highly vilified for racist tweets. In Bolivia, the government forced three Japanese tourists who had not displayed any symptoms into quarantine (Roberto, Johnson and Rauhaus 370). Evidently, the pandemic is not only a public health problem; it is also a cultural phenomenon.

The state of panic during the COVID-19 pandemic is not only manifested in the flagrant acts of racism against people of different ethnicities, but also against objects. Manipulated by misinformation, people reacted collectively and irrationally by attacking 5G towers in the belief that there was a link between them and the spread of coronavirus. Videos shared on YouTube and Facebook of such incidents created outrage at the damage caused to such infrastructure.

The situation in Morocco is not entirely different. According to *Morocco World News*, vendors at a fish market in Tetouan harassed an Asian tourist by shouting the word 'corona' at her. Angry at them, the woman filmed the incident and shared it on YouTube. Moroccan citizens vilified the incident as offensive and racist (Kasraoui 2020). Social media also circulated news of an American tourist beaten in Marrakech by individuals who considered tourists the source of the virus. Additionally, Moroccans informally boycotted Chinese restaurants at the beginning of the pandemic. Another video of a woman claiming that the virus was detected in a Chinese restaurant in Fez went viral online. The Moroccan authorities denounced this incident, and the woman was arrested.

Such 'misinfodemics' may be more dangerous than the COVID-19 pandemic itself as they create panic and fear in society. They exacerbate the risk in an attempt, ironically, to address or alleviate other forms of risk. For example, a resident of Arizona died after consuming Chloroquine, a malaria treatment, thinking it would also be a good treatment for COVID-19. As Krause et. al. show, 'misinformation can literally be a matter of life and death' (1).

COVID-19 has also demonstrated the vulnerability and the precariousness of masses of people. The 'epidemio-economics' will affect several societal sectors and have consequences on generations in ways that reflect the failure of neoliberal capitalism (Peters 755). For instance, COVID-19 revealed educational disparities among students globally and among Moroccan students specifically. Given the pandemic, schools and universities closed their doors but continued to work online. The pandemic forced the Moroccan Ministry of Education to attempt to digitize education. However, the pandemic reflected the precarity of so many students who could not afford electronic devices, while many in rural areas struggled with internet access. These two shortcomings demonstrate the disparities that were already apparent in the education sector in Morocco. This is only one aspect of education vulnerability during the COVID-19 pandemic in Morocco, witnessed in other countries as well. Other factors pose questions about ethics and societal behaviour across the globe. Fighting against the intense racism caused by the COVID-19 pandemic, the World Health Organization struggled to raise awareness about the disease. A common anti-discrimination slogan that circulated during the pandemic '"We're all in the together"' (Wong and Wong 569), sought to protect social health, but also attempted to instil confidence in old social and cultural norms. It is evident, then, that 'the ongoing spread of the coronavirus epidemic has also triggered vast epidemics of ideological viruses which were laying dormant in our societies: fake news, paranoiac conspiracy theories, explosions of racism' (Žižek, 'Communism' 2020). Indeed, the post-pandemic period will not only need to address existing racisms, but, since these new ideological viruses have spread, with social and technological viruses feeding off each other, existing and growing forms of discrimination would be all the harder to eradicate.

COVID-19 and Social Change in Morocco: Between Ethics and Un/ethics

With the rise of the pandemic in Morocco, as news about its devastating impact in Italy and Spain spread across the world, Moroccans' attitude shifted from sarcasm to a state of shock. The Moroccan state closed its borders and all institutions, including the religious ones. Suddenly, all events were cancelled, cafés and restaurants were forced to close or to adopt new practices, and individuals changed not only their views about the pandemic but also their social and cultural behaviours, opting for a more western and individualistic approach. COVID-19 prompted new behaviours in Moroccan society. These modes of behaving may be described not only in terms of human weakness and fragility in times of catastrophe, but also by greed and self-interest at the expense of solidarity and collective well-being. As the state imposed a state of emergency and quarantine, people realized the gravity of the situation. Some decided to abide by the safety instructions, while others ignored the quarantine and the state of emergency, not making any effort to protect themselves and each other.

Though Moroccan culture is based on collective well-being, during the pandemic these norms were often overridden by selfishness. The Moroccan people began endangering the lives of people working in the health sector who, in the case of Morocco and the world over, already 'experience ethical conflicts with separation from family and long hours, as well as the possibility of deadly exposure' (Peters 755). Such behaviour demonstrated self-centred attitudes to care that ignored the collective sacrifice of the medical community in confronting the pandemic.

Caring about one's own movement and freedom at the expense of others who are either obliged to work in such challenging times, or at the expense of those who follow the precautions, points to a form of social irresponsibility that reflects the perennial ruptures in the dream of a cohesive community. Such deeds were often challenged by those who respect social and legal norms, and by those who refused to associate with such 'bad' citizens. Such behaviour demonstrated how some individuals were susceptible to global norms and principles regarding the pandemic.

Another act of social irresponsibility was apparent in the state of panic that followed the announcement of social distancing measures. The panic around the protocols of self-isolation and social distancing generated disruptive and careless behaviour as people panic-bought essential items. Moroccans mirrored the panic-buying depicted in media reports about Australia, New Zealand and the United States.

Such behavioural mirroring of peoples and communities abroad reflects both the pandemic's global reach and its tendency towards homogenizing, in some respects, global behaviour, particularly in matters of public safety. The sense of community and solidarity became no more than slogans; self-interest superseded local collective culture. From this, we learn that behaviour that is fostered by fear and panic unveils the ugly face of individualism and consumerism. By buying huge quantities of goods, 'bad' citizens created shortages and deprived other people of access to some essential products. So, despite the government's advice not to rush and buy huge quantities of products, which would create shortages, people competitively moved towards consumerism to guarantee their own safety. This shows how consumers 'in a particular socio-cultural location have expressed their corporealism, which refers to the circumstances that allow a person to have a solid grasp of the present situation of his body and predict its future' (El Maarouf, Belghazi and El Maarouf 78–79).

These behavioral patterns reflect what Peters refers to as 'collective irrationality' that is based on 'competitive individualism'; it is here that humanitarian values vanish (756). Such individualistic behaviour seems correct, and even rational, from the individual's point of view, but are decidedly irrational from a collective, public viewpoint (Peters 756). In such circumstances, collective awareness, rationality and responsibility become fragile, and even subsumed, as individuals become motivated by their desire for personal safety and parochialism, not only in their thinking but also in their self-management, during the pandemic. Such un/ethics of care are also manifested in the breaking of instructions stated by the government. So, despite the state's warning about the need to observe social distancing and limit the size of gatherings, some people remained complacent.

In Morocco, there were certainly several instances of individuals thinking only of themselves instead of the collective. Yet there were other moments in which communities demonstrated solidarity (but still ignored social distancing protocols in doing so). When individuals received negative COVID-19 test results, neighbours often gathered outside in the streets and celebrated in the Moroccan way (as seen in figure 1). These occurrences demonstrated collective irrationality, irresponsibility and even disrespect for social distancing protocols advised during

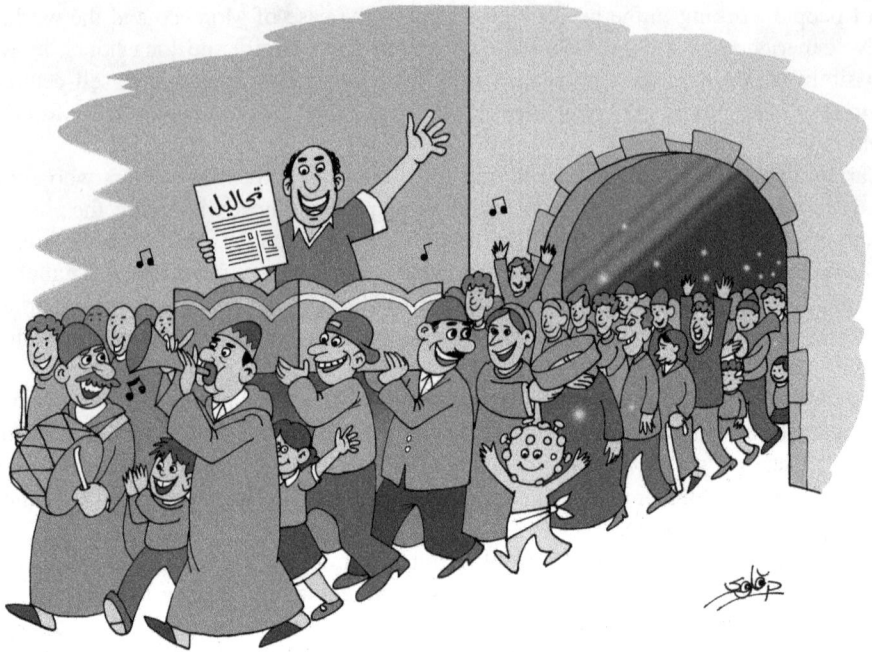

Figure 1:   A crowd in the street celebrating a negative COVID-19 result. Image by Abdellah Derkaoui.

the pandemic. Communities would celebrate as a collective, while, ironically, endanger themselves and the larger society by doing so. The emblematic celebration is in fact a misguided false triumph over the pandemic.

Another example of unethical and irrational behaviour was witnessed in Morocco when the state closed all institutions, including religious ones. These closures provoked demonstrations in different Moroccan cities like Fez, Sale and Tangier. In these demonstrations, people expressed their anger towards both COVID-19 and the state. Similar protests were reported elsewhere. Mosques in Tunisia, according to Joffé, 'were forced to close, despite protests that this would inhibit seeking divine protection' (2). Some believed that the coronavirus was a punishment from God, and so demanded the opening of religious spaces so as to do right by their beliefs, ignoring rules of self-isolation and social distancing that would inevitably be ignored should religious spaces open.

Attempts to enforce self-isolation by different states were criticized and led to demonstrations. Those people were a minority, but were nonetheless (and continue to be) a huge threat to society, endangering not only public safety but also ignoring the fact that lockdown is a 'patriotic duty' (Joffé 5). Collective irrational behaviour is not a local syndrome but a global one. Such scenes of un/ethics were manifested in different parts of the world. In Egypt, for example,

> people took to the street, burning flags with the coronavirus emblem, denouncing its coronialism of the world. In Germany people organized corona parties. In Brazil, people filled the streets declaring their extreme nihilist faith in the existence of COVID-19. (El Maarouf, Belghazi and El Maarouf 84–85)

These patterns of irrational behaviour across the world reflect the ugly face of neoliberal globalization. The unprecedented un/ethical scenes demonstrate many cultures are not immune to panic, individualism, consumerism and un/ethics of self-care and self-protection.

At the same time, during the pandemic, illegal Moroccan migrants attempted to cross borders into Europe. Despite all the struggles they went through to get to Spain, migrants, paradoxically, risked their lives to get back to Morocco to escape intense waves of the pandemic and to protect themselves from possible death in Spain. This situation forced migrants into human trafficking networks, seeking their help to return to Morocco: 'According to Spanish media, around 100 Moroccans illegally left the Spanish coast in late March on boats that set sail towards Morocco' (Alaoui 2020). Also, Moroccan migrants in Spain paid 'human smugglers about €5,400 to clandestinely return home to Morocco' for a journey that ordinarily costs between €400 to €1 000 (Idnes.cz 2020). Similarly, when Morocco closed its borders, many Moroccans remained in the Moroccan colonized city Ceuta; but many later attempted to swim from Ceuta to Tarajal beach in Morocco, in fear of the escalating infection rates (Goodman 2021). The new phase of counter-migration of undocumented migrants from Spain to Morocco raises difficult questions about the concept of transition and transnational mobility. Morocco is thus a receiving country that has to deal with different types of counter-migration (Moumni, 'Migration' 26; Moumni, 'Crisis' 158). In response to this return migration, the Moroccan police sought to quarantine these returnees to manage the possible spread of the virus in Morocco.

Conclusion

Panic during the pandemic produced various acts of worldwide racism in which the 'other' became the 'face of coronavirus' (Haokip 4). Racist acts fluctuated, moving across global and local spaces. Despite all measures taken by the state to restrict the virus and ensure people's safety by regulating behaviour. In reality these measures were commonly thwarted.

Some people failed in their 'patriotic duty' and behaved according to their own neoliberal convictions, ignoring social solidarity. Such actors provoked resentment and a feeling of uncertainty among those who respected the state's instructions; and their behaviour was representative of the huge societal changes that appeared during confinement. In fact, the pandemic unveiled not only the face of solidarity and nationhood among some people but also the problematic faces of individualism, globalization and self-centeredness among others. It is still not clear when we will get back to our 'normal' lives. However, this should push us to consider our uncertain futures, in which we should reflect on our cultural and social values and revisit and revise our 'selves' so that we can transcend this state of uncertainty.

Acknowledgement

This article has benefited a lot from the rigorous peer reviewing process. The author is greatly indebted to the editors and to the journal's anonymous reviewers for their valuable comments and suggestions and also for their critical interaction with the article. Special thanks to the Moroccan Cartoonist Abdellah Derkaoui for giving me permission to use his outstanding cartoon in my paper.

ORCID

Omar Moumni ⏺ http://orcid.org/0000-0003-2749-949X

Works Cited

Alaoui, Mohamed. 'Pandemic Sparks Reverse Migration from Spain to Morocco'. *The Arab Weekly*. 29 Apr. 2020. https://thearabweekly.com/pandemic-sparks-reverse-migration-spain-morocco. Accessed on 21 Aug. 2021.

Atkinson, Paul. 'Social Distancing'. *The Design Journal* 23(3), 2020: 327–30.

BBC News. 'Coronavirus: Boy sentenced for racist street attack'. *BBC News*. 27 Jan. 2021. https://www.bbc.com/news/uk-england-london-54048546. Accessed on 21 Aug. 2021.

Benslimane, Leila. 'Acts of Racism Against the Chinese because of Corona'. *Morocco Jewish Times*. 8 Feb. 2020. https://www.mjtnews.com/2020/02/08/acts-of-racism-against-the-chinese-because-of-corona/. Accessed on 21 Aug. 2021.

Bora, Papori. 'The Problem Without a Name: Comments on Cultural Difference (Racism) in India, South Asia'. *Journal of South Asian Studies* 42(5), 2019: 1–16.

Coetzee, J. M. *White Writing: On the Culture of Letters in South Africa*. New Haven: Yale University Press, 1988.

Clair, Judith, Joy Beatty and Tammy Maclean. 'Out of Sight but not Out of Mind: Managing Invisible Social Identities in the Workplace'. *Academy of Management Review* 30(1), 2005: 78–95.

Demertzis, Nicolas and Ron Eyerman. 'Covid-19 as Cultural Trauma". *American Journal of Cultural Sociology* 8, 2020. 428–50.

El Maarouf, Moulay Driss, Taieb Belghazi and Farouk El Maarouf. 'COVID – 19: A Critical Ontology of the Present'. *Educational Philosophy and Theory* 53(1), 2020: 71–89.

Goodman, Al. 'Thousands of Migrants Swim from Morocco to Spanish Enclave of Ceuta'. *CNN*. 19 May 2021. https://edition.cnn.com/2021/05/18/europe/migrants-swim-morocco-spanish-enclave-ceuta-intl/index.html. Accessed on 21 Aug. 2021.

Halkitis, Perry N. 'Discrimination and Homophobia Fuel the HIV Epidemic in Gay and Bisexual Men'. *Psychology & AIDS Exchange* 2012: n. pag.

Haokip, Thongkholal. 'From "Chinky" to "Coronavirus": Racism against Northeast Indians During the Covid-19 Pandemic'. *Asian Ethnicity* 22(2), 2020: 353–73.

Huang, Peter H. 'Pandemic Emotions: The Good, the Bad, and the Unconscious – Implications for Public Health, Financial Economics, Law, and Leadership'. *Northwestern Journal of Law and Social Policy* 16(2), 2021: 1–54.

Idnes.cz. 'Migrants Paying Smugglers €5,400 to go back to Africa During Coronavirus Crisis'. *Remix*. 27 Apr. 2020. https://rmx.news/article/migrants-paying-smugglers-5-400-to-go-back-to-africa-during-coronavirus-outbreak/. Accessed on 21 Aug. 2021.

Joffé, George. 'COVID-19 and North Africa.' *The Journal of North African Studies* 25(1), 2020: 515–22.

Kasraoui, Safaa. 'Coronavirus: Moroccan Vendors Harass Asian Tourist in Market'. Morocco World News. 25 Feb. 2020. https://www.moroccoworldnews.com/2020/02/294567/coronavirus-moroccan-vendors-harass-asian-tourist-in-market. Accessed on 21 Aug. 2021.

Krause, Nicole M., Isabelle Freiling, Becca Beets and Dominique Brossard. 'Fact-checking as Risk Communication: The Multi-layered Risk of Misinformation in Times of COVID-19'. *Journal of Risk Research* 23, 2020: 7–8.

Martín-Brufau, Ramón, Carlos Suso-Ribera and Javier Corbalán. 'Emotion Network Analysis During COVID-19 Quarantine – A Longitudinal Study'. *Frontiers in Psychology* 11 (559572), 2020: 1–10.

Monson, Sarah. 'Ebola as African: American Media Discourses of Panic and Otherization'. *Africa Today* 63(3), 2017: 3–27.

Moumni, Omar. 'Between Global Financial Crisis and Arab Spring: A Paradox in the Vision of Migration'. In *Migration, Human Rights and the Politics of Identity in a Globalized World*. Edited by Said Graiouid and Taieb Belghazi. Rabat: Faculté des Lettres et Sciences Humaines de Rabat, 2014. 153–63.

Moumni, Omar. 'Migration and the Post "Arab Spring" Era: A Transition Towards a New Security Nexus'. In *Dynamics of Inclusion and Exclusion in the Mena: Minorities, Subalternity and Resistance*. Edited by Hamza Tayebi and Jochen Lobah. Rabat: Hanns Seidel Foundation Morocco, 2019. 25–36.

Moyer, Eileen and Emmy Igonya. 'Queering the Evidence: Remaking Homosexuality and HIV Risk to "end AIDS" in Kenya'. *Global Public Health* 13(8), 2018. 1007–19.

Nduna, Mzikazi and Jacky Mendes. 'Negative Stereotypes Examined through the HIV and AIDS Discourse: Qualitative Findings from White Young People in Johannesburg, South Africa' *SAHARA-J: Journal of Social Aspects of HIV/AIDS* 7(3), 2010: 21–27.

Neilson, David. 'Epistemic Violence in the Time of Coronavirus: From the Legacy of the Western Limits of Spivak's "Can the Subaltern Speak" to an Alternative to the "Neoliberal Model of Development"'. *Educational Philosophy and Theory*, 2020: 760–65.

The North Africa Post, 'COVIDE-19: Moroccan Lawyers Sue French Doctors for Racist, Colonialist Statements on Africans'. *The North Africa Post*. 3 Apr. 2020. https://northafricapost.com/39648-covide-19-moroccan-lawyers-sue-french-doctors-for-racist-colonialist-statements-on-africans.html. Accessed on 21 Aug. 2021.

Oelze, Sabine. 'China Angry over Coronavirus Cartoon in Danish Newspaper'. *Deutsche Welle*. 30 Jan. 2020. https://www.dw.com/en/china-angry-over-coronavirus-cartoon-in-danish-newspaper/a-52196383. Accessed on 21 Aug. 2021.

Peters, A. Michael. 'Love and Social Distancing in the Time of Covid-19: The Philosophy and Literature of Pandemics'. *Educational Philosophy and Theory* 53(8), 2020: 755–759.

Roberto, Katherine J., Andrew F. Johnson and Beth M. Rauhaus. 'Stigmatization and Prejudice During the COVID-19 Pandemic'. *Administrative Theory & Praxis* 42(3), 2020: 364–78.

Siu, Judy Yuen-man. 'Influence of Social Experiences in Shaping Perceptions of the Ebola Virus Among African Residents of Hong Kong During the 2014 Outbreak: A Qualitative Study'. *International Journal for Equity in Health* 14(88), 2015: 1–11.

Smith, L. T. (2012). Decolonizing Methodologies: Research and Indigenous Peoples., 2nd ed. Zed Books.

South China Morning Post. 'Coronavirus: French 'Corona Pizza' Video Outrages Italians, Prompting Apology'. *South China Morning Post*. 4 Mar. 2020. https://www.scmp.com/news/world/europe/article/3064848/coronavirus-french-corona-pizza-video-outrages-italians-prompting. Accessed on 21 Aug. 2021.

Stillwaggon, Eileen. 'Racial Metaphors: Interpreting Sex and AIDS in Africa.' *Development and Change* 34(5), 2003: 809–32.

Wichers, Marieke and Johanna Wigman and Inez Myin-Germeys. 'Micro-level Affect Dynamics in Psychopathology Viewed from Complex Dynamical System Theory'. *Emotion Rev.* 7, 2015: 362–67.

Wong, Wendy H. and Eileen A. Wong. 'What COVID-19 Revealed about Health, Human Rights, and the WHO'. *Journal of Human Rights* 19(5), 2020: 568–81.

Žižek, Slavoj. 'Coronavirus is "Kill Bill"-Esque Blow to Capitalism and Could Lead to Reinvention of Communism'. *Ikaro.* 19 Mar. 2020. https://www.revistaikaro.com/slavoj-zizek-coronavirus-is-kill-bill-esque-blow-to-capitalism-and-could-lead-to-reinvention-of-communism/. Accessed 21 Aug. 2021.

Žižek, Slavoj. 'There will be no return to normality after Covid. We are entering a post-human era & will have to invent a new way of life'. RT. 8 Dec. 2020. https://www.rt.com/op-ed/508940-normality-covid-pandemic-return/. Accessed 21 Aug. 2021.

Tick Tock

Sonia Fanucchi

Tick Tock goes the clock
In the old oak hall.
One long, luxurious minute.
Outside I watch the palm leaves crinkle, pop
Once, again, as before.
'Nel mezzo del cammin' …
In the middle, the middle of the walk.
'Nel mezzo,' the in between.
Against the clock, against the clock.

The sky is very blue today; the grass is very green.
The freshest, sweetest afternoon, is in between
The morning and the night.
Far, far away the voices hum, locked in an endless fight.
'Fee fie foe fum,' they lie, 'we are right, we are right.'
Tick tock, tick tock. Goes the clock, goes the clock.

'Nel mezzo,' I reread the words.
I pause forever on their sense.
Voices cry, 'Have you heard, have you heard?'
No. Hush. Don't shatter the pretence.

'Sickness is catching' … .

'Nel mezzo,' 'Nel Mezzo'
Knock, Knocking in my head.
Tick tock, goes the clock.
Another one is dead.

Re-imagining a New Normal: COVID-19 Pandemic and the Changing Face of Social Interaction

Josiah Nyanda

Future communities have been imagined. When such communities confront us, we respond not by imagining but re-imagining the emerging communities so that we can cope with the new reality. But are there new realities, or is what we imagine as new a case and curse of historical recurrence? The COVID-19 pandemic has disrupted communities as we have known them. Disruptions enable transformation through creativity. Disruptions introduce a semblance of newness that requires new ways of doing, seeing, reading and telling reality. This paper discusses how, in the face of global lockdown, quarantine and social distancing rules – the new normal – the creative impulse of humans has responded and adapted to COVID-19 pandemic-induced change.

Introduction

Change is upon us. Grand, radical and revolutionary. On the face of it, science seems to have conquered theology. Otherwise, how do we explain the momentary dumbness of theologians and modern-day prophets and seers, most of whom have, like their flock and followers, retreated into hibernation at the threat of a plague? At the time of writing this paper, the COVID-19 pandemic had claimed over 2 500 000 lives globally. This was a hard knock to a world that, from the late 1940s, has been thrilled with post-World War II apocalyptic narratives in print and digital format, and whose obsession with the possibility of a nuclear holocaust – a World War III – predicted human extinction at the touch of a button. Full-scale wartime vocabulary of curfews, lockdowns and alert levels found its spot among the list of popular 'Words of an Unprecedented Year' (Mallika 2020). The United Kingdom, one of the global forerunners in mass vaccination against COVID-19, was debating the proposition of a future travel regime controlled by a Covid vaccine passport, further entrenching future possibilities of new forms of national-isms and international relations. The UK had also joined the bandwagon of nation states in establishing quasi-prisons in the form of quarantine hotels and centres. The institutions operated on the official policy of segregating people based on the colour zone travel itin-erary, with red representing tougher immigration strictures. These tough restrictive measures inadvertently institutionalized people and reflected dehumanizing, prison-style solitary confinement and a radical, startling, shift in travel. A new world order, best described by its uncanny resemblance to the prison conditions shown in *The Shawshank Redemption* (Darabont), was subtly establishing itself like the inconspicuous aquatic elodea. In the wake of the deterioration of culture, art, politics and economics, history was 'bearing out … imagined communities' (Anderson xi) at a pace faster than we ever imagined a year ago. This sudden implosion was a precursor to the emerging and imaging of new ways of seeing, reading and telling – a new aesthetics in the expression of the human condition.

Yet, plagues – in their literal and metaphoric sense – have always been a part of humanity, where they not only expose the reality of human mortality, but also create a platform for human creativity to flourish, especially in how we respond to calamitous situ-ations. Time and space have failed to heal the apprehensions that come with deadly con-tagious diseases. Hence, the seemingly harsh, demeaning and callous language of isolation, lockdown, segregation, solitary confinement, separation and sequestration, as we use it today in response to the COVID-19 context, is an old habit that defines human-ity's quest for survival in the face of life-threatening situations. I have in mind the instruc-tive, theological narrative in the book of 'Leviticus,' which prescribes a seven-day isolation for anyone with symptoms of a dreaded skin disease. We could also recollect the way Chinua Achebe's 1958 debut novel *Things Fall Apart* recreates a pre-colonial lifestyle in Africa that takes isolation and sequestration to a level that outsiders might view as inhumane and unjust. The evil forest is, more than just a geographical space, also a graveyard that betrays human frailty. It is the final resting place, a piece of land beyond the village, reserved for all persons condemned by society as plagued by infec-tious diseases. Again, we see another of humankind's responses to death and life-threaten-ing pestilences. In what could be described as a prophetic and futuristic telling of lockdowns and lockups as restrictive measures that not only respond to the spiralling virus but reshape and redefine our lives, Albert Camus's *The Plague* (1947) resonates with the present reality under COVID-19 restrictions. When a plague hits Oran, claiming lives in droves, 'Emergency measures are rushed in. The city gates are shut, and martial law declared. Oran's commercial harbour is closed to sea traffic. Sporting competitions cease. Beach bathing is prohibited' (Sharpe 2020). Reading Sharpe recounting the moments and character of lockdown of the city of Oran is like reading, living and reliving the Alert Level 5 lockdown rules in South Africa, or the equivalent in Zimbabwe or the United Kingdom during the COVID-19 pandemic, seventy-four years after the publication of *The Plague*.

Clearly, we are condemned to history repeating itself; especially the way we respond, deal with and react to disasters when they strike. What appears to have changed is that now the touch of a button enables transcendence. We now live in the paradox of the moment. We are able to travel without travelling. To see the world like sands through the hourglass. To meet without meeting. To party while apart. Such is the new reality. The new normal that made me question, during a Postgraduate Webinar hosted by Wits University's Academic Development Unit, whether we are seeing and hearing the last of the word 'abnormal,' since the abnormal is and will always be the normal prefixed with the word 'new'.

It is for this reason that the focus of my disquisition is how we can begin to re-imagine lived experiences in the context of the COVID-19 pandemic, experiences that speak to and reflect the changing face of social interaction, while simultaneously challenging and shaping a future reality that expresses human desire for freedom. I will, therefore, be using the descriptor new normal with considerable latitude that borders on the reckless abandon of a poet given to poetic license. New normal refers to new ways of seeing, reading, and telling the everyday doings that have defined who we are and how we act individually and as collectives. Arguably, the COVID-19 pandemic has force-marched us into accepting a new reality. This sudden metamorphosis from mundane and routine behaviour has created a community of behaviours that transformed the year 2020 in ways so shockingly unforeseen that it earned itself a host of descriptors: 'the year from hell'; 'the stolen year'; 'a year that never happened'; and 'the pandemic year'. While it eludes easy summary to define the year 2020, what became patently clear, even as Zoom and webinars took centre stage, was that 2020 was the year of being human. And being human meant combining reflective thinking with reflexivity to shape new interactive means. It also meant embracing the winds of change and demonstrating the human creative potential to adapt to the harsh reality of a year gone rogue.

In my proposition for the re-imagination of new ways of reading, seeing and telling COVID-19 and post-COVID-19 narratives of our life experiences, I apply notions of imagined, new, coming, emerging and changing communities to explore how we have been forced into accepting the realities of a new normal. The pandemic changed the way human beings communicate and interact. Alongside the transformation of communities, and societies being permanently damaged and changed, communities of ideas have also emerged.

These ideas were prompted by two personal experiences. The first was my chance encounter with death on 1 May 2020, after an acute coronary syndrome (ACS) resulted in a heart attack, hospitalization and subsequent surgery. The second was a picture, a 'selfie' taken and sent to me by a colleague, Professor Robert Muponde, on 16 July 2020 (Figure 1). The picture is reproduced here with the express permission of the photographer.

The two moments seem miles apart in that one is a picture and the other is a narrative. However, what brings the two together is that they are both personal narratives. Though different, the texts are bound by context, time and narratorial intentionality. They are both narratives of survival in the face of life and death situations. They are also narratives of loss, expression of a life that has lost meaning. The meaninglessness is in the realization that when one encounters death and survives to tell the story, or when the grim reaper takes lives at the rate and pace of COVID-19, we all are truly candles in the wind. Waiting to be

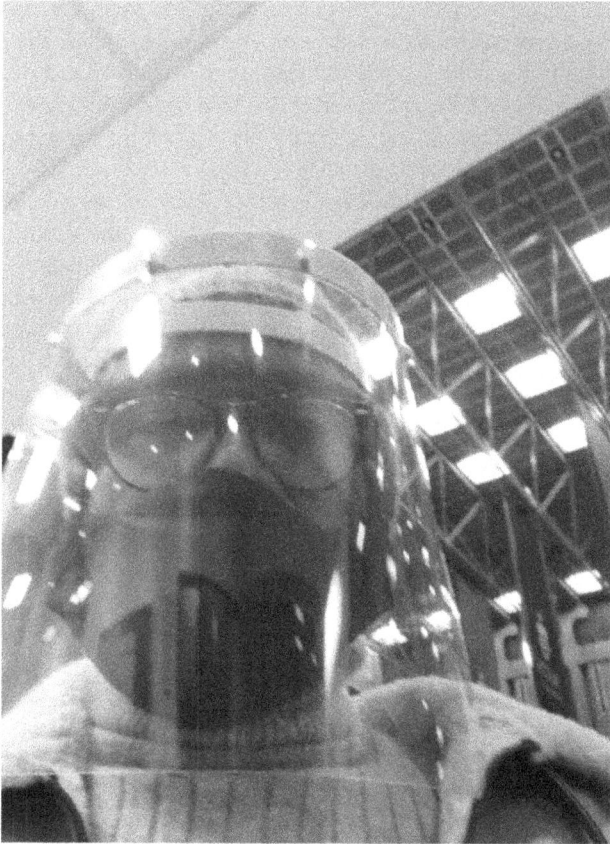

Figure 1.   A 'selfie' by Professor Robert Muponde, taken on 16 July 2020. Reproduced with permission.

blown away any time. But life is not just the ability to breathe. It is given meaning by the way we interact with other humans. The picture above is testament of how life, as we knew it before the plague struck, has vanished; new cultures and new communities have emerged, and thus new ways of reading, seeing and telling.

Thus, what follows is a discussion of face masks, facial make-up and everyday encounters; hospitalization and hospital visits; funerals and marriage ceremonies; and foreign diplomacy and international presence.

Face Masks, Facial Make-up and Everyday Encounters

There is no doubt that a post-COVID-19 pandemic time will come. While we have been warned that we may well learn to live with the pandemic, the same way we have lived with the flu virus, the radical changes that have thus far taken place have left a trail of obituaries, raising questions about the condition and state of humans post-COVID-19. Besides the many lives lost to the pandemic, humanity has been robbed of its sense of self-worth. Human perception of attractiveness and beauty, which often relies on the neo-classical principles of geometric proportions of facial features, has been challenged by time and circumstances. Fear of death has made alterity a reality. Overnight, the selves we knew had transformed, becoming unrecognizable others. Where once lay a bare face with a full chin, lips, nose, cheek and cheek bones exposed and often innervated with diverse beautifiers, now sits a face mask covering the chin, mouth and nose. Depending on the threat of the environment, the mouth and nose may be covered by a respiratory face mask. On top of the common face mask and, circumstantially, a respiratory face mask, sits a transparent or clear face shield covering the entire face. What is left of the face that we have known all along is the eyes. Even these could be hidden under spectacles. Like the earlier picture, the above reminds us of a *Star Wars* Rebel helmet. Except, the description is that of a person on Earth ready to go into a shop to purchase groceries; or a colleague going to the office, as in the above picture that was taken at the Wits University concourse in Solomon Mahlangu House.

We can only imagine the facial features lurking beneath the COVID-19 paraphernalia. This resonates with the Italian philosopher Giorgio Agamben's claims about humanity's propensity to transcend its natural limits, especially in the artificiality of recreational clubs and other such spaces that are stages on which one conceals a version of the self to real another:

> [T]he girls, the hairdresser's salon, ... will all be just as it is, irreparably, but precisely this will be its novelty ... . Irreparable means that these things are consigned without remedy to their being-thus, ... but irreparable also means that for them there is literally no shelter possible, that in their being-thus they are absolutely exposed, absolutely abandoned. (Agamben 39)

Are we to imagine, as did Agamben, the possibility of the pandemic age bringing to an end what we have always known, seen, and worshipped as facial beauty? I have here in mind a bewhiskered chin and moustaches or a clean-shaven face. The foundations, spot-correcting concealers, bronzers, blushers, face powders and lipstick – all hidden under face masks and face shields. Is this the beginning of the end of facial beauty treatments, the absolute abandonment of a cultural art that has been a part of us?

Equally lost under face masks, but remaining an absolute necessity in shaping the course of human interaction, is the art of facial expressions. The host of hardware covering faces today have redefined the way we interact with each other. The smile and sneer have suffered sudden deletion. For marketers and real estate agents, who rely on reading people's faces to gauge customer reactions to their goods and services, reading the tone of voice and eye expression is the new stratagem. Lip reading has vanished under the face-covering accoutrements, putting undue pressure on people with hearing impediments, who have had to improvise in order to cope with the new modus operandi and emerging communities.

Also interesting is that the age of the plague has demystified the way we interact with financial institutions such as banks. In the pre-pandemic period, it was unimaginable to enter a banking hall wearing a face mask and not attract the attention of the bank security, especially in South Africa where cash-in-transit heists have been described as 'an epidemic' (BBC 2018). Enter the pandemic, and a new stage has been set. Now, one cannot enter the banking hall without wearing a face mask. We can speculate about all the security risks this new normal of masked faces poses to bank personnel and banking clients but, elsewhere, project leader in artificial intelligence and machine learning at the World Economic Forum, Lofred Madzou (2020), proposes the use of facial recognition technology as the new way of doing business in the post-pandemic period. Admittedly, the winds of change are blowing, forcing humans to explore their creative potential for adaptation to ensure survival. Beyond facial make-up and human encounters, other cultural practices like marriage ceremonies and funerals have shown fluidity by adapting to pandemic-induced strictures as the ensuing section will show.

Covid-style Marriage Ceremonies and Funeral Rites

The COVID-19 pandemic has stolen the aesthetics of traditional African marriages, also known as customary marriages, and funerals. Marriage ceremonies and funerals in Africa draw meaning from their ritualistic performativity which includes song, dance, grieving, mourning and burial rites. The rituals are rooted in age-old traditions that have survived the test, trials and tribulations of time, space, religion, science and history. Even as the dynamism of culture is both a socio-logical fact and a living reality, marriage ceremonies and funerals are the bedrock of family bonds in African cultures. The two events – one usually done as an expression of maturation into adulthood, and another as a celebration of life lived regardless of one's age at the time of death because of death's untimely and unselective nature – are momentous cultural rituals that bring families, friends and foes together. Aptly captured in two African proverbs – 'if you have no relatives, get married' and 'it is astonishing how important a person becomes when they die' – marriage ceremonies and funerals have the potential to create tightly knit com-munities where personal relationships within those communities become intense, so wide and all encompassing. Nevertheless, the same events can bring the best and worst out of families. This celebration of life lived and a new stage in life about to begin has, over time, made funerals and marriage ceremonies collective cultural practices that continuously inscribe and re-write the reality of the everyday. But all this was upended when the ides of March of the year 2020 brought forth a global pandemic. Age-old traditions that had established themselves with a sense of permanence have had to mutate into forms we never imagined. We have begun to see, participate in, and experience virtual marriage ceremonies and funerals.

In his heartening piece titled 'I've Said Goodbye to *"Normal."* You Should, Too' wherein the author dismisses the possibility of a return to what we assumed was normal, Roy Scranton (2021), without being fatalistic nor sounding defeatist, says, 'we won't see "normal" again in our lifetimes'. However, it is his recollection of the time spent on call of duty in Iraq that I find sig-nificant for my discussion here. He recollects,

> I saw what happens when the texture of the everyday is ripped apart. I realized that what we call social life was a vast and complex game, with imaginary rules we all agree to follow, fictions we turned into fact through institutions, stories, and daily repetitions. Some of the rules were old, deeply ingrained, and resilient. Some were so tenuous; they'd barely survive a hard wind. What I saw in Iraq was that every time you shock the system, something breaks. Sometimes those breaks never heal. ... But sometimes those breaks are openings. Sometimes those breaks are opportunities to do things differ-ently. (2021)

My fascination with Scranton's narrative arises from its malleability and applicability to the pan-demic moment. Even though Scranton's recollections represent the haunting spectre of the horrors of war, they also capture the spirit and reality of the COVID-19 pandemic moment. The pandemic has induced a deathly fear in humans, forcing them into thinking creatively, prompting their genius to flourish.

A case in point is the first-ever publicized virtual traditional *lobola* (bridewealth) negotiations involving two families in South Africa, one in the Eastern Cape, another in KwaZulu
Natal. Five months in lockdown triggered a creative moment that challenged the cultural tradition of two families meeting in real space for *lobola* negotiations. The ritual, which would,
under normal circumstances, render dramatically moments such as clearly defined clapping of
hands to produce a particular sound, kneeling and genuflection, the counting and exchange of
money, the exchange of cattle, the slaughtering of a goat or sheep for feasting, was conducted
virtually using Zoom. Conducting the marriage ceremony virtually was a creative and convenient way of responding to and coping with a life in lockdown, which prohibited intercity
and interprovincial travel at its most stringent levels. It showed that in consuming and
burning up the 'normal,' an emergent new normal, characterized by new ways of doing,
seeing, and telling, was taking shape.

The event garnered widespread media attention. One staff writer at *Moziak News* raised this
question: 'Virtual *lobola* negotiations, the way forward or a convenient solution for now?'
(2020). The writer added that while birthdays, funerals, weddings and marriage proposals
have all had to adapt to our new normal, 'one couple broke even more boundaries when they
conducted their *lobola* negotiations over Zoom' (2020). There is no doubting that a face-to-
face interactive meeting creates a platform for spectacle and performance that is lost in a
virtual meeting. The diction used to describe the event shows that this was a groundbreaking
moment for both the two families involved, and also for a cultural practice and tradition that
has held and preserved its authenticity for centuries. The range of signifiers included 'the
making of history,' 'the way forward,' 'adjustment to new COVID-19 normal' and 'first
virtual *lobola* negotiations,' all of which speak to the seeding of a new aesthetics, the fluidity
of human interaction and the emergence of new, mediated cultural practices faced with
threats of loss of tradition.

It is also worth mentioning that *lobola* negotiations have been responding not only to pandemic threats, but also to the forces of the capital economy. The custom has gradually transformed from some controversial ways of marriage such as abductions (forced marriage) and
paying *lobola* through manual labour. Presently, cash is also acceptable as a negotiation currency
in lieu of cattle. Except, the virtual negotiations rob the moment of the pleasures of counting real
money, which in this case would have to be transferred electronically, thus turning the whole
event into an online business transaction in which the bride is inadvertently a commodity to
be purchased online.

A traditional African marriage is defined by live cattle, robust real-space negotiations, and a
cultural dress code for both families. Virtual means electronic, cyber, mechanized, high-tech and
computerized. Full human presence is lost. Enter the detached, impassive and matter-of-fact,
emotionless deadpan of the touch of a button that is the electronic funds transfer. Live cattle
add to the human. Their mooing and bellowing add to the meaning, drama and theatricality
of a union that is to begin.

It is common for face-to-face *lobola* negotiations to break down due to misunderstanding
between two families. However, there is always a mediator to calm the storm. It is equally
hard to imagine how virtual *lobola* negotiations can be mediated in the face of a misunderstanding. The touch of a button can bring virtual *lobola* negotiations to a close, while the mute and
unmute buttons can be exploited, which means there is no real freedom of expression. Visibility
plays a part in *lobola* negotiations. It gives impression and regulates negotiations through physical human faces, voices, bodies and traditional dress. This gets lost in the cyber world as mostly

the head is visible through video calling, thus compromising the cultural beauty and complexity of a normal *lobola* negotiation.

Likewise, the pandemic has robbed communities of the intimacy, glitz, glamour and dramatic performance of funerals. Take South Africa for instance, where hundreds, if not thousands of people might attend an individual funeral service, the aftermath of which is a drinking and eating binge called 'after tears'. The classification of funerals as superspreaders of COVID-19, thus limiting funeral attendance to fifty people, changed how we view and respond to death. It also marked a transformative moment in how we participate in burying the dead. Even as President Ramaphosa pronounced the new measures and declared that 'funerals have become a death trap for many of our people' (2021) – paradox intended – he acknowledged the multiple rituals that would be lost to the lockdown restrictions. In a long and winding speech that bordered on negotiating with and cajoling the citizens, coupled with a pleading tone, Ramaphosa expressed his clear understanding of how stifling and rupturing to cultural practice the restrictions were:

> Providing a fitting send-off for a departed loved one is deeply ingrained in all of us. There are certain rituals that we perform in line with our respective cultures and traditions; not just at the funeral itself but in the days leading up to the burial. But these are all things we simply cannot do at this time … . We are in the grip of a deadly pandemic and all these activities that would normally take place are just increasing our exposure to risk – for ourselves, for the bereaved family and for our own families at home. There will be a time when we can go to the home of the deceased to pay our respects, and to sympathise properly with our neighbours, friends and relatives. Funerals have become a death trap for many of our people. For now, it is best and safer to stay at home. (2021)

The restrictions have called for innovative ways of coping with the death of a family member through virtual attendance at burials. Again, Zoom has come to the rescue. Others have resorted to shooting a video that will be shared with family members across the globe. However, in the absence of body viewing, even those who attend the burial can neither confirm nor deny that they buried the right corpse.

Funerals under pandemic conditions in South Africa have also exposed the double standards and hypocrisy in the application of COVID-19 regulations. For example, the admission by the police minister that 'it was difficult for the police to control the mourners' at the funeral service of King Goodwill Zwelithini shows that religious gatherings are controlled on the basis of class, hierarchy and power dynamics (Times Live 2021).

Also buckling under the strain of the pandemic, Zimbabwe banned traditional funerals. Taking the cue from Italy, the transportation of corpses between cities was also banned – unless the corpse was contained in an expensive, hermetically sealed coffin. Regardless of where the deceased's family were located, the Zimbabwean dead would have to be buried in the location where they passed away. This locking down and locking in of dead bodies muffled the brief eulogy and 'the usual body-viewing ceremonies, sung prayers and speeches' (France24 2021). One aggrieved citizen averred: '"It is against our culture to be buried by strangers in the midst of strangers. We want to be buried among our ancestors … . The respect for our dead relatives is all we had (left)' (France24 2021). One could argue that the apparent insensitivity of the measures taken by governments can only be accepted if we consider the pandemic a war situation. Faced with death and extraordinary circumstances of a global crisis, extraordinary

measures needed to be taken. This included radical sacrilege and defilement of custom and tradition. These are some of the pitfalls of lawlessness and martial law in war and emergencies.

Italy was not unaffected by the change in custom and mourning brought on by the pandemic,
made stark by the country's strong Roman Catholic values that dictate how the dead should be
buried. Sofia Bettiza chronicles 'How COVID-19 is Denying Dignity to the Dead in Italy'. She
recreates the indignity of dying alone in isolation, without family or friends, and being buried in
the 'grim anonymity of a hospital gown' (2020). However, it is the emotive words of Andrea
Cerato, a funeral home employee, that vividly capture the mood of the moment when he says,
"'This pandemic kills twice … . First, it isolates you from your loved ones right before you
die. Then, it doesn't allow anyone to get closure'" (Bettiza 2020). The double tragedy captured
by Cerato shows the devastation caused by the pandemic. The sense of loss transcends the physical loss of a loved one. It is emotional and psychological. Analysts have warned of years of post-
traumatic stress disorders (PTSD) in the aftermath of the COVID-19 pandemic. Even as the story
by Bettiza suggests a dire situation, a story of a wall between the dead and the living imposed by
a pandemic, the human desire to save and feel the connection between death and life is shown by
the creative responses of the living to a situation that deprives them the freedom to mourn and
bury their loved ones. We are told through the undertaker that they "'put the clothes the family
gives us on top of the corpse as if they were dressed … . A shirt on top, a skirt below' (2020). In
the absence of family members, the undertakers act as 'replacement families, replacement
friends, even replacement priests' (2020). In all this, we see communities we never imagined
come into existence, communities that have emerged as a result of, and a response to, the pandemic. It is the ability of humanity to adapt to change by devising new ways of doing things that
is important. It shows that humans can survive the vicissitudes of life through alternate means.
Yet, despite our surprising creativity in a time of crisis, COVID-19 has also exposed the fragility
of international relations.

Foreign Diplomacy and International Presence

Noting the virus's globally indiscriminate spread, the World Health Organization gave it
'global pandemic' status. The declaration by WHO was a call to action, for all nations –
rich and poor – to put hands on deck in the fight against a plague that was proving to be bor-
derless. As has come to define human relations, whenever there is a crisis, vultures prey on the
weak. The call by WHO exposed global fissures, the 'them' and 'us' attitude that has always
defined the rider and horse relationship of conflict – oppressor and oppressed – between rich
nations and poor nations, the global north and the global south. A new nationalism emerged –
new in the sense that the currencies that defined it and gave it character were no longer guns
and whips, nor the World Bank or International Monetary Fund (IMF). It was measured and
defined by the few drops of vaccine. The Oxford Dictionary definition was the same: 'identification with one's own nation and support for its interests, especially to the exclusion or det-
riment of the interests of other nations'. Motive too was the same – domination, control and
self-enrichment. The newness of the nationalism at play was the trading currency – the
vaccine.

Closing borders, suspending air transport by grounding planes and placing a ban on foreign
travel meant that international relations and foreign diplomacy were no longer decided at the
World Economic Forum in Davos. It also meant that leaders from the global south would
have to contend with their average-to-poor health systems, with no option of seeking medical

treatment in developed nations. Therefore, the vaccine became the trump card, the diplomatic currency shaping international relations.

That the pandemic exposed glaring inequalities among nations is undebatable. This was made even clearer by what appeared like a deliberate and calculated move aimed at denying weak nations access to the vaccine by creating an artificial shortage so that poor nations could come abegging. Another case of 'he who pays the piper calls the tune' was unfolding. Take for instance the drama of vaccine wars coming to Europe with the 'E.U. and U.K. Fight [ing] Over Covid Vaccines' (Mueller and Stevis-Gridneff 2021). Shocking reports revealed that for months, 'wealthy countries [had] been clearing the world's shelves of coronavirus vaccine, leaving poorer nations with little hope of exiting the pandemic in 2021' (2021). Clearly, the pandemic had set the stage for rich nations to show their true colours by exposing the fallacy of an interdependent world.

History has on record the Berlin Conference of 1884–1885 as a precursor to the scramble for Africa; a conference that divided and conquered Africa. Similarly, the fault lines emerging 'in the scramble for vials, opening a new and unabashedly nationalist competition that could poison relations and set back collective efforts to end the pandemic' are setting the stage for a possible scramble for not only Africa but all poorer nations (Mueller and Stevis-Gridneff 2021). This time not through the might of the gun but drops of vaccine. The potential for the new scramble to cultivate and sow a new culture in foreign diplomacy and international relations speaks to the new ways of doing, reading and seeing international relations unfolding in the face of the pandemic.

Hospitals, Hospitalization and Hospital Visits

When one confronts mortality and lives to tell the story, only a personal, subjective narrative can capture the moment. Autoethnography allows for such personal analysis and commentary.

The day is 1 May 2020, the day the working worker is on holiday observing Workers' Day in lockdown. One worker, the messenger of mortality, sent by the grim reaper, violently knocked on my door, leading to hospitalization. Standing on guard were the gods of our time – paramedics, doctors, nurses, support staff, friends and relatives. Paramedics were the first to arrive. Their masked faces spoke of the strange pandemic times. At the hospital, my cousin, the only close relative present, was denied entry due to COVID-19 precautionary restrictions. Already traumatized by the incident, six hours of waiting for an update from the resuscitation room must have been a lifetime for him. The waiting period was worse for my family in the United Kingdom and Zimbabwe. Having last been in hospital as a patient 42 years back, the strange feeling of being surrounded by masked doctors and nurses, whose dress code could be mistaken for astronaut gear, was overwhelming. With no family member present in my room, no friend either, the cardiac resuscitation machine and all the medical staff around me were the family I had. I surrendered to them – the gods of our time.

But what has this got to do with the disquisition on re-imagining new communities in the way COVID-19 has transformed social interaction? Hospitals have become home to hundreds of millions of patients infected with COVID-19. Homes away from home. In keeping with its original definition, hospital, from the Latin noun 'hospes,' meaning guest or visitor, is and should be warm, welcoming and homely. Other words related to hospital are hospice, hospitality, hospitable – all of which point to the hospital as a place of respite, even as one is getting medical care. This respite is made possible by a combination of things: the medical care one receives from specialized medical staff, as well as moral support and love from family, relatives and friends. This explains why hospitals have visiting times. Visiting times enable interaction between the hospitalized patient and their loved ones. Those who came up with visiting times knew that medical treatment alone would not be enough for one's well-being.

COVID-19 has turned the tide on hospital visits. Not only was my cousin denied entry to the hospital, but this also meant that he could not contact and update my family in different parts of the world. The United Kingdom was on full lockdown and my family could not travel to be with me in South Africa. Zimbabwe was on full lockdown and my children could not travel. South Africa, itself, was on full lockdown making international travel in and out of the country impossible. It was heart-warming when the paramedics paid me a visit a day after my admission into hospital to check on my condition. The doctors, nurses and support staff, the gods, had become an improvised family for me and other patients.

When Motorola engineer Martin Cooper invented the first handheld mobile phone in 1973, he ushered in a cultural shift in the way we communicate and do business, which in 2020, the year of the pandemic, has conveniently overcome physical distance. Coping with lockdown rules has been made bearable because of the mobile phone – an additional mode facilitating social interaction. After six hours in the resuscitation room, the first thing I asked for when I came to was my phone. The first message I sent was to my wife in the UK – then to my cousin who had been waiting outside the hospital. I was certain that the two would know I was alive – the message would travel at the touch of a button. Again, minutes after coming out of theatre, I requested my mobile phone. The family had to know that the surgical procedure was a success. Evidently, it is now the duty of the hospital patient to contact and update family members. The changing times have ushered in virtual hospital visits. While this has its own limitations such as robbing people of the intimate moments of a handshake, a reassuring pat or squeeze on the shoulder, it also exposes glaring social and economic inequalities that have been lurking beneath the surface.

Conclusion

While I have limited the scope of 'plague' to the current COVID-19 pandemic times, I am aware of the vast literal, moral and metaphoric meanings of the word. Plagues are as old as humanity and thus definitions and their emotional effects cannot be confined into a straight-jacket. Pandemics bring out the best and worst in humans. Other kinds of opportunistic plagues such as corruption and political rot, violence, social inequalities, poverty and lies have manifested due to COVID-19. Focusing on the new normal that emerges as humans respond to plagues such as COVID-19 has enabled me to explore the creative impulse that has come to define humanity.

Times of crisis are fertile ground for all forms of creativity. This is part of what defines humanity and its desire to survive by taming nature. The age-old adage that, when winds of change come, you either build a windmill or perish, gives impetus for adaption and problem-solving. Even as I narrowed my discussion to the re-imagination of a new normal, the possible issues that this lens inspires are vast. One such issue is how creative arts such as live musical performances have taken to the digital stage on YouTube. This is a rich area that others could also explore. What this discussion has done is to open the stage for further exploration of how the pandemic has birthed and shaped imagined and coming communities in ways that reveal the power of being human.

Works Cited

Achebe, Chinua. *Things Fall Apart*. London: William Heinemann, 1958.

Agamben, Giorgio. *The Coming Community: Theory Out of Bounds*. Translated by Michael Hardt. Minneapolis: U of Minnesota P, 2003.

Anderson, Benedict. *Imagined Communities: Reflections on the Origins and Spread of Nationalism*. London: Verso, 2006.

BBC News. 'South Africa's Cash-in-transit Heists: A National Emergency?'. *BBC News*. 18 Jan. 2018. https://www.bbc.com/news/world-africa-44328938. Accessed 22 Jan. 2021.

Bettiza, Sofia. 'Coronavirus: How Covid-19 is Denying Dignity to the Dead in Italy'. *BBC World Service*. 25 Mar. 2020. https://www.bbc.com/news/health-52031539. Accessed on 28 Jan 2021.

Camus, Albert. *The Plague*. Hamish: Hamilton, 1947.

Darabont, Frank, dir. *The Shawshank Redemption*. Perf. Morgan Freeman. 1994. itv DVD, 2008. Blu-ray DVD.

France24. '"Buried by Strangers": Funeral Curbs Raise Ire in Zimbabwe'. *France24*. 18 Jan. 2021. https://www.france24.com/en/live-news/20210118-buried-by-strangers-funeral-curbs-raise-ire-in-zimbabwe Accessed 10 Aug. 2021.

Madzou, Lofred. 'Facial Recognition can Help Re-start Post-pandemic Travel. Here's How to Limit the Risks'. *World Economic Forum*. 16 Dec. 2020. https://www.weforum.org/agenda/2020/12/facial-recognition-technology-and-travel-after-covid-19-freedom-versus-privacy/. Accessed on 29 Dec. 2020.

Mallika, Soni. 'Oxford English Dictionary Couldn't Pick just One 'Word of the Year' for 2020'. *The Hindustan Times*. 23 Nov. 2020. https://www.hindustantimes.com/world-news/oxford-english-dictionary-couldn-t-pick-just-one-word-of-the-year-for-2020/story-1Y1szWG3uWJ8YkaTeFHFPN.html. Accessed on 22 Feb. 2021.

Moziak. 'Virtual Lobola Negotiations the Way Forward or a Convenient Solution for Now?'. *Moziak*. 13 Aug. 2020. https://moziak.africa/virtual-lobola-negotiations-the-way-forward-or-a-convenient-solution-for-now/. Accessed on 25 Feb. 2021.

Mueller, Benjamin and Matina Stevis-Gridneff. 'E.U. and U.K. Fighting Over Scarce Vaccines'. *The New York Times*. 27 Jan. 2021. https://www.nytimes.com/2021/01/27/world/europe/eu-uk-covid-vaccine.html. Accessed on 21 Feb. 2021.

Ramaphosa, Cyril. 'Statement by President Cyril Ramaphosa on Progress in the National Effort to Contain the Covid-19 Pandemic, 11 January 2021'. *The Presidency: Republic of South Africa*. 11 Jan. 2021. http://www.thepresidency.gov.za/speeches/statement-president-cyril-ramaphosa-progress-national-effort-contain-covid-19-pandemic%2C-11-january-2021. Accessed on 15 Jan. 2021.

Scranton, Roy. 'I've Said Goodbye to "Normal." You Should, Too'. *The New York Times*. 25 Jan. 2021. https://www.nytimes.com/2021/01/25/opinion/new-normal-climate-catastrophes-html. Accessed on 15 Feb. 2021.

Sharpe, Matthew. 'Guide to the Classics: Albert Camus' *The Plague*'. *The Conversation*. 6 Apr. 2020. https://theconversation.com/guide-to-the-classics-albert-camus-the-pague 2020. Accessed on 25 Feb. 2021.

Times Live. 'Dozens Throng Gates outside the Royal Palace during Memorial Service of Kind Zwelithini'. 18 Mar. 2021. *Times Live*. https://www.timeslive.co.za/news/south-africa/2021-03-18-dozens-throng-gates-outside-the-royal-palace-during-memorial-service-for-king-zwelithini/. Accessed on 9 May 2021.

Index

Note: Page numbers followed by "n" denote endnotes.

For Product Safety Concerns and Information please contact our EU
representative GPSR@taylorandfrancis.com
Taylor & Francis Verlag GmbH, Kaufingerstraße 24, 80331 München, Germany

* 9 7 8 1 0 3 2 2 8 6 8 4 6 *